Stereochemistry of Carbohydrates

Stereochemistry of Carbohydrates

J. F. Stoddart

Lecturer in Chemistry, University of Sheffield, Sheffield, England

WILEY-INTERSCIENCE

a Division of John Wiley and Sons, Inc.

New York • London • Sydney • Toronto

Library of Congress Catalog Card Number: 73–151035

ISBN–O–471–82650–2

Printed in the United States of America

10 9 8 7 6 5 4 3 2 1

Foreword

Carbohydrate chemistry has made important contributions to conformational analysis, a field which has become of great importance to all organic chemists and many biochemists in the last twenty years and which was recognized by the award of the 1969 Nobel Prize in chemistry to Barton and Hassel.

Cellulose is probably the first molecule in which the chair shape of the six-membered ring was detected through X-ray analysis (by Sponsler and Dore in 1926); the term conformation was first introduced in the field of sugar chemistry (by Haworth in 1929); the effect of conformation on reaction rate was probably first recognized in carbohydrates (by Isbell in 1937). Reeves' discussion of the conformations of sugars (1949) antedates Barton's pioneering paper on conformational analysis by a year, and the first major recognition of the importance of conformation in nuclear magnetic resonance spectroscopy is found in a paper by Lemieux, Bernstein, and coworkers in 1958. It is therefore surprising and perhaps a little unfortunate that, by and large, workers in the field of conformational analysis (with a few exceptions, such as Angyal and Lemieux) have not drawn extensively on carbohydrates as examples to illustrate conformational principles. One reason for this lack of firm contact between the two areas may be the fact that, although all recent textbooks on carbohydrate chemistry have included discussion in terms of conformation, such discussion has been incidental rather than systematic, and, as a result, unappealing to those outside the carbohydrate field proper. A second reason is that most textbooks treat carbohydrate chemistry as an isolated aspect of organic chemistry, whereas, in fact, it is conformational ideas and stereochemical principles superimposed on aliphatic and heterocyclic chemistry.

It is here—in the *systematic* application of conformational and stereo-chemical principles—that we think the present book excels. The principles are explained clearly and applied consistently. The book thus provides firm stereochemical and conformational underpinnings for the reader interested primarily in carbohydrate chemistry. At the same time, however, it serves, for the organic chemist interested in stereochemistry and conformational analysis, as a very readable account of the facts—quantitative as well as qualitative—in the carbohydrate field which are pertinent to his own interests. It should stimulate investigators in many areas to turn to carbohydrates as suitable and often readily available models to illustrate or confirm stereochemical principles.

The author has indeed brought about what we consider a happy union between two fields which have always been closely related but which have, in the past, been divided by a lack of overlap of interests. We hope that *Stereochemistry of Carbohydrates* will contribute toward bridging the gap.

Ernest L. Eliel
Professor of Chemistry
University of Notre Dame
Notre Dame, Indiana

J. K. N. Jones
Chown Research Professor
Queen's University
Kingston, Ontario, Canada

Preface

This book has been written out of a belief shared with several colleagues that there is a need for a textbook which attempts to discuss the chemistry of carbohydrate compounds in a manner designed to attract the attention of other organic chemists, whether they be students, teachers, or researchers. I have taken the view that this objective is most likely to be achieved through a presentation which is stereochemical in nature. Recent conceptual advances in stereochemistry, centered around considerations of molecular symmetry, allow the adoption of new approaches to the presentation of the configurational aspects of sugar molecules. At the cost of dispensing with the more conventional introduction, usually of a historical nature, which is characteristic of many textbooks on carbohydrate chemistry, I have attempted to tackle the problem of configurational isomerism among the sugars in terms of the symmetry properties of constitutionally symmetrical isomers, in the hope that such an approach may be of some heuristic value.   This kind of introduction also provides a logical exposition of the basis for the brilliantly deductive arguments employed by Emil Fischer about seventy years ago in his determinations of the relative configurations of all the hexoses. In order that the reader with little previous knowledge of modern stereochemical concepts can follow the discussion throughout the book, I have purposely taken pains to state principles and define terms as clearly as possible, particularly in the first two chapters.

For the remainder, I have endeavored to focus attention on the remarkable interplay among constitutional, configurational, and conformational isomerism, which is almost uniquely characteristic of carbohydrates. Above all, I believe that an appreciation of this theme is all important toward establishing a firm foundation for the understanding of the chemistry of monosaccharide derivatives in general. As far as polysaccharides are concerned, I have purposely integrated a discussion of their stereochemistry with that of other carbohydrate derivatives in the hope that by so doing this developing area of the subject will receive the attention it deserves. Where at all possible, I have tried to discuss concepts rather than simply present facts. As a result, I have made no attempt to be comprehensive in my coverage of the literature, and I am aware that my selection of topics for discussion reflects some bias of personal interest. However, I trust that the reader who has made his way through the pages of this book and wants to look further will be sufficiently well equipped to do so.

Fortunately, in the early stages of the preparation of the manuscript, I was convinced of the wisdom of having it scrutinized by a few international authorities in the general areas of organic stereochemistry and carbohydrate chemistry.* In this regard, I am particularly grateful to Professors S. J. Angyal, E. L. Eliel, J. K. N. Jones, W. D. Ollis, A. S. Perlin, and S. Wolfe and to Dr. D. A. Rees. Not only did these people bring much constructive criticism to bear on various drafts of the manuscript, but also, in some instances where their recent research had relevance to the subject matter of the book, they kindly made their results available to me in advance of publication. Other friends and colleagues, including Professors G. O. Aspinall, G. W. Hay, Sir Edmund Hirst, and W. A. Szarek, and Drs. T. B. Grindley, J. C. P. Schwarz, and P. Toft, read portions of the manuscript and offered many useful comments.

Much of the manuscript was written while I was a NRC Postdoctoral Fellow in the Department of Chemistry, Queen's University, Kingston, Ontario. It was completed on my coming to Sheffield as an ICI Postdoctoral Research Fellow. Accordingly, I wish to acknowledge financial support from the National Research Council of Canada and from Imperial Chemical Industries Limited.

The foreword by Professors Eliel and Jones is but one manifestation of the goodwill which was accorded to me by many during the preparation of the manuscript. For this, and for the rest, I am grateful.

J. F. STODDART

December 1970
Sheffield, England

---

* I am grateful to Professors W. D. Ollis and S. Wolfe for making allowances out of their research grants to meet expenses of producing numerous copies of the manuscript.

Contents

Stereochemistry of Carbohydrates

Introduction

1.1 General Remarks and Definitions

In the study of carbohydrates, many of the problems which arise are stereochemical in nature. Consequently, the answers are often to be had from a knowledge of the structural and dynamic aspects of stereochemistry. Whereas structural stereochemistry is concerned with a description of the spatial arrangements of atoms in molecules, the dynamic aspect deals with the interpretation of equilibria and rate processes in terms of changes in these spatial arrangements.

Before attempting to discuss some aspects of the stereochemistry of carbohydrates, it will be helpful to indicate the breadth of definition that will be given to some familiar stereochemical terms. As a glance at some of the recent pronouncements shows (1–7), much discussion and debate presently surrounds the definition of terms such as *constitution, configuration, conformation,* and *structure.* Consideration of these terms is highly relevant to the treatment of carbohydrate stereochemistry which will be presented within these covers, and the following definitions will be used.

1. The term *constitution* refers to the nature and sequence of the bonding between the atoms in a molecule.

2. The *configuration* of a molecule is a particular spatial arrangement of its atoms without regard to arrangements which differ only on torsion about single bonds. In carbohydrate molecules, configurational differences are usually associated with different spatial arrangements of tetrahedrally disposed ligands[1] attached to *chiral carbon atoms.*[2] Thus, the three forms of tartaric acid shown in Figure 1.1 have nonidentical arrangements of

---

[1] The term *ligand* includes (*cf.* refs. 7–9) both atoms and functional groups.
[2] This term supersedes (6) the term *asymmetric carbon atoms,* which has been used (*cf.* ref. 10) in the past. A carbon atom is said to be *chiral* if exchange of any two of the four tetrahedrally disposed ligands gives a nonidentical molecule.

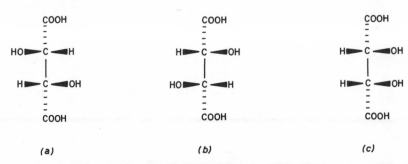

Figure 1.1   The three forms of tartaric acid.

ligands around their chiral carbon atoms and so have nonidentical configurations.

3. The term *conformation* denotes the different spatial arrangements of atoms in a molecule obtained on torsion about one or more single bonds. Thus, as shown in Figure 1.2, *n*-butane may exist in an infinite number of nonidentical conformations by virtue of torsion around its C_2-C_3 bond. However, consideration is usually limited (*cf.* ref. 11) to particular conformations which correspond to energy minima (the three staggered conformations) or to energy maxima (the three eclipsed conformations). The discipline which makes use of these considerations to interpret, understand, and explain the physical and chemical behavior of compounds is often called *conformational analysis.*

4. *Structure* comprises constitution, configuration, and conformation (*cf.* ref. 6). For some molecules, such as methane, chloroform, dichloromethane, and chlorobromoiodomethane, a knowledge of the configuration as well as the constitution is required to define the structure,[3] whereas with other molecules [e.g., tartaric acid (Figure 1.1) and *n*-butane (Figure 1.2)] the structure is defined only when the conformation, configuration, and constitution are all known.

Stereochemistry is concerned with the properties of kinds of molecules called *isomers*, which, although different in structure, have the same molecular formulas. Molecules related in this manner are said to exhibit *isomerism.* It will be convenient to distinguish among three types of isomerism called *constitutional isomerism, configurational isomerism,* and *conformational isomerism.*

[3] Note that chlorobromoiodomethane contains a chiral carbon atom and so has two configurations; hence two structures are possible. The other compounds (i.e., methane, chloroform, dichloromethane) have one configuration and one structure.

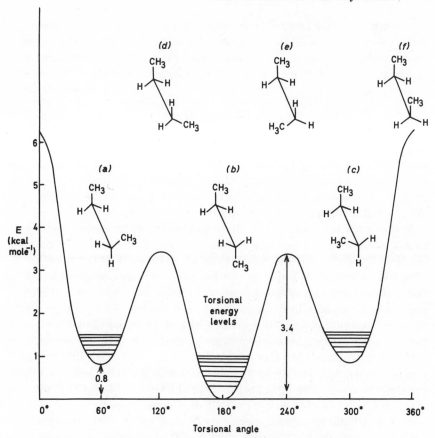

Figure 1.2 The potential energy profile for *n*-butane.

1. *Constitutional isomerism* occurs when the atoms of two or more molecules with the same molecular formulas are arranged in a different order, as in *n*-butane and isobutane. In other words, *constitutional isomers* have the same molecular formulas, but nonidentical constitutions.[4]

2. *Configurational isomerism* is exhibited by molecules which have the same molecular formulas and constitutions but nonidentical configurations. Such molecules are called *configurational isomers.*

[4] A distinction is often drawn (*cf.* refs. 12 and 13) between the types of constitutional isomers like *n*-butane and isobutane, and the class of readily interconvertible constitutional isomers known as *tautomers,* of which the keto and enol forms of acetoacetic ester are examples. In this book, no effort will be made to distinguish between *tautomerism* and constitutional isomerism. All isomers which have the same molecular formulas but nonidentical constitutions will be referred to as constitutional isomers.

3. *Conformational isomerism* is exhibited by molecules which have the same molecular formulas and constitutions (and if capable of exhibiting configurational isomerism, the same configurations) but nonidentical conformations. Such molecules are called *conformational isomers* or *conformers*.[5]

Configurational isomers and conformers are often (*cf*. refs. 7 and 15) referred to collectively as *stereoisomers*. If two stereoisomers are related as an object and its mirror image, they are said to be *enantiomers*.[6] For example, tartaric acids (*a*) and (*b*) in Figure 1.1 and conformers (*a*) and (*c*) of *n*-butane in Figure 1.2 are enantiomers. Stereoisomers which are not related in this manner (*cf*. refs. 12 and 16) are called *diastereomers*. For example, tartaric acids (*a*) and (*c*) in Figure 1.1 and conformers (*a*) and (*b*) of *n*-butane in Figure 1.2 are diastereomers.

Mislow (15) has pointed out that the concept of isomerism becomes a practical one only when there is some means of distinguishing between isomers. In particular, interconversion of conformers is often occurring at a fast rate, and in order to observe them the measurement must be faster than their rate of interconversion. Thus, the time scale is all important in being able to distinguish between isomers. The minimum half-life required for this purpose decreases with the method of observation in the following order: physical isolation; magnetic resonance spectroscopy; torsional, vibrational, and electronic spectroscopy; and diffraction measurements (*cf*. ref. 16). It follows that isomers which can be isolated will in principle be observable by all other methods. On the other hand, isomers which are too unstable to be isolated may sometimes be observable by nuclear magnetic resonance spectroscopy or, if not, by infrared spectroscopy. Consequently, the unsatisfactory aspect of regarding isomerism as a practical concept resides in the paradox that molecules which are isomers on one time scale of observation may not qualify on a slower one.

Isomerism may be regarded as a theoretical concept, however, if it is agreed that only molecules in their lowest electronic, vibrational, and

---

[5] An arbitrary distinction is often drawn between conformers and the conformational isomers called *atropisomers* (*cf*. ref. 14), which are separated by a sufficiently high torsional energy barrier to permit isolation of isomers. In this book, no distinction will be drawn between conformers and atropisomers. All conformational isomers will be referred to as conformers, regardless of the magnitude of the energy barrier to interconversion.
[6] Enantiomers rotate the plane of polarized light in opposite directions but have the same absolute numerical values for their specific rotations. In the past, *stereoisomerism* has included *optical isomerism* and *geometrical isomerism*. However, in view of the fact that enantiomers may exhibit immeasurably small optical activities or have different specific rotations (even opposite in sign) in different solvents, the use of terms such as optical isomerism is not recommended. For further discussion of the vagueness attending the use of these terms, see ref. 1.

torsional states qualify to be called isomers. When this restriction is imposed, of all the conformations of *n*-butane represented by the energy profile in Figure 1.2, only the three staggered conformations with zero-point torsional energies may be referred to as conformers. It is noteworthy that all excited states of the molecule corresponding to higher torsional energy levels will have only a momentary existence anyway, and will tend to lose energy in order to revert to one of the conformers (*cf.* ref. 17). Hence, our definition of isomerism will include the additional proviso that it may be exhibited only by molecules in their pertinent ground states.[7]

A consideration of carbohydrate stereochemistry often requires a description of the steric relationships between ligands on vicinal carbon atoms. If we consider the conformations of *n*-butane shown in Figure 1.2, the steric relationships between methyl groups associated with torsional angles of 0°, 60°, 120°, and 180° between projected C-C bonds in conformations (*f*), (*a, c*), (*d, e*), and (*b*), respectively, correspond to the following descriptions: *syn-periplanar* (*cis, syn, cis-coplanar*), *syn-clinal* (*gauche*), *anti-clinal*, and *anti-periplanar* (*trans, anti, trans-coplanar*) (*cf.* ref. 20). Since the older names indicated in parentheses are still in common use, they will be employed interchangeably in this book with the more recent terms.

1.2 Historical Background

Investigations on carbohydrates have played an important role in the development of stereochemistry. A few of the major contributions, some of which have influenced the advancement of our knowledge in other branches of organic chemistry, will now be mentioned.

The stereochemical proofs which allowed Fischer (21; for reviews in English see ref. 22) to assign relative configurations to all the hexoses and pentoses represent one of the outstanding achievements in stereochemistry. Later, the determination of the ring sizes of the monosaccharides by Hirst (e.g., ref. 23) and Haworth (24) prepared the way for the study of the conformational properties of these compounds. Although Sponsler and Dore (25) were the first to discuss puckering of the pyranoid ring when interpreting their X-ray diagrams of cellulose in terms of the chair con-

---

[7] Other authors (e.g., refs. 18 and 19) have drawn similar distinctions. One proposal (18) distinguishes between *conformation* and *form*, whereby the term conformation refers to molecules with minimum torsional energies and all other spatial arrangements are designated as forms.

former of the D-glucopyranoid ring, it was Haworth (26) who introduced the term conformation into the English language and hinted at the consequences of its consideration. Nonetheless, the application of conformational analysis to the sugars had to await developments within cyclohexane systems (e.g., ref. 27). In the light of this knowledge, Hassel and Ottar (28), and later Reeves (29) and Mills (30), put the qualitative aspects of the conformational analysis of pyranoid rings on a sound footing. The unexpected preference for an electronegative substituent on C_1 of a pyranoid ring to assume the axial orientation was first discussed by Edward (31) and was later termed the *anomeric effect* by Lemieux (32). The destabilization of a conformer which places a polar bond between two electron pairs on a vicinal oxygen atom is now a generally recognized phenomenon in the conformational analysis of heterocyclic compounds (e.g., ref. 33). The last decade has seen the development by Angyal (34; see also Section 3.2) of a semiempirical quantitative approach to the conformational analysis of pyranoid derivatives.

The constitutional and configurational features of many polysaccharides have been unraveled mainly by the methods introduced by the Birmingham school in the thirties and forties (for a current appraisal, see ref. 35). More recently, Ramachandran and his associates (36) have indicated how polysaccharide chains may be analyzed for permissible conformations. Undoubtedly, the conformational analysis of polysaccharides is still in its infancy and important advances may be expected in the next few years (*cf.* ref. 37).

The growth of structural carbohydrate stereochemistry has been accompanied (and in some instances made possible) by important advances in physical methods of analysis. For example, the application of the principle of optical superposition by Hudson (38) in formulating his rules of isorotation was of great value in correlating the relative configurations at C_1 of the cyclic forms of the sugars. In more recent times, the observation by Lemieux and his associates (39) that, in ^{1}H nuclear magnetic resonance spectroscopy, the magnitude of the spin-spin coupling constant between protons on vicinal carbon atoms depends on the size of the torsional angle between the projected C-H bonds has greatly facilitated the growth of conformational analysis in other areas of organic chemistry as well as carbohydrate chemistry.

Important observations in the carbohydrate field have also helped to lay the foundations of the dynamic aspect of stereochemistry. Isbell (40), in the course of his investigations on the rates of bromine oxidation of aldoses, was probably the first to realize that the rate of a reaction is often dependent on stereochemical factors. About the same time, he also recognized (41) that neighboring groups may participate in reactions, provided certain steric conditions are fulfilled.

1.3 Scope

The material presented in the next four chapters will be limited to a discussion of a few stereochemical topics which have particular relevance to the chemistry of carbohydrates. The structural stereochemistry of these compounds and the equilibrium aspects of their dynamic stereochemistry will receive special emphasis. By focusing attention on these aspects of the stereochemistry of carbohydrates, it is possible to give an account which is largely unique to this class of organic compounds.

On the other hand, since many of the reactions exhibited by carbohydrates are common to other organic compounds, the temptation to discuss their reactivity from a stereochemical angle has been avoided. Although some excuse could have been found for such an extension of the present treatment, the view has been taken that the stereochemical aspects of reaction rate processes are perhaps best described within the context of a discussion of reaction mechanisms. Indeed, an excellent review by Capon (42) of reaction mechanisms in carbohydrate chemistry has appeared recently and has achieved precisely this purpose. Hence, the limited scope of this book finds some circumstantial, as well as philosophical, justification.

References

1. W. K. Noyce, *J. Chem. Educ.*, **38**, 23 (1961).
2. E. L. Eliel, *Stereochemistry of Carbon Compounds*, McGraw-Hill, New York, 1962.
3. K. Mislow, *Introduction to Stereochemistry*, Benjamin, New York, 1966.
4. R. S. Cahn, Sir Christopher Ingold, and V. Prelog, *Angew. Chem. Intern. Ed.*, **5**, 385 (1966).
5. J. D. Roberts and M. C. Caserio, *Basic Principles of Organic Chemistry*, Benjamin, New York, 1965, p. 137.
6. E. L. Eliel, *Elements of Stereochemistry*, Wiley, New York, 1969.
7. IUPAC 1968 Tentative Rules, Section E, Fundamental Stereochemistry, Information Bulletin No. 35, 25th Conference at Cortina, Italy, June, 1969, Berichthaus Zurich; *J. Org. Chem.*, **35**, 2849 (1970).
8. V. Prelog, *Chem. Britain*, p. 382 (1968).
9. D. Arigoni and E. L. Eliel, in *Topics in Stereochemistry*, Vol. 4, ed. E. L. Eliel and N. L. Allinger, Wiley-Interscience, New York, 1969, p. 127.
10. Ref. 3, pp. 25, 90, and 116.
11. J. McKenna, *Conformational Analysis of Organic Compounds*, The Royal Institute of Chemistry Lecture Series, No. 1, London, 1966.

12. G. W. Wheland, *Advanced Organic Chemistry*, 3rd ed., Wiley, New York, 1960.
13. Ref. 5, p. 498.
14. Ref. 3, p. 78
15. Ref. 3, p. 50.
16. K. Mislow and M. Raban, in *Topics in Stereochemistry*, Vol. 1, ed. E. L. Eliel and N. L. Allinger, Wiley-Interscience, New York, 1967, p. 1.
17. R. H. Pethrick and E. Wyn-Jones, *Quart. Rev.*, **23**, 301 (1969).
18. F. V. Burtcher, Jr., T. Roberts, S. J. Barr, and N. Pearson, *J. Am. Chem. Soc.*, **81**, 4915 (1959).
19. H. H. Lau, *Angew. Chem.*, **73**, 423 (1961).
20. W. Klyne and V. Prelog, *Experientia*, **16**, 521 (1960).
21. E. Fischer, *Untersuchungen über Kohlenhydrate und Fermente*, Verlag Springer, Berlin, 1909.
22 C. S. Hudson, *J. Chem. Educ.*, **18**, 353 (1941); *Advan. Carbohydrate Chem.*, **1**, 1 (1945).
23 E. L. Hirst and C. B. Purves, *J. Chem. Soc.*, p. 1352 (1923).
24. W. N. Haworth, *The Constitution of the Sugars*, Arnold, London, 1929.
25. O. L. Sponsler and W. H. Dore, *Colloid Symposium Monograph*, **4**, 174 (1926).
26. Ref. 24, p. 90.
27. D. H. R. Barton, *Experientia*, **6**, 316 (1950).
28. O. Hassel and B. Ottar, *Acta Chem. Scand.*, **1**, 929 (1947).
29. R. E. Reeves, *J. Am. Chem. Soc.*, **71**, 215 (1949); **72**, 1499 (1950); *Advan. Carbohydrate Chem.*, **6**, 107 (1951).
30. J. A. Mills, *Advan. Carbohydrate Chem.*, **10**, 1 (1955).
31. J. T. Edward, *Chem. Ind.*, p. 1102 (1955).
32. R. U. Lemieux and N. J. Chü, *133rd Meeting Am. Chem. Soc., Abstracts of Papers*, 31N (1958); R. U. Lemieux, *135th Meeting Am. Chem. Soc., Abstracts of Papers*, 5E (1959); *Molecular Rearrangements*, Ed. P. de Mayo, Wiley-Interscience, New York, 1963, p. 713.
33. E. L. Eliel, *Kem. Tidskr.*, **81**, No. 6/7, 22 (1969); S. Wolfe, A. Rauk, L. M. Tel, and I. G. Csizmadia, *J. Chem. Soc.*, B, p. 136 (1971).
34. S. J. Angyal, *Abstracts of Papers, 18th Intern. Congress Pure Appl. Chem.*, Montreal, 1961, p. 275; E. L. Eliel, N. L. Allinger, S. J. Angyal, and G. A. Morrison, *Conformational Analysis*, Wiley, New York, 1965, p. 351.
35. G. O. Aspinall, *Polysaccharides*, Pergamon Press, 1970.
36. G. N. Ramachandran, C. Ramakrishnan, and V. Sasisekharan, in *Aspects in Protein Structure*, Ed. G. N. Ramachandran, Academic Press, New York, 1963, p. 121.
37. D. A. Rees, *The Shapes of Molecules: Carbohydrate Polymers*, Oliver & Boyd, Edinburgh, 1967.
38. C. S. Hudson, *J. Am. Chem. Soc.*, **33**, 66 (1909).
39. R. U. Lemieux, R. K. Kullnig, H. J. Bernstein, and W. G. Schneider, *J. Am. Chem. Soc.*, **79**, 1005 (1957).
40. H. S. Isbell, *J. Res. Natl. Bur. Std.*, **18**, 141, 505 (1937); **20**, 97 (1938).
41. H. S. Isbell, *Ann. Rev. Biochem.*, **9**, 65 (1940); H. L. Frush and H. S. Isbell, *J. Res. Natl. Bur. Std.*, **27**, 413 (1941).
42. B. Capon, *Chem. Rev.*, **69**, 407 (1969).

Constitution and Configuration

2.1 Introduction

A consequence of the constitutional properties of the carbohydrates is often the existence, for a given constitution, of a number of configurational isomers. In view of recent conceptual advances in stereochemistry, it will be convenient and, hopefully, instructive to approach a consideration of the configurational isomerism of the sugars through an examination of the symmetry properties of the *constitutionally symmetrical* acyclic carbohydrate molecules (e.g., $CH_2OH \cdot CHOH \cdot CHOH \cdot CH_2OH$). In this manner, it will become evident how the stereoisomeric relationships among different ligands in these molecules determine the way in which they are related to the *constitutionally unsymmetrical* acyclic carbohydrate molecules (e.g., $CHO \cdot CHOH \cdot CHOH \cdot CH_2OH$).

Since the stereoisomeric relationships among different ligands in molecules are dependent on symmetry properties, we shall preview a presentation of the configurational aspects of carbohydrate chemistry in terms of these relationships with a brief discussion of molecular symmetry.

2.2 Symmetry and Point Groups

The symmetry properties of a molecule may be discussed (1,2) in terms of the *symmetry elements* of a particular structure of the molecule. In the majority of cases, this means that a molecular conformation has to be selected before a molecule may be examined for its symmetry elements. After a molecular conformation has been chosen and hence a structure defined for the molecule, the existence of a symmetry element is demonstrated by a *symmetry operation*. The principal symmetry elements and operations are summarized in Table 2.1. Molecules which have a plane of symmetry (σ or S_1), a center of symmetry (i or S_2), or other rotation-reflection axes of symmetry (S_n with $n > 2$) are said to have *reflection symmetry*. Molecules with reflection symmetry are superimposable on their mirror images and are said to be *achiral*. Molecules without reflection symmetry are not superimposable on their mirror images and are said to be *chiral*. Chiral molecules that possess no elements of symmetry whatsoever, except for the C_1 axes which are always present, are said to be *asymmetric*. An asymmetric molecule is necessarily also chiral, but a chiral molecule need not also be asymmetric, since it may posses $C_n(n > 1)$ axes.

Table 2.1   Symmetry Elements and Symmetry Operations

Symmetry Elements	Symmetry Operations
$C_n{}^a$ (axis of symmetry)	Rotation about an axis through $360°/n$
σ^b (plane of symmetry)	Reflection in a plane
i^c (center of symmetry)	Inversion through a center
S_n (rotation-reflection axis of symmetry)	Rotation about an axis through $360°/n$, followed by reflection in a plane perpendicular to the axis

[a] All molecules have the trivial C_1 axis which constitutes the identity element, E.
[b] A plane of symmetry is a special case of S_n with $n = 1$.
[c] A center of symmetry is a special case of S_n with $n = 2$.

Each molecule may be allocated to a *point group*, depending on the combination of symmetry elements which are present. A summary of some important point groups, each defined by an assembly of certain specified symmetry elements, is presented in Table 2.2. It will be noticed that the boldface symbol used to denote a point group is based largely on the principal element of symmetry within the group, and that the subscripts help to identify other symmetry elements in the group with the point-group symbol.

The presence of symmetry elements and the allocation of point groups will now be illustrated by considering what symmetry operations in Table 2.1 may be carried out on the chair conformers of the nine inositols shown in Figure 2.1. Examination of their symmetry properties shows that *allo*-inositol[1] belongs to point group **C**$_1$ and is therefore asymmetric, D-*chiro*-

[1] It should be noted that enantiomers of the *allo* isomer are rapidly interconverting through conformational inversion of chair conformers. A more detailed discussion of this feature will be given in Section 3.2.2.

Table 2.2   Some Important Point Groups

Point Group	Symmetry Elements	Symmetry Number
C_1	E	1
$C_2{}^a$	E, C_2	2
D_2	$E, 2C_2$	4
C_s	E, σ	1
C_i	E, i	1
S_4	E, C_2, S_4 (coincident with the C_2 axis)	2
$C_{2v}{}^b$	$E, C_2, 2\sigma_v$	2
C_{3v}	$E, C_3, 3\sigma_v$	3
$C_{\infty v}$	$E, C_\infty, \infty\sigma_v$	1
$C_{2h}{}^c$	E, C_2, σ_h, i	2
$D_{2d}{}^d$	$E, 3C_2$ (mutually perpendicular), $2\sigma_d, S_4$ (coincident with one of the C_2 axes)	4
D_{3d}	$E, C_3, 3C_2$ (all perpendicular to the C_3 axis), $3\sigma_d, i, S_6$ (coincident with the C_3 axis)	6
D_{2h}	$E, 3C_2$ (mutually perpendicular), 3σ (mutually perpendicular), i	4
D_{3h}	$E, C_3, 3C_2$ (all perpendicular to the C_3 axis), $3\sigma_v, \sigma_h$	6
$D_{\infty h}$	$E, C_\infty, \infty C_2$ (all perpendicular to the C_∞ axis), $\infty\sigma_v, \sigma_h, i$	2
T_d	$E, 4C_3, 3C_2$ (mutually perpendicular), $6\sigma, 3S_4$ (coincident with the C_2 axes)	12

[a] Although molecules belonging to point groups C_n where $n > 2$ are not very common, some are known to exist; for example, cyclohexaamylose belongs to point group C_6.
[b] If there is only one C_n axis, and if n σ planes intersect at that C_n axis, then the planes are designated σ_v (where v means vertical).
[c] If there is only one C_n axis and no intersecting σ planes, but instead a σ plane perpendicular to the C_n axis, then the plane is designated σ_h (where h means horizontal).
[d] When a set of σ planes bisect the angles between a set of C_2 axes, the planes are designated σ_d (where d means diagonal).

and L-*chiro*-inositol each have only a C_2 axis and hence belong to point group C_2 and are chiral, and *myo*-, *epi*-, and *muco*-inositols all contain only a σ plane and so belong to point group C_s and are achiral. Of the others, all of which are achiral, *neo*-inositol has a σ plane perpendicular to a C_2 axis in addition to having a S_2 axis and so belongs to point group C_{2h}, and *cis*-inositol has three σ planes which intersect at a C_3 axis and so belongs to

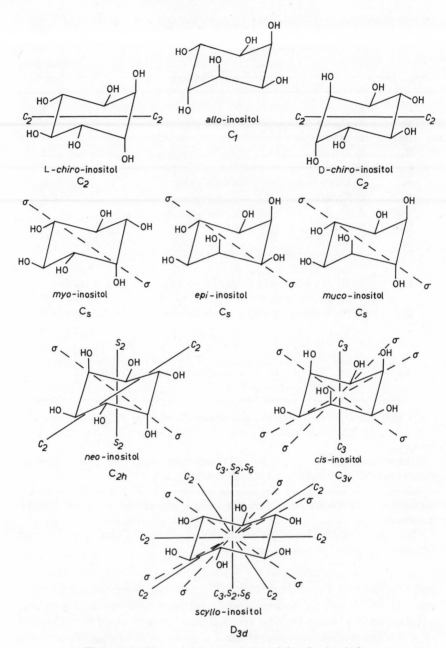

Figure 2.1   The symmetry properties of the nine inositols.

point group C_{3v}. Finally, in *scyllo*-inositol, the most highly symmetrical of the isomers and comparable in this respect to cyclohexane, three σ planes intersect at a C_3 axis and bisect the angles between the three C_2 axes. With this combination of symmetry elements, in addition to having a center of symmetry and a S_6 axis coincident with the C_3 axis, *scyllo*-inositol belongs to point group D_{3d}. Since it is an example of a molecule having a principal C_n axis with n C_2 axes in a plane perpendicular to the principal axis, it is said to have *dihedral symmetry* (hence D).

The number of indistinguishable but nonidentical positions through which a molecule may be rotated is known as the *symmetry number*. The symmetry numbers associated with different point groups are indicated in Table 2.2. Inspection reveals, for example, that while *scyllo*-inositol has a symmetry number of 6, *cis*-inositol has one of only 3. Such differences have important consequences when assessing the contributions of entropy factors toward the free energy contents of configurational isomers such as the inositols (Section 3.2.2).

2.3   Stereoisomeric Relationships

One of the more recent developments in stereochemistry has been the recognition that the stereoisomeric relationships among ligands in molecules may be defined (3) in terms of molecular symmetry operations.

Ligands are termed *equivalent* if they can be interchanged by a C_n symmetry operation on the molecule. Thus, the two hydroxymethyl groups in 1,3-propanediol (**1**) are equivalent on account of rotation about a C_2 axis. Figure 2.2 shows that transformation of each hydroxymethyl group in turn to a formyl group leads to the *same* aldehyde (**2**).

Ligands are termed *enantiotopic* when they may be interchanged only by a S_n symmetry operation on the molecule. Thus, the two hydroxymethyl groups in glycerol (**3**) are enantiotopic on account of reflection in a σ plane. Figure 2.3 shows that transformation of each hydroxymethyl group in turn to a formyl group leads to *enantiomeric* aldehydes (**4** and **5**).[2] Although enantiotopic ligands are indistinguishable in achiral circumstances, they are in principle distinguishable under the influence of a chiral environment. An enzyme is a chiral reagent and so has the ability to distinguish between enantiotopic ligands. Thus, as shown in Figure 2.4, ATP: glycerophosphotransferase catalyzes (1, 4, 5) the phosphorylation of glycerol (**3**) by adenosine triphosphate (ATP) at only one of the hydroxymethyl groups

---

[2] A carbon atom which bears enantiotopic ligands is sometimes (4) referred to as a *prochiral* carbon atom, for example, C_2 in glycerol.

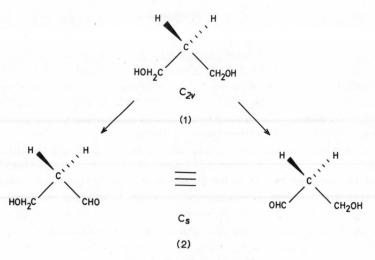

Figure 2.2   Equivalent ligands.

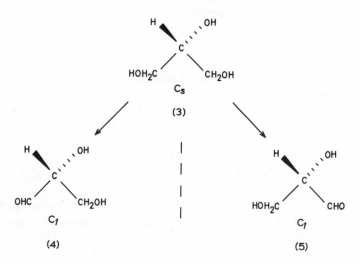

Figure 2.3   Enantiotopic ligands.

14

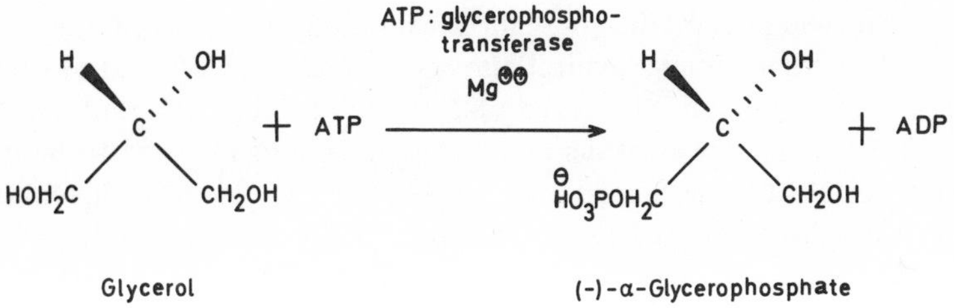

Figure 2.4   Enzyme-catalyzed phosphorylation of glycerol to $(-)$-α-glycerophosphate.

to give $(-)$-α-glycerophosphate (**6**)—but no $(+)$-α-glycerophosphate—and adenosine diphosphate (ADP).

Ligands are termed *diastereotopic* when they cannot be interchanged by any symmetry operation on the molecule. Thus, the two hydroxymethyl groups in **7** are diastereotopic on account of the absence of any symmetry operation that will interchange them. Figure 2.5 shows that transformation of each hydroxymethyl group in turn to a formyl group leads to *diastereomeric* aldehydes (**8** and **9**).

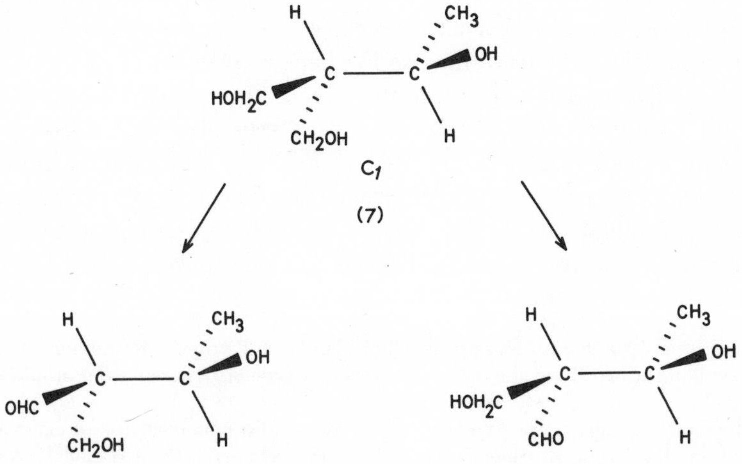

Figure 2.5   Diastereotopic ligands.

Under nuclear magnetic resonance examination in chiral or achiral solvents, equivalent nuclei exhibit the same chemical shift and are said to be *isochronous*, whereas diastereotopic nuclei exhibit different chemical shifts, barring accidental coincidence of signals, and are said to be *anisochronous*. Enantiotopic nuclei are isochronous in achiral solvents but may be anisochronous, at least in principle, in chiral solvents.

2.4 Fischer Projection Formulas and Configurational Nomenclature

Historically, the particular configurations for enantiomers **4** and **5** shown in Figure 2.3 were assigned arbitrarily to (+)-glyceraldehyde (dextrorotatory) and (−)-glyceraldehyde (levorotatory), respectively. However, in 1951, evidence (6) that this assignment was the correct one came from a crystal structure analysis of sodium rubidium (+)-tartrate, employing the method of anomalous X-ray scattering. The Fischer projection formulas for **4** and **5** are shown in Figure 2.6.[3] They are obtained (9) by orientating **4** and **5** so that the chiral carbon atom is in the plane of the projection, the formyl and hydroxymethyl groups are inclined equally below the plane of the projection, and the hydroxyl group and hydrogen atom are inclined equally above the plane of the projection. It is important to remember that Fischer projection formulas should not be lifted out of their projection plane. Also, although they may be rotated in the projection plane through 180°, it is not permissible to rotate them through 90° or 270°, since horizontal bonds must be projected above the plane and vertical bonds below the plane according to Fischer's convention.

One configurational nomenclature convention employed to distinguish between (+)-glyceraldehyde (**4**) and (−)-glyceraldehyde (**5**) assigns the descriptor D to (+)-glyceraldehyde, since it has the hydroxyl group on the *right* in the Fischer projection formula (9). The descriptor L is assigned to (−)-glyceraldehyde (**4**), since it has the hydroxyl group on the *left* in the Fischer projection formula.[4] Hence, the descriptors D and L specify the *absolute configuration*.

---

[3] Although these representations are usually called Fischer projection formulas, they are in fact modifications (7) of the original tetrahedral type of representation proposed by Fischer (8).

[4] In the early literature, the symbols *d* and *l* were also employed as configurational descriptors. However, occasionally they were confused with the rotational symbols (+) and (−) through the abbreviation of the terms *dextrorotatory* and *levorotatory* to *d* and *l*, respectively. Nonetheless, a racemic form is still referred to as a *dl*-pair or *dl*-modification. In this context, there is no ambiguity.

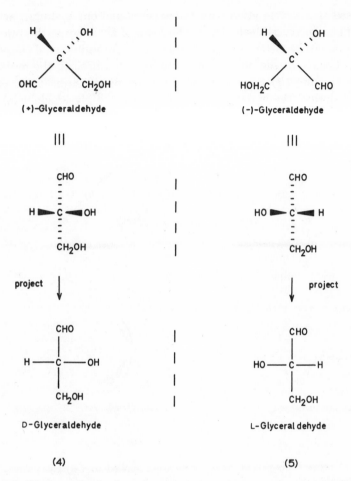

Figure 2.6   Fischer projection formulas of (+)-glyceraldehyde and (−)-glyceraldehyde.

Although the DL convention is usually employed with carbohydrates for reasons that will soon become apparent, a nomenclature convention which has more general applicability in organic chemistry as a whole is that devised by Cahn, Ingold, and Prelog (10). This convention is based on a sequence rule, which gives to the atoms attached to the chiral center a priority that decreases with decreasing atomic number. If the atoms attached to the chiral center are the same, the priority is determined by the atomic numbers of the atoms further away. Multiple bonds are considered formalistically as multiple single bonds, so that a formyl group, for example, is treated as a carbon atom with *two* oxygens and one hydrogen attached to it. Thus, in glyceraldehyde, on the basis of these rules, the priority is as follows: OH > CHO > CH_2OH > H. After the sequence of the substituents attached to the chiral center has been established, the molecule is viewed (Figure 2.7) from the position most remote from the ligand of lowest priority (the hydrogen atom in the case of glyceraldehyde) along

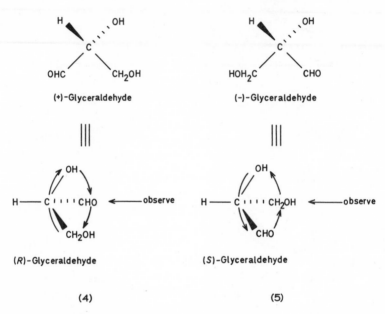

Figure 2.7 The Cahn-Ingold-Prelog convention applied to (+)-glyceraldehyde and (−)-glyceraldehyde.

the axis coincident with the bond joining it to the chiral center, and, according to whether the order of decreasing priority of the three remaining ligands is clockwise or anticlockwise, the absolute configuration is specified as (*R*) or (*S*), respectively. Thus, (+)-glyceraldehyde (**4**) has the (*R*)-configuration, and (−)-glyceraldehyde (**5**) has the (*S*)-configuration.

A knowledge of the Cahn-Ingold-Prelog convention is useful when discussing the symmetry properties of constitutionally symmetrical molecules, which is the next topic to be considered.

2.5   Constitutionally Symmetrical Acyclic Carbohydrates

When we consider acyclic carbohydrate molecules with more than one chiral carbon atom, the specification of the absolute configuration at all the carbon atoms is a less simple task. First, we shall examine the constitutionally acyclic polyhydric alcohols or *alditols*,[5] which have the general constitutional formula $CH_2OH \cdot (CHOH)_n \cdot CH_2OH$ (when $n = 2$, we have the *tetritols*; when $n = 3$, the *pentitols*; when $n = 4$, the *hexitols*; when $n = 5$, the *heptitols*; etc.). When n is even, the number of chiral configurational isomers is 2^{n-1} and the number of achiral configurational isomers or *meso* isomers[6] is $2^{(n-1)/2}$. When n is odd, the number of chiral configurational isomers is $2^{n-1} - 2^{(n-1)/2}$ and the number of *meso* isomers is $2^{(n-1)/2}$ (Table 2.3).

Table 2.3   *Configurational Isomerism among the Alditols*

Alditols	n	Number of Chiral Configurational Isomers	Number of *meso* Isomers	Total Number of Isomers
Tetritols	2	2	1	3
Pentitols	3	2	2	4
Hexitols	4	8	2	10
Heptitols	5	12	4	16

There are only three tetritols (Figure 2.8), two (**10** and **11**) with C_2 symmetry and one (**12**) with C_s symmetry. In their case, as in the remainder of the sugar series, the carbon chain of the Fischer projection formula is numbered from top to bottom and it is the absolute configuration of the *highest-numbered chiral carbon atom* which determines the nature of the configurational descriptor. Specification of the *relative configurations* at the other chiral carbon atoms is given by the *generic prefix*.[7] Thus, the name *threo* indicates that the hydroxyl groups are on opposite sides of the

---

[5] The term *glycitol* is also used.

[6] The term *meso* is specifically used in reference to isomers which are achiral when there also exist isomers which are chiral.

[7] When the DL convention is used, the generic prefix specifies the relative configuration and the configurational descriptor distinguishes between the two enantiomers, that is, it specifies the absolute configuration. Although employment of the Cahn-Ingold-Prelog convention requires specification of the absolute configuration at each chiral carbon atom, it does permit the use of IUPAC nomenclature. For example, D-threitol is $(2R, 3R)$-2,3,4-trihydroxy-butanol according to the Cahn-Ingold-Prelog convention and IUPAC nomenclature rules.

Fischer projection formula,[8] whereas the name *erythro* indicates that they are on the same side. With *meso* isomers, such as erythritol (**12**), configurational descriptors are not required.

There are four pentitols (Table 2.3), and their Fischer projection formulas are shown in Figure 2.9. Two (**13** and **14**) are enantiomers and asymmetric, and two (**15** and **16**) have C_s symmetry. It is interesting that in both D-arabinitol (**13**) and L-arabinitol (**14**),[9] C_3 is *not* a chiral carbon atom. This comes about because C_2 and C_4 have the same absolute configuration [(R) in **13** and (S) in **14**], making the two $CH_2OH \cdot CHOH$ groups attached to C_3 identical. Therefore, exchange of any two ligands on C_3 gives a molecule indistinguishable from the original and shows that C_3 is not a chiral carbon atom.[10] In the case of both ribitol (**15**) and xylitol (**16**),

---

[8] The extension of Fischer projection formulas to molecules with two chiral carbon atoms is illustrated in Figure 2.8. In those with three or more chiral carbon atoms, the conformation which is projected onto the plane is the one in which the carbon atoms are coplanar and form a loop:—

Although a Fischer projection formula corresponds to a conformation of high symmetry and is a useful configurational representation, we shall see in Section 3.3 that acyclic carbohydrate molecules do in fact exist as *zigzag* or *sickle* conformers in solution as well as in the crystalline state.

[9] If the Fischer projection formula shown in Figure 2.9 for D-arabinitol (**13**) is rotated through 180° in the plane of the projection (which is allowed), the nomenclature convention dictates that **13** be named D-lyxitol. Thus, D-arabinitol and D-lyxitol are synonyms. The same observation holds, of course, for the enantiomer (**14**). It is a general rule that asymmetric alditols have alternative Fischer projection formulas and names.

[10] The situation may be viewed in another way. Examination of the symmetry properties of the 3-deoxy derivative (**A**) shows that the two hydrogens on C_3 are equivalent on

(A)

account of a C_2 symmetry operation. Thus, replacement of either by a hydroxyl group gives the same compound.

D-Threitol (10) | L-Threitol (11) | Erythritol (12)

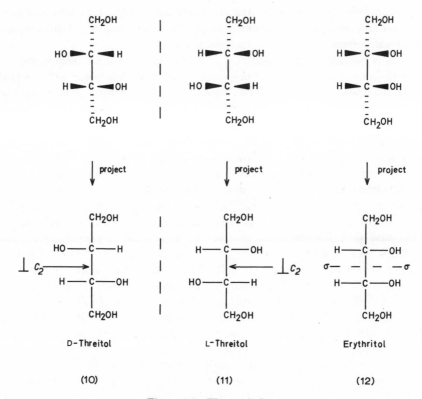

Figure 2.8 The tetritols.

D-Arabinitol
D-Lyxitol
(13)

L-Arabinitol
L-Lyxitol
(14)

Ribitol
(15)

Xylitol
(16)

Figure 2.9 The pentitols.

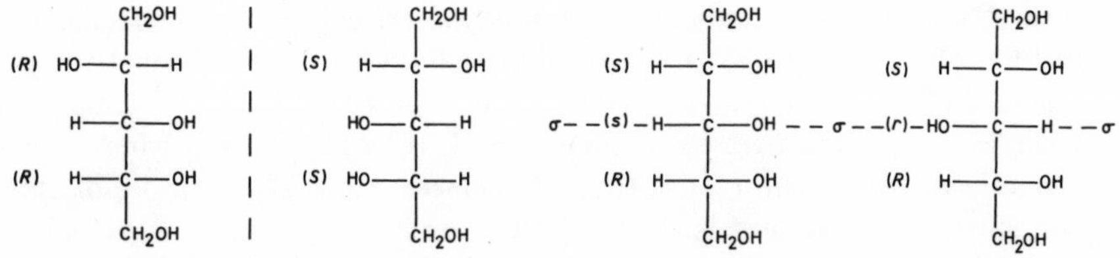

the two $CH_2OH \cdot CHOH$ groups (L) attached to C_3 are of opposite configuration and it is a chiral carbon atom, since exchange of any two ligands
on C_3 interconverts the two diastereomers. However, since C_3 lies on a σ
plane, it constitutes a special case of a chiral center and is sometimes referred to as a *pseudoasymmetric* carbon atom (11). When the subrule (10)
that L_R precedes L_S in priority is employed, the absolute configuration at
C_3 of **15** and **16** is specified by (s) and (r), respectively, in a manner
similar to the specification of absolute configuration at chiral centers by
(S) and (R). It is worthwhile noting that, whereas the generic prefixes
ribo and *xylo* specify the relative configuration at three chiral carbon atoms,
the generic prefixes *arabino* and *lyxo* specify it at only two chiral carbon
atoms in constitutionally symmetrical molecules.[11]

There are ten hexitols (Table 2.3), and their Fischer projection formulas
are shown in Figure 2.10. Four (**17–20**) have C_2 symmetry, two (**21 and
22**) have C_s symmetry, and the other four (**23–26**) are asymmetric. The
generic prefixes *manno, ido, allo, galacto, gluco, gulo, talo,* and *altro* specify
the relative configuration at the four chiral carbon atoms. The asymmetric
hexitols (**23–26**) have alternative Fischer projection formulas and names.

Of the sixteen heptitols (Table 2.3), four have C_s symmetry and twelve
are asymmetric. The reader is invited to satisfy himself that in four of the
twelve asymmetric isomers C_4 is *not* a chiral center, whereas in the four
meso isomers C_4 is a pseudoasymmetric carbon atom.

Another important class of constitutionally symmetrical acyclic carbohydrates consists of the *aldaric acids,*[12] which have the general constitutional formula $COOH \cdot (CHOH)_n \cdot COOH$. Their symmetry properties are
identical with those of the corresponding alditols.

2.6   Constitutionally Unsymmetrical Acyclic Carbohydrates

When one of the hydroxymethyl groups of an alditol is replaced by a
formyl group, the constitutionally unsymmetrical acyclic molecule that
results is termed an *aldose.* Thus, aldoses have the general constitutional
formula $CHO \cdot (CHOH)_n \cdot CH_2OH$ (when $n = 1$, we have the *aldotrioses*;
when $n = 2$, the *aldotetroses*; when $n = 3$, the *aldopentoses*; when $n = 4$,
the *aldohexoses*; when $n = 5$, the *aldoheptoses*; etc.). The number of chiral
configurational isomers is 2^n, and the number of enantiomeric pairs is
2^{n-1} (Table 2.4). The configuration of an aldose is specified for the Fischer

---

[11] However, in constitutionally unsymmetrical molecules the generic prefixes *arabino*
and *lyxo* specify the relative configuration at three chiral carbon atoms.
[12] The terms *glycaric acid* and *saccharic acid* are also used.

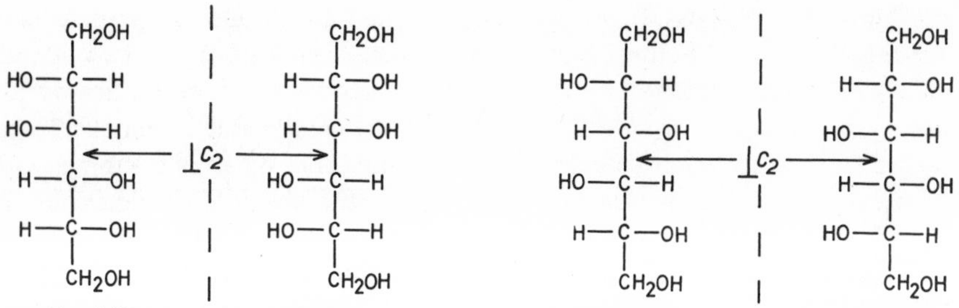

D-Mannitol (17) | L-Mannitol (18) | D-Iditol (19) | L-Iditol (20)

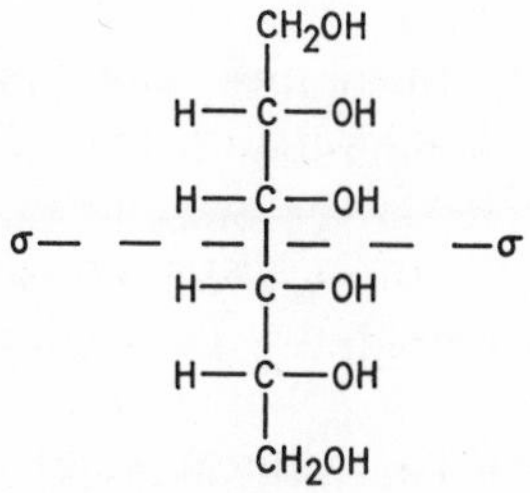

Allitol

(21)

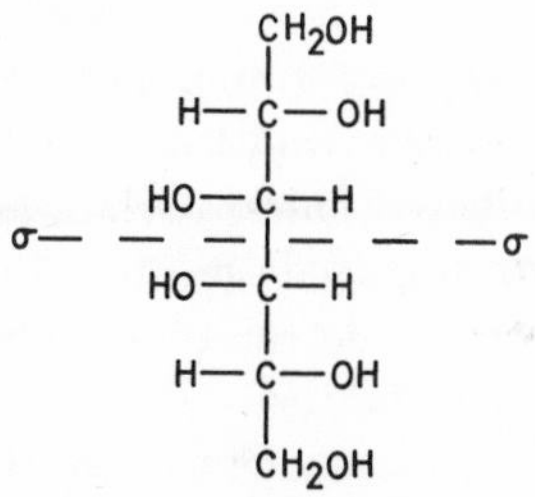

Galactitol

(22)

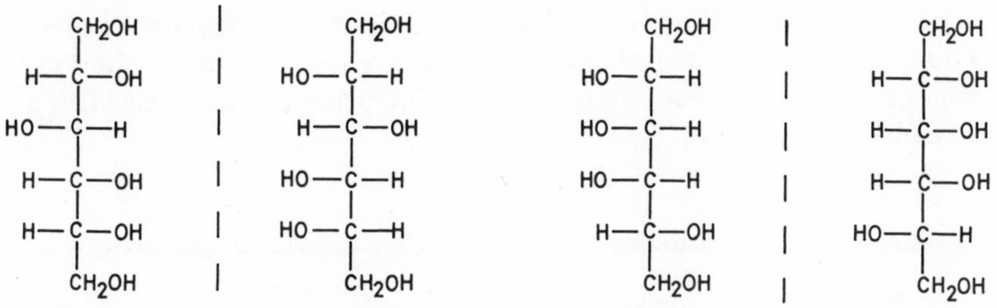

D-Glucitol, L-Gulitol (23) | L-Glucitol, D-Gulitol (24) | D-Talitol, D-Altritol (25) | L-Talitol, L-Altritol (26)

Figure 2.10 The hexitols.

Table 2.4   Configurational Isomerism among the Aldoses

Aldoses	n	Number of Chiral Configurational Isomers	Number of Enantiomeric Pairs (i.e., *dl*-pairs)
Trioses	1	2	1
Tetroses	2	4	2
Pentoses	3	8	4
Hexoses	4	16	8
Heptoses	5	32	16

projection formula with the formyl group at the top and the carbon atoms numbered from top to bottom. The absolute configuration of the highest-numbered chiral carbon atom determines the nature (D or L) of the configurational descriptor, and the generic prefix (*threo, ribo, gluco,* etc.) specifies the relative configurations at the other chiral carbon atoms (*cf.* the alditols).

It is convenient to consider the relationship between the aldoses and the alditols in terms of the symmetry properties of the latter. A classification of the alditols according to their symmetry properties leads to the following observations:

1. Alditols with **C₂** symmetry have *equivalent* hydroxymethyl groups. Thus, replacement of each hydroxymethyl group in turn by a formyl group leads to the *same* aldose. This manipulation is illustrated in Figure 2.11 for D-threitol (**10**).

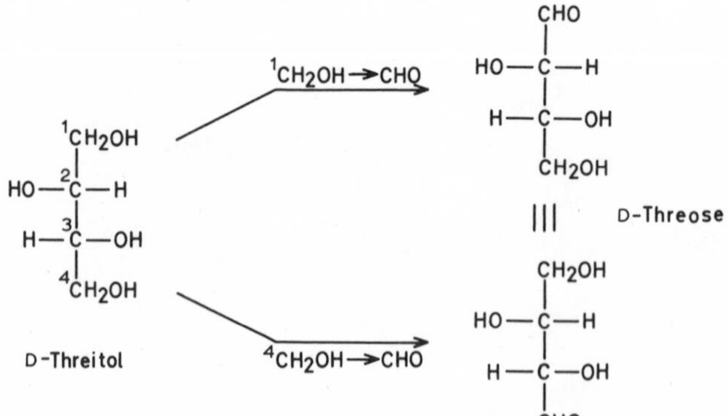

Figure 2.11   Aldoses related to alditols with **C₂** symmetry, for example, threitol (**10**).

2. Alditols with C_s symmetry have *enantiotopic* hydroxymethyl groups. Thus, replacement of each hydroxymethyl group in turn in such alditols (*cf.* glycerol) by a formyl group leads to *enantiomeric* aldoses. This manipulation is illustrated in Figure 2.12 for xylitol (**16**).

3. Alditols which are asymmetric (i.e., belong to point group C_1) have *diastereotopic* hydroxymethyl groups. Thus, replacement of each hydroxy-

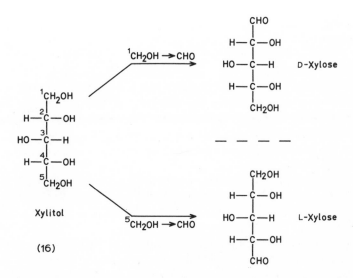

Figure 2.12   Aldoses related to alditols with C_s symmetry, for example, xylitol (**16**).

methyl group in turn in such alditols by a formyl group leads to *diastereomeric* aldoses. This manipulation is illustrated in Figure 2.13 for D-glucitol (**23**).

The symmetry-based correlation of the aldoses with the alditols is summarized in Figure 2.14. It is this correlation between the aldoses and their constitutionally symmetrical acyclic derivatives, such as the alditols and the aldaric acids, that helped Fischer to elucidate the relative configurations of all the hexoses (9, 12).

When the CHOH group at C_2 of an alditol is replaced by a carbonyl group, the constitutionally unsymmetrical molecules that result are termed *ketoses* and have the general constitutional formula $CH_2OH \cdot CO \cdot (CHOH)_n \cdot CH_2OH$. When $n = 3$, we have the *ketohexoses*, of which there are 2^3 or 8. Their Fischer projection formulas are shown in Figure 2.15, along with

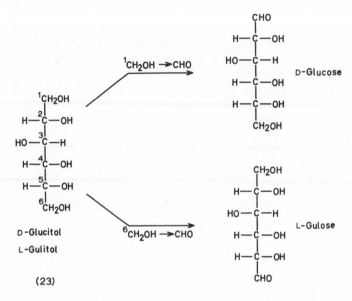

Figure 2.13   Aldoses related to asymmetric alditols, for example, D-glucitol (**23**).

their generically based systematic names and their trivial names (in parentheses). Reduction of a ketohexose leads to the formation of a new chiral center, and the two diastereomeric hexitols which are obtained and which differ in configuration at *one*, and *only* one, chiral center are referred to as *epimers*.[13]

In weakly basic aqueous solutions, an aldose (e.g., D-glucose) is partially converted via a 1,2-enediol intermediate as shown in Figure 2.16 into its C_2 epimeric aldose (e.g., D-mannose) and its corresponding constitutionally isomeric ketose (e.g., D-fructose). The transformations are reversible, but side reactions are usually so preponderant that equilibrium is never in fact established.

2.7   Lactols

When certain aldehydes and alcohols are mixed together, heat is evolved, and there is evidence (13) that 1 mole of aldehyde reacts almost quantita-

[13] An isomerization involving a change in configuration at one, and only one, chiral center is usually called an *epimerization*.

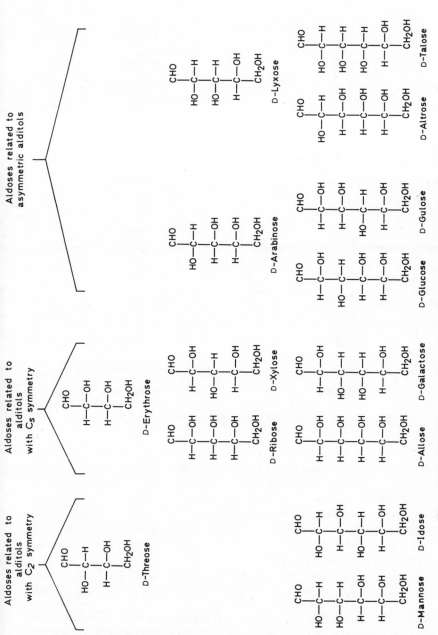

Figure 2.14 The symmetry-based correlations of the aldoses with the alditols.

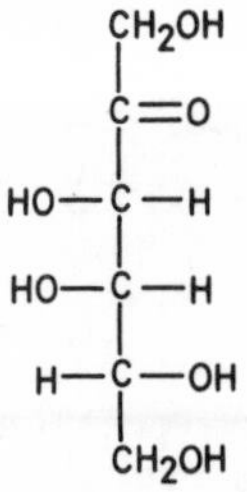

D-*Lyxo*hexulose

(D-Tagatose)

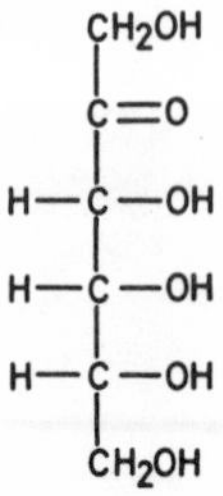

D-*Ribo*hexulose

(D-Psicose)

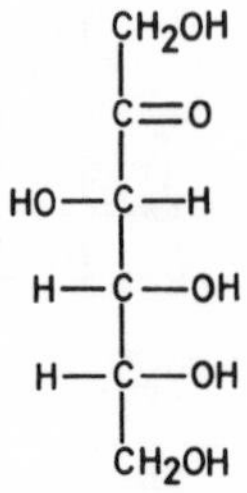

D-*Arabino*hexulose

(D-Fructose)

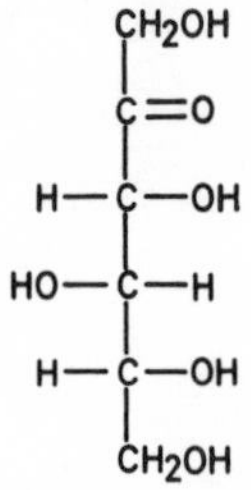

D-*Xylo*hexulose

(D-Sorbose)

Figure 2.15 The ketohexoses.

tively with 1 mole of alcohol to form a *hemiacetal* (Figure 2.17). For example, the heat of solution of gaseous formaldehyde in methanol at 23° is 15 kcal mole^{-1} of formaldehyde (14). Although the position of equilibrium between a hemiacetal and its precursors is dependent on the size of the substituent on the formyl group, derivatives of *aldehydo*-D-galactose (15) and *aldehydo*-D-galacturonic acid (16)[14] are known to form stable hemiacetals with a number of alcohols.

It is useful to consider the symmetry designations of the H—C=O faces of an aldehyde when it reacts with an alcohol to form a hemiacetal.

[14] A *uronic acid* is an aldose in which the hydroxymethyl group has been replaced by a carboxyl group. It is also worth noting here that, when the formyl group of an aldose is replaced by a carboxyl group, we have an *aldonic acid*. The corresponding lactones, which in some instances may be derived from these two acids, are termed *uronolactones* and *aldonolactones*, respectively.

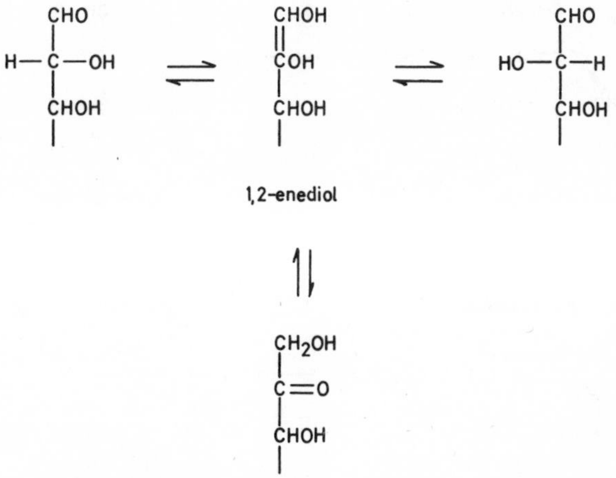

$$\begin{array}{ccc} \text{CHO} & \text{CHOH} & \text{CHO} \\ | & || & | \\ \text{H—C—OH} & \text{COH} & \text{HO—C—H} \\ | & | & | \\ \text{CHOH} & \text{CHOH} & \text{CHOH} \\ | & | & | \end{array}$$

1,2-enediol

$$\begin{array}{c} \text{CH}_2\text{OH} \\ | \\ \text{C}=\text{O} \\ | \\ \text{CHOH} \\ | \end{array}$$

Figure 2.16   The base-catalyzed interconversions of C_2 epimeric aldoses and their corresponding constitutionally isomeric ketoses.

On account of $\mathbf{C}_{2v}$ symmetry, the faces above and below the H—C=O plane in formaldehyde are *equivalent*, and therefore the addition of an alcohol (e.g., methanol) from either side yields the *same* hemiacetal (Figure 2.17a). In aldehydes which have $\mathbf{C}_s$ symmetry (e.g., acetaldehyde), the faces above and below the H—C=O plane are *enantiotopic*, so that addition of an achiral alcohol such as methanol yields *enantiomeric* hemiacetals (Figure 2.17b). If the aldehyde is asymmetric, the faces above and below the H—C=O plane are *diastereotopic*, and addition of an alcohol yields *diastereomeric* hemiacetals. Two diastereomeric hemiacetals (Figure 2.17c) of the methyl ester (**27**) of *aldehydo*-2,3,4,5-tetra-*O*-acetyl-D-galacturonic acid have been obtained as crystalline compounds.

In view of the propensity for hemiacetal formation, it is not surprising that appropriate hydroxyaldehydes and hydroxyketones form cyclic hemiacetals and hence exhibit constitutional isomerism between their acyclic and cyclic forms. In fact, both 4-hydroxybutanal (**28**) and 5-hydroxypentanal (**29**) exist (17) predominantly as cyclic hemiacetals, which are often referred to as *lactols*. Since both hydroxyaldehydes have $\mathbf{C}_s$ symmetry (*cf.* Figure 2.17b), they exist in equilibrium (Figure 2.18) with their enantiomeric lactols.

In the case of the asymmetric aldoses and ketoses, not only do they form diastereomeric lactols, but they also exhibit constitutional isomerism between different sizes of lactol rings. Although five-membered and six-membered lactol rings form (17) quite readily, other lactol rings are not so

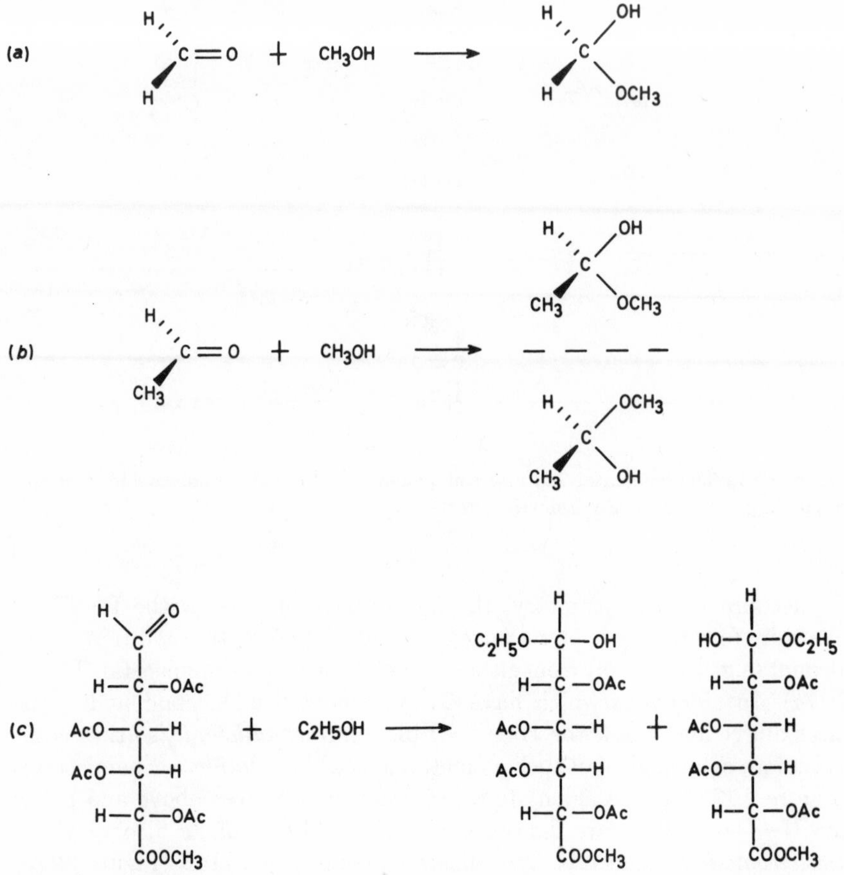

Figure 2.17 Hemiacetal formation, involving aldehydes with (a) equivalent faces, (b) enantiotopic faces, and (c) diastereotopic faces.

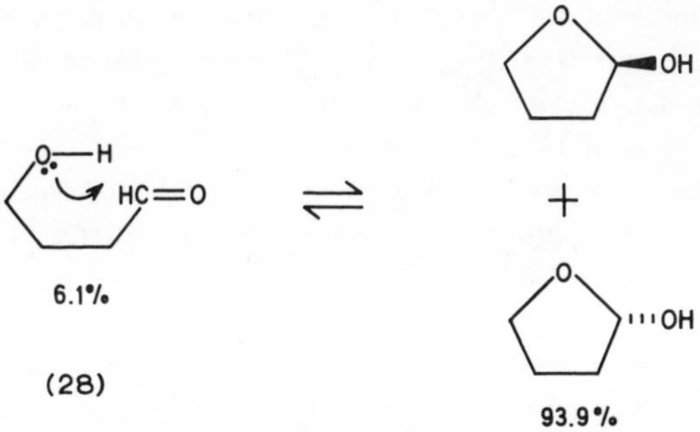

Figure 2.18 Lactol formation.

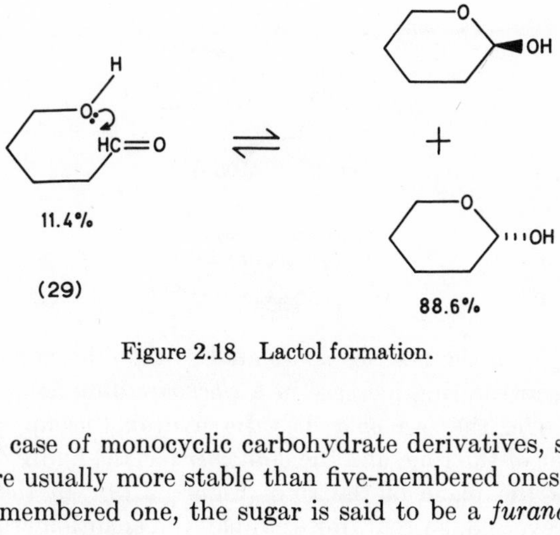

stable. In the case of monocyclic carbohydrate derivatives, six-membered lactol rings are usually more stable than five-membered ones. If the lactol ring is a five-membered one, the sugar is said to be a *furanose*;[15] if a six-membered one, a *pyranose*.

[15] These names were introduced by Haworth (18), who suggested that five-membered lactol rings may be related to furan (**A**) and six-membered lactol rings to pyran (**B**):

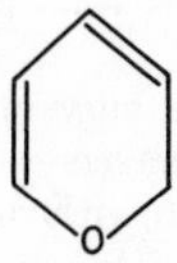

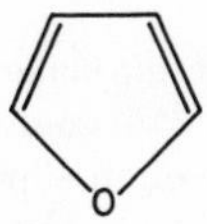

The names are now employed in a purely operational sense and may refer to lactol rings with heteroatoms other than oxygen in the ring.

In aqueous medium at about pH 6.9, an equilibrium solution of D-glucose contains[16] only 0.0026% of the *aldehydo* form, as determined by a polarographic method (19). Although the proportion of furanoses in an equilibrium solution of D-glucose is small (20), *aldehydo*-D-glucose (**30**) is shown in Figure 2.19 in equilibrium with its diastereomeric furanoses (**31** and **32**) and diastereomeric pyranoses (**33** and **34**). Diastereomers such as **31** and **32**, and **33** and **34**, which differ in configuration at C_1, and *only* C_1, are referred to as *anomers*.[17]

Although the most common lactol rings encountered are the furanoses and the pyranoses, seven-membered lactol rings called *septanoses* may be formed if the hydroxyl groups of an aldose or ketose are suitably substituted. Thus, 2,3,4,5-tetra-*O*-methyl-D-glucose exists (21) to some extent in both water and chloroform solutions as one (**35**) of its septanose forms.

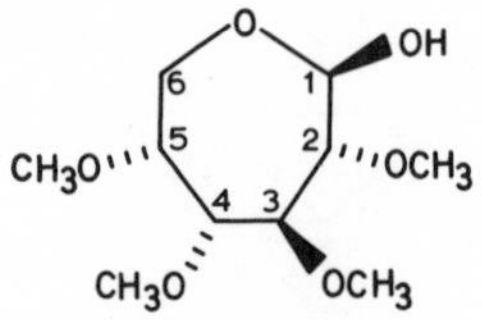

2,3,4,5-Tetra-*O*-methyl-
β-D-glucoseptanose

(35)

When a sugar in the D-series is oriented so that the numberings on the carbon atoms in the ring increase in a *clockwise* direction, looking at the ring from above, the α-*anomer* has the hydroxyl group on C_1 inclined *below* the plane of the ring, and the β-*anomer* has the hydroxyl group on C_1 inclined *above* the plane of the ring (Figure 2.19). In the L-series, this definition is reversed, so that, for example, the enantiomer of α-D-manno-pyranose (**36**) becomes α-L-mannopyranose (**37**) (Figure 2.20). The nature of the symbol (α or β) used to denote the relative configuration at the anomeric center is governed by the absolute configuration at C_5. Thus, the heptopyranose shown in **38** is L-*glycero*-β-D-*allo*-heptopyranose.[18]

---

[16] Reasons for the very much lower concentration of the *aldehydo* form of D-glucose compared with the concentrations of 4-hydroxybutanal (**28**) and 5-hydroxypentanal (**29**) in equilibrium with their lactols are given and discussed in Chapters 3 and 5.

[17] An isomerization involving a change in configuration at C_1, the so-called *anomeric center*, is usually termed an *anomerization*.

[18] The generic prefixes *glycero* and *allo* define the relative configurations at C_6, and at C_2, C_3, C_4, and C_5, respectively. The descriptors D and L establish the absolute configurations at C_5 and C_6, respectively.

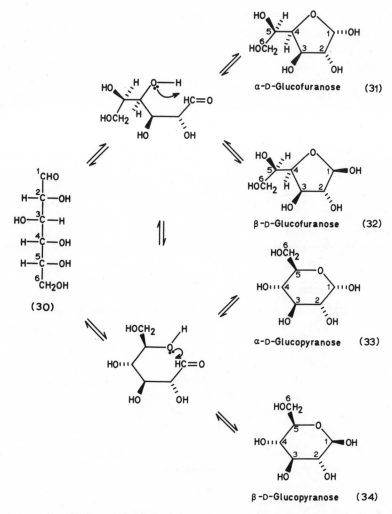

Figure 2.19   Some of the possible constitutional and configurational isomers present in an aqueous solution of D-glucose.

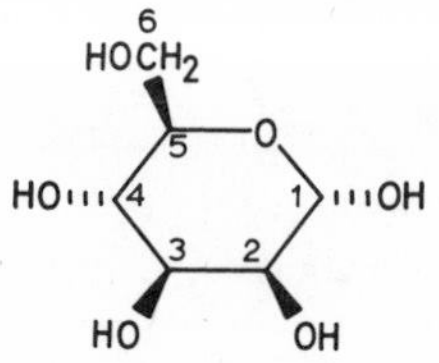

α-D-**Mannopyranose**

(36)

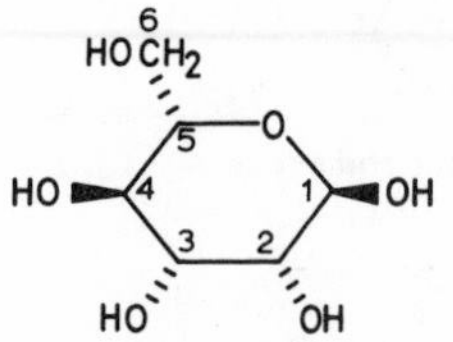

α-L-**Mannopyranose**

(37)   Figure 2.20   The enantiomeric α-mannopyranoses.

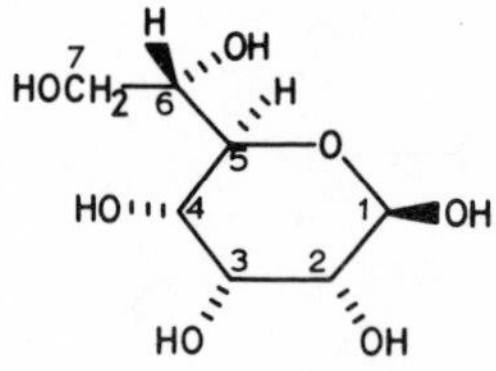

L-*Glycero* -β-D-*allo* -
heptopyranose

(38)

Finally, we shall consider an instance in which acyclic-cyclic constitutional isomerism leads to the formation of equimolar proportions of enantiomers. This occurs after the D-galactose : O_2 oxidoreductase (D-galactose oxidase) catalyzed (22) oxidation of D-galactose (**39**) at C_6 (Figure 2.21), when the initially formed product, D-*galacto*hexodialdo-1,5-pyranose (**40**), isomerizes via the acyclic form with C_s symmetry to L-*galacto*hexodialdo-1,5-pyranose (**41**). An equimolar mixture of enantiomers is called a *dl-pair, dl-modification,* or *racemic form,* and the process which leads to its formation is usually referred to as *racemization.*[19]

[19] Racemization is an irreversible process since formation of a *dl*-pair is favored by an entropy of mixing of $R \ln 2$ (see Section 3.1.1).

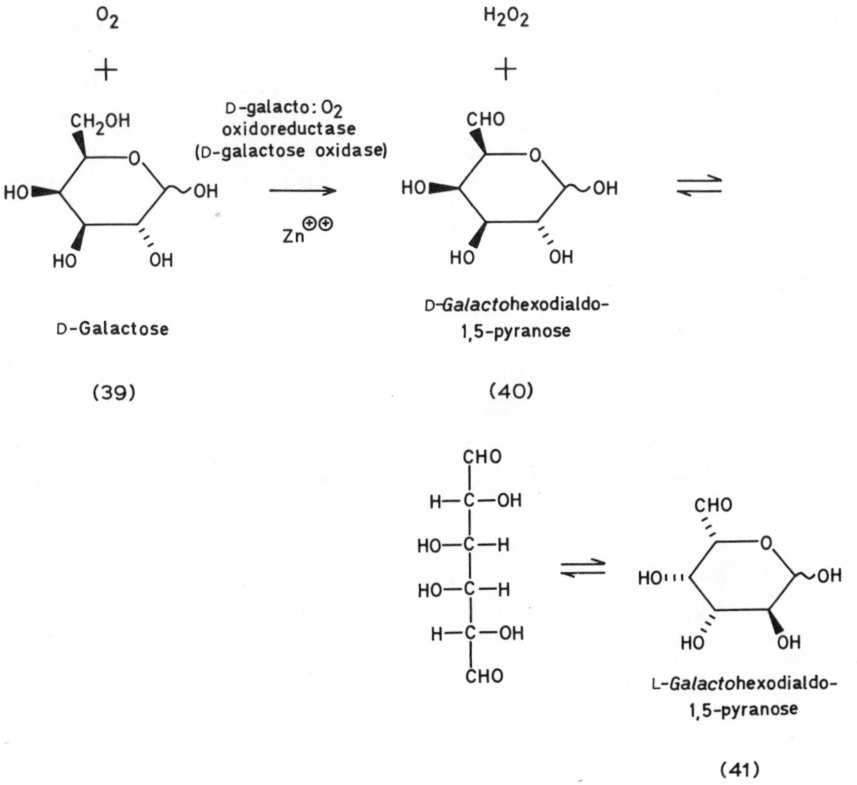

O_2

$+$

CH$_2$OH

HO

HO   OH

D-Galactose

(39)

D-galacto: O_2
oxidoreductase
(D-galactose oxidase)

$\longrightarrow$

$Zn^{\ominus\oplus}$

H_2O_2

$+$

CHO

HO   OH

HO   OH

D-*Galacto*hexodialdo-
1,5-pyranose

(40)

$\rightleftharpoons$

CHO

H—C—OH

HO—C—H

HO—C—H

H—C—OH

CHO

$\rightleftharpoons$

CHO

HO   OH

HO   OH

L-*Galacto*hexodialdo-
1,5-pyranose

(41)

Figure 2.21   DL-*Galacto*hexodialdose.

2.8   Perspective Formulas

In this book the convention suggested by Mills (23) has been used for representing cyclic carbohydrates,[20] whereby they are drawn as perspective formulas with the ring (or rings) projected into the plane of the paper, and the orientation of the substituents above or below the ring (or rings) is represented by solid or broken lines, respectively. Although perspective formulas may be rotated in the plane of the paper at will, furanose and pyranose rings will be drawn where possible in this book with the same orientations as those in Figure 2.19. The adoption of this type of perspective

[20] Wherever possible, conformational formulas will be used to represent cyclic compounds known to exist predominantly as one conformer. However, in this chapter and subsequently, if a cyclic compound is known to be conformationally mobile and only a constitutional and configurational representation is required, perspective formulas will be used.

formula by carbohydrate chemists would bring the constitutional and configurational representation of carbohydrates into line with that of other cyclic natural products, including steroids, terpenoids, and alkaloids. Moreover, as Mills (23) has pointed out, the alternative Haworth perspective formulas (18), which show the ring at right angles to the plane of the paper with substituents placed above or below this plane, are suitable only for the representation of monocyclic systems and a few simple polycyclic systems. Nonetheless, they are widely used by carbohydrate chemists. In the past, Fischer projection formulas have also been employed to represent cyclic compounds; however, they are not found very often in the present-day literature.

Examples of both Haworth perspective formulas (**31a** and **33a**) and Fischer projection formulas (**31b** and **33b**) are given in Figure 2.22. The decision to adopt a specific convention in this book does not preclude the necessity for the reader to be conversant with other conventions.

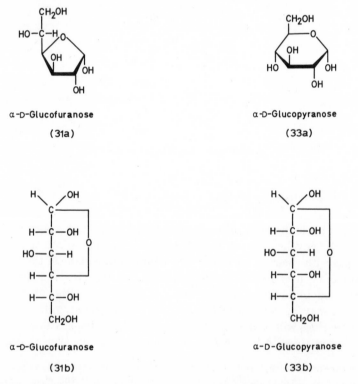

Figure 2.22 Haworth perspective formulas (**31a** and **33a**) and Fischer projection formulas (**31b** and **33b**).

2.9   Homomorphous Sugars

Aldoses and ketoses are often described collectively as *free sugars* or *reducing sugars*,[21] and perhaps less frequently as *glycoses*. Reducing sugars (containing five or more carbon atoms), which have the same configurations at corresponding carbon atoms around the pyranose ring, often have very similar physical, chemical, and enzymic properties and have been termed (24, 25) *homomorphous sugars* or *homomorphs*.

Figure 2.23 shows that the aldopentopyranoses, aldohexopyranoses, and

[21] Aldoses and ketoses have been referred to as reducing sugars, since they have the property of being able to reduce an alkaline solution of copper(II) sulfate (Fehling's solution).

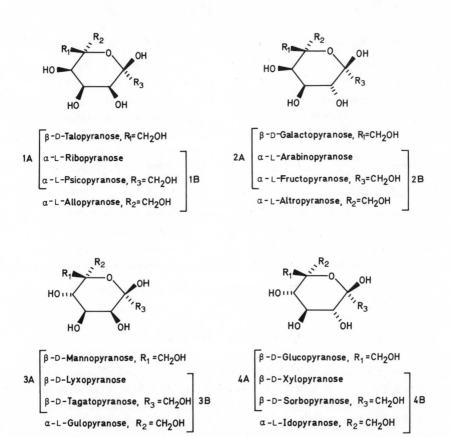

Figure 2.23   The four pairs of homomorphous pyranoses. R_1, R_2, and R_3 are H unless otherwise stated.

ketohexopyranoses may be considered to form eight groups (1A, 1B, 2A, 2B, 3A, 3B, 4A, and 4B) of homomorphs.[22] These groups have been considered as four pairs in Figure 2.23, since aldohexopyranoses which differ in configuration at C_5, and only C_5, are related to the same aldopentopyranoses and ketohexopyranoses. Therefore, if this classification of these sugars into homomorphs is considered in terms of those which have the same configurations at the corresponding carbon atoms around the furanose ring, there are only four groups (1, 2, 3, and 4 in Figure 2.24) of homomorphs,[22] corresponding to the four pairs in the pyranose series.

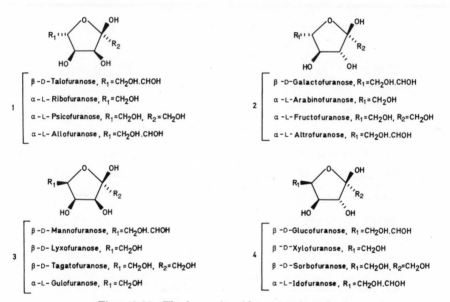

Figure 2.24   The four pairs of homomorphous furanoses.

2.10   Glycosides and Glycosidic Anhydrides

In the presence of an acid catalyst and an alcohol, reducing sugars form mixed cyclic acetals which are referred to as *glycosides*. Thus, two of the products obtained on treatment of D-glucose with dry methanolic hydrogen chloride are methyl α-D-glucopyranoside (**42**) and methyl β-D-gluco-

---

[22] In classifying these homomorphs only one anomer has been considered. If we chose to consider the other anomer, the number of groups of homomorphs would be doubled.

pyranoside (**43**). The substituent on O$_1$ (the methyl group in **42** and **43**) is called the *aglycone*.

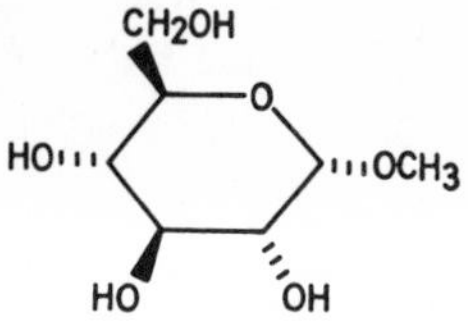

Methyl-α-D-glucopyranoside

(42)

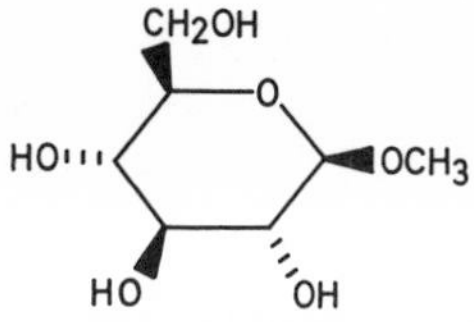

Methyl-β-D-glucopyranoside

(43)

Reducing sugars also undergo intramolecular condensations in the presence of an acid catalyst to give internal glycosides or *glycosidic anhydrides*. Thus, D-idose is partially converted into 1,6-anhydro-β-D-idopyranose (**44**) in weakly acidic solutions (see Section 5.6).

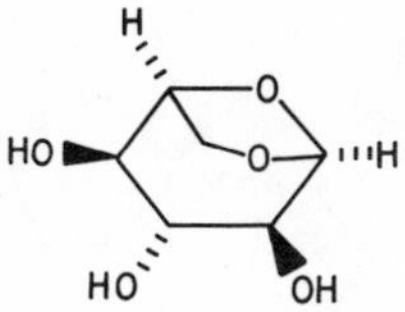

1,6-Anhydro-β-D-idopyranose

(44)

2.11 Oligosaccharides

Reducing sugars, glycosides, glycosidic anhydrides, and their derivatives are referred to collectively as *monosaccharides*. When the aglycone is another monosaccharide unit, the dimeric product which results is called a *disaccharide*. Furthermore, disaccharides may be classified as *reducing* (lactol hydroxyl group present) or *nonreducing* (lactol hydroxyl group absent). Both 4-*O*-α-D-glucopyranosyl-D-glucose (maltose, **45**) and 4-*O*-β-

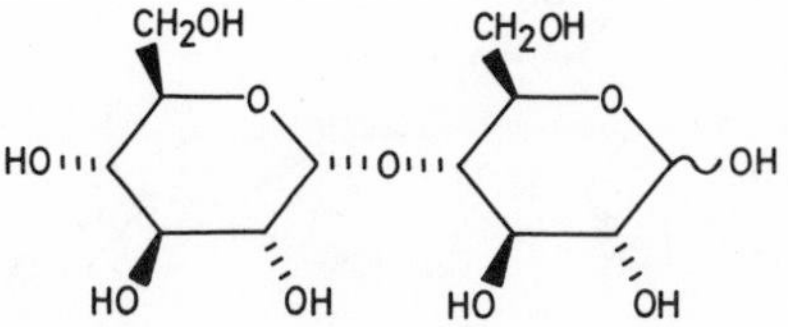

Maltose

(45)

D-glucopyranosyl-D-glucose (cellobiose, **46**) are reducing disaccharides, which differ in configuration at the anomeric carbon atom of their non-

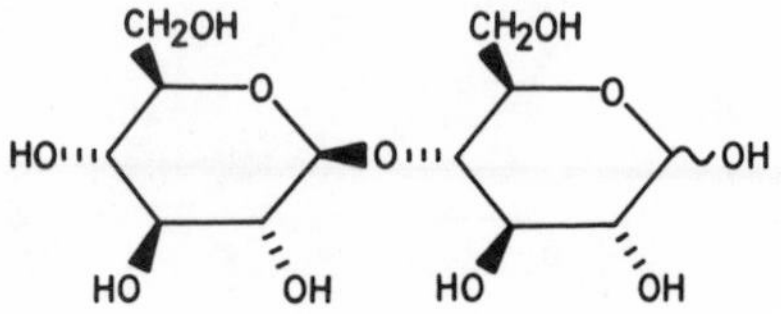

Cellobiose

(46)

reducing D-glucose residue. Maltose contains an α(1→4)-glycosidic linkage, and cellobiose a β(1→4)-glycosidic linkage. In α-D-glucopyranosyl-β-D-fructofuranoside (sucrose, **47**), the lactol hydroxyl groups of each mono-

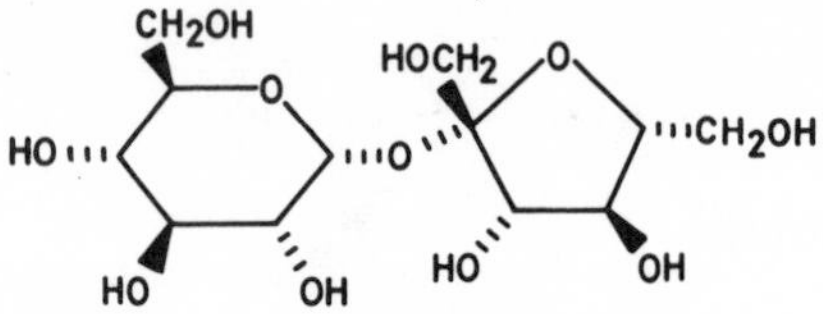

Sucrose

(47)

saccharide unit are involved in glycoside formation and hence the di-saccharide is nonreducing. When a uronic acid residue is linked glycosidically to a neutral monosaccharide unit as in 6-*O*-β-D-glucopyranosyluronic acid-D-galactose (**48**), the acidic disaccharide is usually called an *aldobiouronic acid*.

In addition to being either reducing or nonreducing, a *trisaccharide*—the next higher homolog—may be *branched*, for example, *O*-β-D-gluco-

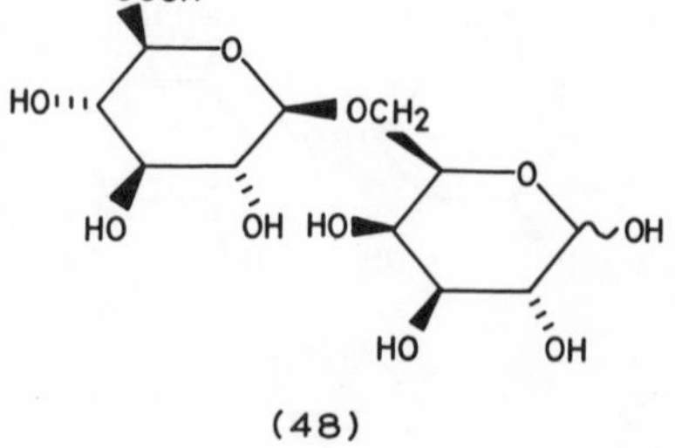

(48)

pyranosyl-(1→6)-*O*-[β-D-glucopyranosyl(1→3)]-D-glucose (**49**), or, of course, it may be *linear*.[23]

(49)

Disaccharides, trisaccharides, and higher homologs up to about decasaccharides are often referred to collectively as *oligosaccharides*.

2.12   Polysaccharides

Carbohydrate polymers of glycosidically linked monosaccharide units are called *polysaccharides*. If a polysaccharide contains one kind of monosaccharide unit, it is termed a *homopolysaccharide;* if it contains more than one kind, a *heteropolysaccharide*.

The constitutional and configurational properties of a polysaccharide define its *primary structure*. In other words, a knowledge of polysaccharide primary structure implies a knowledge of the constitution of the polysaccharide and of the configurations at all the chiral carbon atoms associated with the monosaccharide residues which comprise the polysaccharide chains.[24]

[23] A reducing trisaccharide is said to be *branched* if each of two non-reducing monosaccharide residues is linked glycosidically to the reducing sugar residue. In a *linear* trisaccharide, the monosaccharide residues are linked glycosidically to each other in a head-to-tail fashion.

[24] The term *chain* is often used to describe linear portions of polysaccharides, when monosaccharide residues are glycosidically linked to each other in a head-to-tail fashion. Polysaccharides may be linear or branched. In this context, the terms linear and branched are used only in a primary structural sense (*cf.* the description of linear and branched trisaccharides) and do not imply any description of the conformation of the polysaccharide.

Before entering into a discussion of the primary structures of some polysaccharides, it is important that the reader should appreciate the concept of polydispersity (26) in regard to polysaccharide preparations. There is good evidence to suppose that polysaccharides which have been elaborated biosynthetically are unlikely to be composed of truly identical molecules. The variation in molecular architecture is manifest in both their physical and their chemical properties.

It is customary in synthetic polymer chemistry to distinguish between monodisperse and polydisperse preparations, and these distinctions may be extended (26) to natural polymers such as polysaccharides. If the preparation contains identical molecules, it is said to be *monodisperse*, that is, there are no variations in *all the measurable* physical and chemical properties, as shown in Figure 2.25a. If, however, there is a variation in some of the physical and chemical properties of the separate molecules that comprise the polymer preparation, and if this variation is unimodal, that is, the distribution curve has one minimum and two points of inflection, as shown in Figure 2.25b, the preparation is said to be *polydisperse*. If the preparation contains two or more monodisperse polymers (Figure 2.25c), or if the distribution curve for any measurable property is bimodal or polymodal (Figure 2.25d), the polymer is said to be *heterogenous*.[25] To date, no naturally occurring polysaccharides have been shown to be monodisperse.

Although it may be argued that polydispersity could be a consequence of degradative changes brought about during isolation from the natural source, present evidence (26) indicates that some variation in primary structure is to be expected from the fact that polysaccharide biosynthesis is more remote from gene control than is protein biosynthesis; polysaccharide biosynthesis is gene controlled only in so far as enzymes involved in the biosynthetic pathways along the route to polysaccharides are under primary gene control. A consequence is that many of the more complex heteropolysaccharide molecules, in particular, probably have molecular architectures which are characterized by regions associated with various degrees of primary structural order and disorder.[26]

One of the manifestations of polydispersity in polysaccharide preparations is *molecular weight distribution*. As a result, we may only obtain an *average* molecular weight for a polysaccharide, There are different types of averages, and the actual average obtained depends (28) on the method of molecular weight determination.

[25] The term *homogeneous* is often used to describe a preparation which is polydisperse.
[26] This is an expression of opinion, since, strictly speaking, we cannot distinguish between irregularity *within* a molecule and *between* molecules (27).

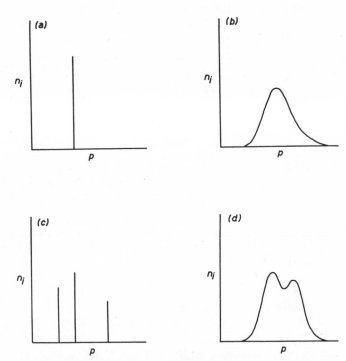

Figure 2.25   Some typical distribution curves (26) where n_i is the number of molecules having a quantity p of a physical or chemical property for (*a*) monodisperse, (*b*) polydisperse, and (*c*) and (*d*) heterogeneous preparations.

The primary structure of glycogen, the reserve polysaccharide of the animal kingdom, is that of a branched glucan (i.e., it is composed of glucose) containing chains with an average of about twelve $\alpha(1\rightarrow4)$-linked D-glucose residues in a highly ramified tree-like structure. The branch points involve $(1\rightarrow6)$-glycosidic linkages and also have the α-configuration. The chains have been termed A-chains, B-chains, and C-chains (Figure 2.26), depending on their location within the molecule. It should be appreciated that, in any particular glycogen preparation, the length of the chains of $\alpha(1\rightarrow4)$-linked D-glucose residues and the precise position of the $\alpha(1\rightarrow6)$ branch points on the chains that carry branch points are subject to a certain amount of random variation. Furthermore, when it is considered that the number of theoretically distinguishable glycogen molecules (26) in a preparation of molecular weight 10^7 is greater than 10^{2000} (!), we can appreciate that any sample of glycogen is almost certainly chemically polydisperse in addition to being physically polydisperse.

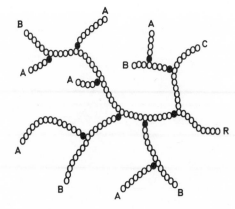

Figure 2.26 Diagrammatic representation of the primary structure of
glycogen. O = α(1→4)-linked D-glucose
residues, ● = α(1→6)-linked D-glucose
residues, and R = reducing D-glucose
residue. A-chains are α(1→6)-linked to
B-chains, which are designated as such
because they carry A-chains. C-chains
(one per molecule) are terminated by a
reducing residue and carry B-chains
and (less probably) A-chains.

Some linear heteropolysaccharides exhibit a regular primary structural pattern along their polyscacharide chains,[27] and in their case it is permissible to discuss their primary structures in terms of *repeating units*. This regularity is a feature of many animal and bacterial polysaccharides. For example, isolation of the aldotetrauronic acid, *O*-β-D-glucopyranosyluronic acid-(1→4)-*O*-β-D-glucopyranosyl-(1→4)-*O*-α-D-glucopyranosyl-(1→4)-D-galactose, together with some other evidence, has established (29) fragment **50**[28] as the repeating unit in Type VIII pneumococcus-specific

(50)

polysaccharide. Primary structural regularity is not always obvious. For example, some linear heteropolysaccharides isolated from seaweeds have a masked repeating type of primary structure (30). Carrageenan, which may be extracted with water from certain red seaweeds, is often a mixture of several polysaccharides. One component, κ-carrageenan, has a primary structure of this masked repeating type, based on an alternating sequence

[27] They are sometimes called *regular polysaccharides*.
[28] Since the polysaccharide has a high positive value ($[\alpha]_D + 121°$) for its specific rotation, the $(1 \rightarrow 4)$-glycosidic linkages between the D-galactose and D-glucuronic acid residues have been tentatively assigned (29) the α-configuration (Section 4.7).

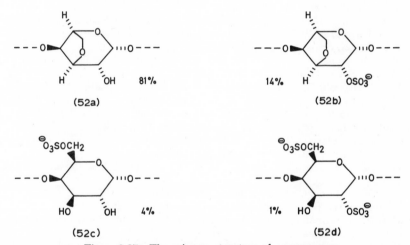

$$-A-B-A-B-A-B-A-E-A-B-$$

where A is :— (51)

and B may be one of the following :—

(52a) 81%

(52b) 14%

(52c) 4%

(52d) 1%

Figure 2.27 The primary structure of κ-carrageenan.

(Figure 2.27) of 3-*O*-substituted *O*-4-sulfato-β-D-galactopyranose residues (**51**) and 4-*O*-substituted α-D-galactopyranose residues, which are present as the 3,6-anhydride (81%; **52a**), the 3,6-anhydride-2-sulfate (14%; **52b**), the 6-sulfate (4%; **52c**), and the 2,6-disulfate (1%; **52d**). The carrageenans have interesting conformational properties, but a discussion of these is reserved for Section 3.6 of the next chapter.

References

1. K. Mislow, *Introduction to Stereochemistry*, Benjamin, New York, 1966.
2. F. A. Cotton, *Chemical Applications of Group Theory*, Wiley-Interscience, New York, 1963.
3. K. Mislow and M. Raban, in *Topics in Stereochemistry*, Vol. 1, ed. E. L. Eliel and N. L. Allinger, Wiley-Interscience, New York, 1967, p. 1.
4. K. R. Hanson, *J. Am. Chem. Soc.*, **88**, 2731 (1966).
5. H. Hirshmann, in *Comprehensive Biochemistry*, Vol. 12, ed. M. Florkin and E. H. Stotz, Elsevier, Amsterdam, 1964, p. 236.
6. J. M. Bijvoet, A. F. Peerdeman, and A. J. Van Bommel, *Nature*, **168**, 271 (1951).
7. C. S. Hudson, *Advan. Carbohydrate Chem.*, **3**, 1 (1948).
8. E. Fischer, *Ber.*, **40**, 102 (1907).
9. *Cf.* E. L. Eliel, *Stereochemistry of Carbon Compounds*, McGraw-Hill, New York, 1962.
10. R. S. Cahn, C. K. Ingold, and V. Prelog, *Experientia*, **12**, 81 (1956); R. S. Cahn, *J. Chem. Educ.*, **41**, 116 (1964); R. S. Cahn, Sir Christopher Ingold, and V. Prelog, *Angew. Chem. Intern. Ed.*, **5**, 385 (1966).
11. IUPAC 1968 Tentative Rules, Section E, Fundamental Stereochemistry, Information Bulletin No. 35, 25th Conference at Cortina, Italy, June, 1969, Berichthaus Zurich; *J. Org. Chem.*, **35**, 2849 (1970).
12. C. S. Hudson, *J. Chem. Educ.*, **18**, 353 (1941); *Advan. Carbohydrate Chem.*, **1**, 1 (1945).
13. H. Adkins and A. E. Broderick, *J. Am. Chem. Soc.*, **50**, 499 (1928).
14. J. F. Walker, *Formaldehyde*, Reinhold, New York, 1944, p. 138.
15. M. L. Wolfrom, *J. Am. Chem. Soc.*, **53**, 2275 (1931); M. L. Wolfrom and W. M. Morgan, *J. Am. Chem. Soc.*, **54**, 3390 (1932).
16. R. J. Dimler and K. P. Link, *J. Am. Chem. Soc.*, **62**, 1216 (1940).
17. C. D. Hurd and W. H. Saunders, *J. Am. Chem. Soc.*, **74**, 5324 (1952).
18. W. N. Haworth, *The Constitution of the Sugars*, Arnold, London, 1929.
19. J. M. Los, L. B. Simpson, and K. Wiesner, *J. Am. Chem. Soc.*, **78**, 1564 (1956).
20. S. J. Angyal, *Angew. Chem. Intern. Ed.*, **8**, 157 (1969).
21. E. F. L. J. Anet, *Carbohydrate Res.*, **8**, 164 (1968).
22. G. Avigad, D. Amaral, C. Asensio, and B. L. Horecker, *J. Biol. Chem.*, **237**, 2736 (1962).
23. J. A. Mills, *Advan. Carbohydrate Chem.*, **10**, 1 (1956).
24. W. Pigman and H. S. Isbell, *Advan. Carbohydrate Chem.*, **23**, 11 (1968).
25. E. L. Eliel, N. L. Allinger, S. J. Angyal, and G. A. Morrison, *Conformational Analysis*, Wiley-Interscience, New York, 1965, p. 362.
26. R. A. Gibbons, *Nature*, **200**, 665 (1963): in *Glycoproteins*, ed. A. Gottschalk, Elsevier, Amsterdam, 1966, p. 27.
27. D. A. Rees, *The Shapes of Molecules: Carbohydrate Polymers*, Oliver & Boyd, Edinburgh, 1967, p. 79.
28. C. T. Greenwood, in *Physical Methods in Organic Chemistry*, ed. J. C. P. Schwarz, Oliver & Boyd, Edinburgh, 1964.
29. J. K. N. Jones and M. B. Perry, *J. Am. Chem. Soc.*, **79**, 2787 (1957).
30. N. S. Anderson and D. A. Rees, *J. Chem. Soc.*, p. 5880 (1965): N. S. Anderson, T. C. S. Dolan, and D. A. Rees, *J. Chme. Soc.*, C, p. 596 (1968).

Conformation

3.1 Introduction and Theoretical Considerations

For most molecules, including carbohydrate ones, a knowledge of conformation as well as constitution and configuration is required to define their shape, and hence their structure. In conformational analysis, consideration is usually limited to the conformations which correspond to either energy minima or energy maxima (*cf.* Section 1.1 and ref. 1). These two types of conformations correspond, respectively, to the stable conformers defined in Section 1.1 and to the transition states between stable conformers. Whereas the positions of conformational equilibria are determined by the relative magnitudes of the energy minima associated with conformers along the conformation coordinate, interconversion rates between conformers are controlled by the energy differences between the ground states occupied by the conformers and the transition states between the different conformers.

3.1.1 Conformational Equilibria

In any equilibrium between two states,[1] the equilibrium constant K is related to the standard free energy difference $\Delta G°$ between the two states by the expression

$$\Delta G° = -RT \ln K \tag{1}$$

where R is the universal gas constant and T is the absolute temperature.[2] The standard free energy difference is a complex quantity which is related

---

[1] The states may, of course, be comprised of different chemical entities, of constitutional isomers, or of configurational isomers, as well as of conformers.

[2] For example, at 25°, equilibrium constants K of 2, 5, 10, and 100 correspond, respectively, to $-\Delta G°$ values of 0.41, 0.95, 1.4, and 2.7 kcal mole^{-1}.

to the standard enthalpy difference $\Delta H°$ and the standard entropy difference $\Delta S°$ according to the relationship

$$\Delta G° = \Delta H° - T\, \Delta S° \qquad (2)$$

Combining equations 1 and 2 gives

$$\ln K = -\Delta H°/RT + \Delta S°/R \qquad (3)$$

so that, if the equilibrium constant is determined at a series of different temperatures and $\ln K$ is plotted against $1/T$, a straight-line graph is obtained. The value of $\Delta H°$ is calculated from the slope of this line, which is equal to $\Delta H°/R$, and the value of $\Delta S°$ is then deduced most conveniently from equation 2.

It is possible (*cf.* ref. 2), in principle at least, to calculate the structure and the energy of a given molecule by a quantum-mechanical approach through solution of the appropriate Schrödinger equation. However, in practice the complexities of the problem are enormous; and although considerable progress has been achieved (3) in recent years, calculations based on classical mechanical principles must still be employed with relatively large molecules such as monosaccharides. In this approach the relative intramolecular potential energies or so-called *molecular strain energies* of different conformers are compared. The total molecular strain energy E_T is given by the expression

$$E_T = E_d + E_\theta + E_t + E_r + E_e \qquad (4)$$

where E_d is the sum of the strain associated with bond deformation, E_θ is the sum of the bond-angle-bending strain, E_t is the sum of the torsional strain about single bonds, E_r is the sum of the nonbonded interactions, and E_e is the sum of any electronic interactions, which are usually found to be solvent dependent. A number of assumptions are involved in equating the potential energy difference ΔE with $\Delta H°$; these include:

1. Other potential energy terms are the same for each conformer.
2. Zero-point energies are the same for each conformer.
3. pV terms (where p = pressure and V = volume) are the same for each conformer.

The most important entropy differences between two states which may be estimated quantitatively arise because of the following factors:

1. A state containing a conformer with a symmetry number σ higher than unity will have its relative entropy reduced by $R \ln \sigma$. This will increase its relative free energy by $RT \ln \sigma$.

2. A state containing a conformer which exists in admixture with another distinguishable conformer will have its relative entropy increased according to the general theory of the entropy of mixing by $R(N_1 \ln N_1 + N_2 \ln N_2)$, where N_1 and N_2 are the mole fractions of the two conformers. This will decrease the relative free energy of the state by $RT'(N_1 \ln N_1 + N_2 \ln N_2)$; for example, for a *dl*-modification the reduction in relative free energy will amount to $RT \ln 2$.

It should be noted from equation 2 that the relative influence of entropy factors on the free energy becomes more pronounced as the temperature is increased. Other entropy differences occur between states, and certain ones of them may be estimated qualitatively as follows:

1. A state associated with the more flexible of two conformers will have a higher entropy.

2. A state associated with the more solvated of two conformers will have a higher entropy.

3. When a conformer is involved in either intermolecular or intramolecular hydrogen bonding, the entropy of the state will be reduced.

It is usually assumed that differences in entropy from sources (e.g., translational, electronic, vibrational, and torsional) are small enough to be ignored.

3.1.2 Conformational Interconversion

The rate constant k for conformational interconversion is determined by the magnitude of the free energy difference $\Delta G\ddagger$ between the conformer and the transition-state conformation according to the Eyring equation:

$$k = (\kappa k_B T/h) \exp\ (-\Delta G\ddagger/RT) \qquad (5)$$

where κ is the transmission coefficient (usually taken as unity), k_B is Boltzmann's constant, and h is Planck's constant. The free energy of activation $\Delta G\ddagger$ is related to the enthalpy of activation $\Delta H\ddagger$ and the entropy of activation $\Delta S\ddagger$ by the expression

$$\Delta G\ddagger = \Delta H\ddagger - T\Delta S\ddagger \qquad (6)$$

Experimentally, with a knowledge of the rate constant, one can calculate $\Delta G\ddagger$ for each temperature from equation 5 and plot equation 6 to obtain values for $\Delta H\ddagger$ and $\Delta S\ddagger$.

Semiempirical estimates of $\Delta H\ddagger$ and $\Delta S\ddagger$ may be obtained by classical mechanical approaches in the same manner as described previously for $\Delta H°$ and $\Delta S°$.

3.2   Pyranoid Rings

3.2.1   *Introduction and Nomenclature*

An appreciation of the conformational behavior of pyranoid rings is best sought through an understanding of the conformational properties of cyclohexane and its derivatives. It is well known (1, 4) that the rigid or chair conformer with $\mathbf{D}_{3d}$ symmetry is the most stable conformation of cyclohexane. The chair conformer of a cyclohexane ring with idealized tetrahedral geometry is shown in Figure 3.1. The bonds which are parallel

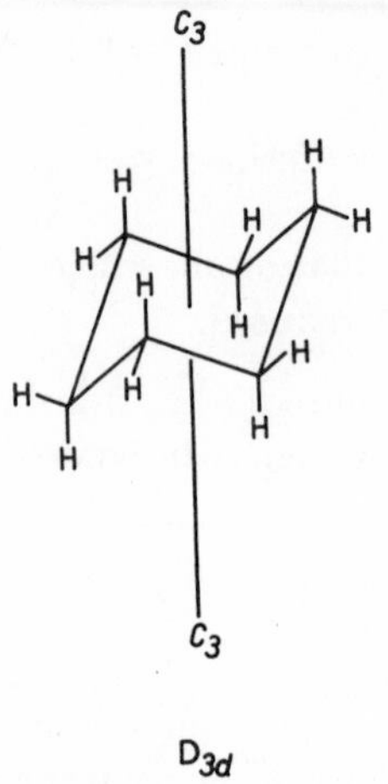

Figure 3.1   The chair conformer of a cyclohexane ring with idealized tetrahedral geometry.

to the C_3 axis are termed *axial* (*a*), and those which, on projection toward this axis, describe tetrahedral angles with it are termed *equatorial* (*e*). However, the cyclohexane ring does not have tetrahedral geometry (5–10), and the endocyclic C—C—C angle has been found to be 111.5° by electron diffraction measurements (5). This endocyclic C—C—C angle θ is related (10) to the torsional C—C—C angle ϕ shown in Figure 3.2 by the relationship

$$\cos \phi = -\cos \theta/(1 + \cos \theta) \tag{7}$$

When θ is 111.5°, ϕ is calculated (10) to be 54.5° from this expression. Thus, the torsional angle between adjacent axial and equatorial bonds is also 54.5°. Since the H—C—H angles in cyclohexane are smaller than tetrahedral, a value for the projected H—C—H angle ω of 118°, rather than 120°,

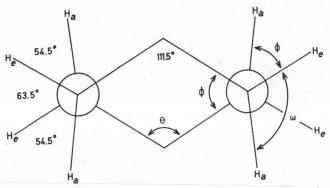

Figure 3.2   A Newman projection of the chair conformer of cyclohexane, showing the flattening of the ring. The angle θ is the endocyclic C—C—C angle, that is 111.5°.

has been used (*cf.* ref. 9) to calculate the torsional angle between adjacent equatorial bonds as 63.5° in Figure 3.2. As a consequence of these geometrical factors, the cyclohexane ring is somewhat flattened, with axial bonds directed away from the principal C_3 axis by almost 4°. These calculations are supported by the results (9) of ¹H nuclear magnetic resonance spectroscopic investigations,[3] as well as X-ray studies (10) on cyclohexane derivatives.

Axial and equatorial bonds are readily interchangeable by the degenerate interconversion shown in Figure 3.3. Such an interconversion involves passage through an infinite number of conformations, all of which are of higher energy than the chair conformer. Interconversion via a planar transition state may be discounted since it would involve (4*a*) an energy

[3] Analysis of the AA'BB' system obtained at low temperatures for the deuterated cyclohexane (**A**) indicated (9) values for J_{ee} and J_{ae} of 2.96 and 3.65 Hz, respectively. From these data a value for ϕ of around 57° was deduced.

(A)

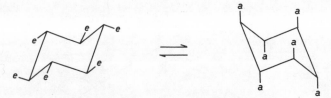

Figure 3.3   The degenerate interconversion of the chair conformer of cyclohexane, showing that axial (*a*) and equatorial (*e*) bonds are interchangeable.

barrier of about 30 kcal mole^{-1}, which is approximately three times that observed experimentally (11).

One of the possible routes to interconversion (Figure 3.4*a*) maintains a σ plane and converts the chair conformer into a boat conformation (point group, **C**$_{2v}$) via a transition state[4] (point group, **C**$_s$) which has five coplanar carbon atoms. The other possible route (Figure 3.4*b*) maintains a C_2 axis of symmetry and converts the chair conformer into the twist-boat conformer (point group, **D**$_2$) via a half-chair (point group, **C**$_2$) transition state[4] which has four contiguous coplanar carbon atoms. Semiempirical strain

[4] Recent semiempirical calculations by Hendrickson (12) suggest that the actual transition states do not correspond exactly to the conformations drawn in Figure 3.4, but occur slightly toward the boat form in the first instance (Figure 3.4*a*) and slightly toward the twist-boat form in the second instance (Figure 3.4*b*).

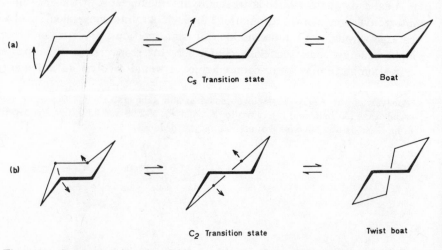

Figure 3.4   Interconversion of cyclohexane (*a*) via a **C**$_s$ transition state, and (*b*) via a **C**$_2$ transition state.

energy calculations indicate (12) that the latter route offers a slightly lower barrier to interconversion. Moreover, there is some experimental support (13) in favor of half-chair transition states. The twist-boat conformers are flexible forms and may be interconverted via boat conformations by a process known as *pseudorotation* (4), which involves a simultaneous and continuous change of torsional angles such that each ring atom subsequently takes up each of the possible ring positions. Although the twist-boat conformer is 5.5 kcal mole^{-1} less stable than the chair, it is the minimum energy conformation on the pseudorotational itinerary which interconverts enantiomeric twist-boat conformers via boat transition-state conformations at 6.4 kcal mole^{-1} above the chair conformers. All the features of ring inversion and pseudorotation which are manifest in the degenerate interconversion of the chair conformers of cyclohexane are summarized by the energy profile shown in Figure 3.5.

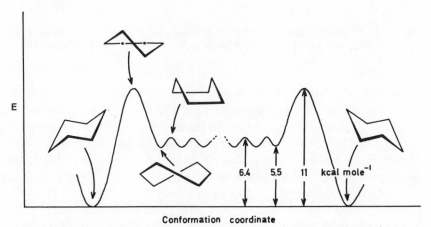

E

6.4   5.5   11   kcal mole^{-1}

Conformation   coordinate

Figure 3.5   The energy profile for the degenerate interconversion of the chair conformers of cyclohexane.

Substituent positions on conformations other than the chair conformer may also be designated as axial or equatorial, except for those associated with a carbon atom lying on a C_2 axis, where they are termed *isoclinal* (*iso*) (4b, 14). The natures of the bond positions on the twist-boat, boat, and half-chair (e.g., cyclohexene) conformations are shown in Figure 3.6. Bulky substituents tend to assume equatorial or isoclinal rather than axial positions.

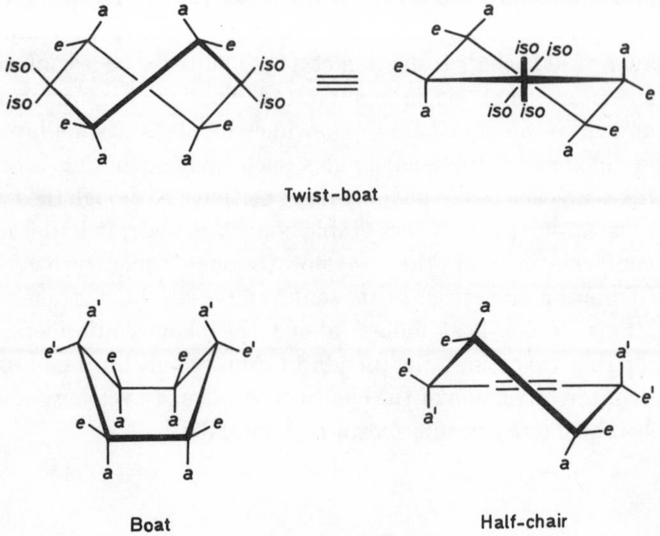

Twist-boat

Boat   **Half-chair**

Figure 3.6   Substituent positions on the twist-boat, boat, and half-chair conformations: *iso* = isoclinal; *a* = axial; *e* = equatorial; *a'* = quasi-axial; *e'* = quasi equatorial.

On account of the lower symmetry of the pyranoid ring, its conformational properties are more intricate than those of cyclohexane. In fact, when the ring carries the familiar arrangement of substituents associated with pyranoid derivatives, the chair conformers are invariably asymmetric. Therefore, in theory at least, two chair conformers are possible for all monocyclic pyranoid derivatives. More often than not, however, and certainly with most naturally occurring pyranoid derivatives, one chair conformer is much more stable than the other. Available data (15, 16) from X-ray crystallographic studies on pyranoid derivatives indicate that C-O bonds (1.42 Å) are about 10% shorter than C-C bonds (1.54 Å) and that endocyclic C—O—C angles (*ca.* 112–114°) are usually larger than tetrahedral. Consequently, just as with the cyclohexane ring, considerable flattening of the pyranoid ring must occur (5, 10), and there is evidence (17) from the results of ^{1}H nuclear magnetic resonance spectroscopy of some pyranoid derivatives that this is indeed the case.

Over the years, a number of different conventions for the representation of pyranoid ring conformations have been proposed (18) since Reeves (19) first enunciated his conformational nomenclature. The convention (*cf.* ref. 20) employed here is based on the following set of rules:

1. Conformations are designated C for chair, B for boat, S for twist-boat, and H for half-chair.

2. The pyranoid ring is numbered as described in Section 2.7, and, in addition, the ring oxygen is numbered 0 (zero).

3. A reference plane is chosen so that it contains four of the ring atoms. When an unequivocal choice is impossible, as with the chair and twist-boat conformers, the reference plane is chosen so that the lowest-numbered carbon atom in the ring is displaced from this plane.

4. Ring atoms which lie above the reference plane (numbering clockwise from above) are written as superscripts and precede the letter, while ring atoms which lie below the reference plane are written as subscripts and follow the letter.

Thus, as shown in Figure 3.7, the reference planes for the two possible chair conformers of the pyranoid ring are chosen so that they contain

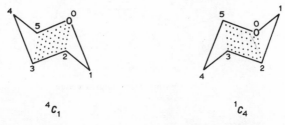

$$^{4}C_{1} \qquad\qquad ^{1}C_{4}$$

Figure 3.7   The $^{4}C_{1}$ and $^{1}C_{4}$ conformers of the pyranoid ring. The reference planes are indicated by dots.

O, C_2, C_3, and C_5. When C_1 is below the reference plane, the chair conformer is designated as $^{4}C_{1}$; when it is above the reference plane, as $^{1}C_{4}$. These descriptors correspond, respectively, to the conformational descriptors $C1$ and $1C$ introduced by Reeves (19) for chair conformers. Although the Reeves convention continues to merit popular support, the descriptors $^{4}C_{1}$ and $^{1}C_{4}$, as defined by the set of rules given above, will be employed throughout this book. A consequence of the present convention—and of the Reeves convention as well, for that matter—is that enantiomeric conformers have different descriptors, that is, the $^{4}C_{1}$ (D) conformer is the enantiomer of the $^{1}C_{4}$ (L) conformer. For this reason conformational descriptors should always be used in reference to either the D- or the L-series.[5]

---

[5] For example, a statement to the effect that methyl α-glucopyranoside exists as the $^{4}C_{1}$ conformer would be ambiguous.

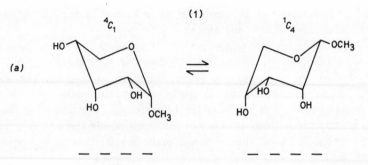

Methyl α-D-ribopyranoside

(1)

(a)

$^4C_1$ $^1C_4$

- - - - -   - - - - -

(b)

$^1C_4$ $^4C_1$

Methyl α-L-ribopyranoside

(2)

Figure 3.8   (a) The $^4C_1$ and $^1C_4$ conformers of methyl α-D-ribopyranoside (**1**), and (b) the $^1C_4$ and $^4C_1$ conformers of methyl α-L-ribopyranoside (**2**).

This point is illustrated in Figure 3.8 for methyl α-D-ribopyranoside (**1**) and methyl α-L-ribopyranoside (**2**).

By analogy with the conformational behavior of the cyclohexane ring, it should be possible for both the $^4C_1$ and $^1C_4$ conformers to be converted into twist-boat conformers via transition states which probably correspond more or less to half-chair conformations. Six different twist-boat conformers, separated by six different boat conformations, may be identified on the boat/twist-boat pseudorotational itinerary of the pyranoid ring; these are shown in Figure 3.9. However, as in the case of the cyclohexane ring, twist-boat conformers are usually found to be much less stable than the $^4C_1$ and $^1C_4$ conformers. Hence any contributions to conformational equilibria from twist-boat conformers will be small; and, apart from providing a plethora of routes for the interconversion between the $^4C_1$ and $^1C_4$ conformers, they may be excluded from consideration in most instances. The

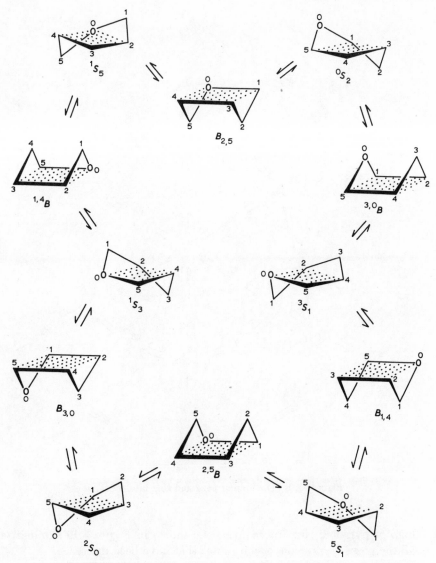

Figure 3.9 The boat/twist–boat pseudorotational itinerary of the pyranoid ring. The reference planes are indicated by dots.

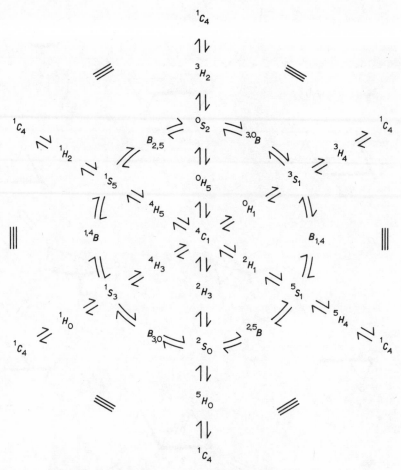

Figure 3.10   The map of pyranoid ring interconversions.

map of pyranoid ring interconversions shown in Figure 3.10 summarizes all the possible interconversion routes that have been discussed.

3.2.2   *Steric and Electronic Interactions*

In order to predict the conformational properties of a pyranoid derivative, a knowledge of the relative free energies of the two chair conformers is required. So far, it has not been possible to obtain accurate free energies, and hence semiquantitative approaches, such as the one developed by Angyal and his associates (21–23) in recent years, have, of necessity, been used. In this approach, estimates of the relative free energies are obtained by taking both steric and electronic factors into consideration.[6] Detailed information regarding nonbonded interactions has been obtained from studies on the conformational properties of the cyclitols (of which the inositols mentioned in Section 2.2 are examples) and of some model pyranose sugars. The results of these investigations will be discussed shortly. At a later stage, the implications of the presence of an oxygen atom in the pyranoid ring, with all the associated effects, both steric and electronic, which it introduces, will be considered.

As an introduction to the semiquantitative treatment, two qualitative observations on the conformational properties of the aldohexopyranoses may be made. First, an axial hydroxyl group, and particularly an axial hydroxymethyl group, will have considerable destabilizing effects (*cf.* ref. 19). As a result, most of the α-D-aldohexopyranoses, which would have an axial hydroxymethyl group in the $^1C_4$ conformer, exist predominantly as the $^4C_1$ conformer (Figure 3.11*a*). Second, the presence of two axial groups

[6] In another approach, the relative potential energies of the sixteen aldohexopyranoses and eight aldopentopyranoses arising from nonbonded interactions were calculated (24) using Kitaigorodsky-type functions (25). However, no account was taken of electronic factors, and the calculated values are not in good agreement with the experimental data (22).

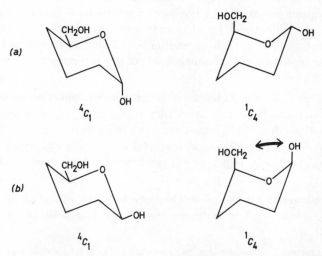

Figure 3.11   (*a*) The $^4C_1$ and $^1C_4$ conformers of the α-D-aldohexopyranoses, and (*b*) the $^4C_1$ and $^1C_4$ conformers of the β-D-aldohexopyranoses. The hydroxyl groups on C_2, C_3, and C_4 have been omitted for the sake of clarity and generalization.

on the same side of the pyranose ring[7] will have an even greater destabilizing effect.[8] Thus, all the β-D-aldohexopyranoses exist predominantly as the $^4C_1$ conformer, since the $^1C_4$ conformer would involve the bulky hydroxymethyl group in *syn*-axial relationship with the anomeric hydroxyl group (Figure 3.11*b*). Since the hydroxymethyl group is absent in the ketohexopyranoses and aldopentopyranoses, some of them might be expected to provide examples of conformational instability and to exist as equilibrium mixtures of $^4C_1$ and $^1C_4$ conformers in solution. This is indeed the case.

The semiquantitative approach to calculating the relative free energies of cyclitols and pyranoses in aqueous solution is based on a number of assumptions, of which three are important:

1. The pyranose ring is assumed to have the same geometry as the cyclohexane ring. The flattening of both rings has already been discussed. The main difference between the two rings is probably caused by the shorter C-O bonds in the pyranose ring.

2. Intramolecular hydrogen bonding is unlikely to be important in influencing conformational equilibria in aqueous solutions and may be ignored in the calculations. There is some evidence (27–30) to indicate that, although intramolecular hydrogen bonding may influence conformational equilibria in chloroform or carbon tetrachloride solutions, in aqueous solutions intermolecular hydrogen bonding with water is much more important than intramolecular hydrogen bonding.

3. The relative free energies of conformers may be obtained by summing the energies associated with nonbonded interactions between ligands (E_r) and making allowances for electronic interactions (E_e) and entropy differences. Considering each interaction separately in this manner is tantamount to assuming that the magnitude of one interaction is not influenced by the others.

None of these assumptions is strictly valid, but the success of the method indicates that the errors they introduce must be relatively small. Contributions from differences in bond deformation strain (E_d), bond-angle-bending strain (E_θ), and torsional strain (E_t) are considered to be negligible, and only two types of nonbonded interactions are taken into account:

1. Nonbonded 1,3-diaxial interactions between *syn*-axial ligands other than those between two hydrogen atoms. This interaction is designated as $(X_a:Y_a)$.

[7] The interaction that results is sometimes called (1*a*) a 1,3-diaxial or *syn*-axial interaction.
[8] The importance of this interaction in pyranose sugars was first recognized by Hassel and Ottar (26) and has been referred to as the *Hassel-Ottar effect*.

2. Nonbonded 1,2-interactions between ligands *gauche* to each other on adjacent carbon atoms apart from those involving hydrogen atoms. Axial-equatorial and equatorial-equatorial interactions are assumed to be equivalent. This interaction is designated as $(X_1:Y_2)$.

Values for all the possible interactions of these types which could conceivably occur in cyclitols and pyranoses have been obtained (22, 23) from studies on equilibria of cyclitols with their borate complexes and from studies on the anomeric equilibria of pyranoses.[9]

When cyclitols with 1,3,5-*syn* hydroxyl groups are added to a borate solution, a 1:1 tridentate complex is formed (31) as shown in Figure 3.12 and the pH of the aqueous solution decreases. From the changes in pH with stepwise addition of cyclitol, equilibrium constants K may be determined from the relationship

$$K = \frac{[\text{complex}]^-}{[\text{borate}]^- \times [\text{cyclitol}]} \tag{8}$$

Thus, the experimentally observed free energy difference may be obtained from equation 1 in Section 3.1.1. The nonbonded interactions for both the cyclitol and its complex are then listed separately and summed. In addition, a term ΔG_F° is added to the expression for the complex to account for its free energy of formation, which is assumed to be the same for all the various cyclitols. In each case, the expression for the difference in relative free energy between the cyclitol and its complex is equated with the experimentally observed free energy difference ΔG°. A set of simultaneous equations results, which may be solved to yield values of 0.35, 0.45, and 1.9 kcal mole^{-1} (at 22°) for $(O_1:O_2)$, $(O_a:H_a)$, and $(O_a:O_a)$, respectively.[10] Although the value for $(O_a:H_a)$ agrees well with the other values[11] in the

[9] The α- and β-anomers of pyranoses equilibrate spontaneously in aqueous solution (*cf.* Section 2.7), and hence it becomes feasible experimentally to obtain their relative free energies.

[10] From Figure 3.12 we see that $K = 5$ for complex formation of *scyllo*-quercitol. This corresponds to a ΔG° value of -0.95 kcal mole^{-1}. The sum of the nonbonded interactions in *scyllo*-quercitol is $4(O_1:O_2)$, and the sum of the nonbonded interactions in the complex is $2(O_a:H_a) + (O_a:O_a)$. Remembering to add on a term ΔG_F° for the free energy of formation to the expression for the complex, we have $\Delta G^{\circ} = 2(O_a:H_a) + (O_a:O_a) + \Delta G_F^{\circ} - 4(O_1:O_2) = -0.95$ kcal mole^{-1}. In analogous fashion, another five equations may be obtained for the other five cyclitols in Figure 3.12, and the set of six simultaneous equations may be solved for $(O_1:O_2)$, $(O_a:H_a)$, $(O_a:O_a)$, and ΔG_F°. (The value found for ΔG_F° is -2.5 kcal mole^{-1}.)

[11] The magnitude of $(O_a:H_a)$ is markedly dependent on the nature of the solvent—aprotic or protic. The value of 0.45 kcal mole^{-1}, which has been obtained in aqueous solution, agrees well with the values (32, 33) obtained in other protic solvents.

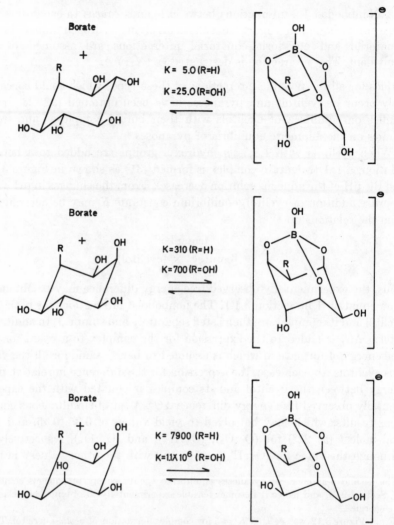

Figure 3.12 Tridentate borate complex formation of *scyllo-*, *epi-*, and *cis*-quercitol (R = H), and *myo-*, *epi-*, and *cis*-inositol (R = OH) in borate solution.

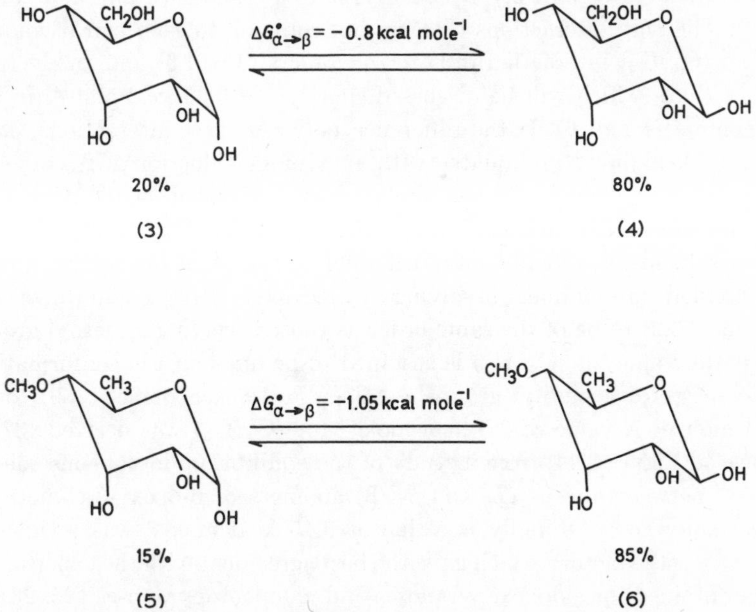

Figure 3.13 The equilibria between the α- (3) and β- (4) anomers of D-allopyranose and between the α- (5) and β- (6) anomers of 6-deoxy-4-O-methyl-D-allopyranose.

literature (32, 33) for this interaction,[12] and also gives good results for pyranoses, the value for $(O_a:O_a)$ seems to be too high when applied to these compounds. This would seem to suggest that the flattening of the pyranose ring (and hence the splaying apart of *syn*-axial substituents) occurs with greater ease than it does with the cyclohexane ring.

A value for $(O_a:O_a)$ on the pyranose ring has been obtained from studies (22, 34) of the equilibria in aqueous solution at 25° between the α- and β-anomers of D-allopyranose (3 and 4 in Figure 3.13) and between the α-

[12] To a first approximation, it may be assumed that $(O_a:H_a)$ corresponds to *one-half* the *conformational free energy* $(-\Delta G^\circ_{OH})$ of a hydroxyl group. The conformational free energy of a group X on a cyclohexane ring is the negative of the standard free energy change $(-\Delta G^\circ_X)$ for the equilibrium:

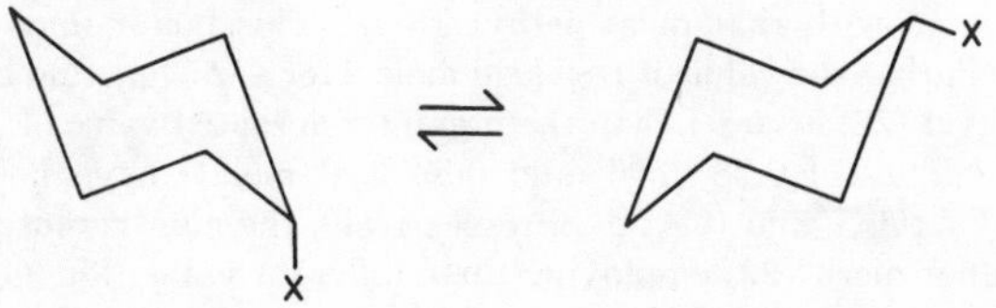

and β-anomers of 6-deoxy-4-O-methyl-D-allopyranose (**5** and **6** in Figure 3.13). The only interactions that are not common to each pair of anomers are an $(O_a:O_a)$ interaction in both α-anomers (**3** and **5**) and an electronic interaction—which will be discussed shortly—of 0.55 kcal mole^{-1} in both β-anomers (**4** and **6**). If the difference between these interactions, $0.55 - (O_a:O_a)$ kcal mole^{-1}, is equated with an average value for $\Delta G^{\circ}_{\alpha \to \beta}$ of -0.95 kcal mole^{-1}, a value of 1.5 kcal mole^{-1} may be derived for $(O_a:O_a)$.

Since the conformational free energy of a hydroxymethyl group in protic solvents is probably not much different from that of a methyl group,[13] nonbonded interactions involving a hydroxymethyl group have been assumed (22) to be of the same order as those involving a methyl group.[14] Thus the value for $(C_a:H_a)$ is assumed to· be one-half the conformational free energy of a methyl group $[-\Delta G^{\circ}_{CH_3} = 1.8$ kcal mole^{-1} (39)] or 0.9 kcal mole^{-1}. A value of 2.5 kcal mole^{-1} for $(C_a:O_a)$ was derived (37), as shown in Figure 3.14, from a study of the equilibrium in aqueous solution at 40° between the α- (**7**) and β- (**8**) anomers of 6-deoxy-5-C-methyl-D-xylohexopyranose. Finally, a value of 0.45 kcal mole^{-1} was assigned to $(C_1:O_2)$ as the factor[15] which gave the best agreement with the experimental data obtained for aldohexopyranoses and aldopentopyranoses (22, 23).

There remains the task of trying to assess the importance of the steric interaction between an axial hydroxyl group on C_2 or C_4 and the *syn*-axial lone pair on the ring oxygen atom, assuming that the nonbonding electrons on the oxygen atom may be pictured as being sp^3 hybridized. From the

---

[13] Published values for $-\Delta G^{\circ}_{CH_2OH}$ range from 1.4 ± 0.25 kcal mole^{-1} in carbon disulfide at room temperature (35) to 2.06 kcal mole^{-1} in isopropyl alcohol at 80° (36).

[14] It has been suggested (22, 37) that this would be the case if the hydroxyl group is "turned away" from the *syn*-axial hydrogen atoms when the hydroxymethyl group is axial. If the rotation of an axial hydroxymethyl group is restricted in this manner, the entropy of mixing will be less for the axial than for the equatorial isomer, and the latter will be favored in regard to entropy (*cf.* ref. 38). If free rotation of an equatorial hydroxymethyl group is assumed, there are three equally populated rotational conformers, and the entropy of mixing is close to $R \ln 3$ or 2.2 cal deg^{-1} mole^{-1}. In the axial isomer, if the "OH-inside" conformer is sterically disfavored, only two "OH-outside" conformers will be populated to any extent. Thus, the entropy of mixing of the axial isomer will be $R \ln 2$ or 1.4 cal deg^{-1} mole^{-1}. Therefore, the equatorial isomer will be favored in respect to entropy (*cf.* ref. 33c) by 0.8 cal deg^{-1} mole^{-1}. At room temperature, this would correspond to an increase of 0.24 kcal mole^{-1} in the conformational free energy of a hydroxymethyl group compared with that of a methyl group. This factor may be taken account of fortuitously in that the value of 1.80 kcal mole^{-1} for $-\Delta G^{\circ}_{CH_3}$, and hence for $-\Delta G^{\circ}_{CH_2OH}$, used by Angyal (22) is larger than the presently accepted value of 1.70 kcal mole^{-1} (32).

[15] Although values of 0.38, 0.66, and 0.83 kcal mole^{-1} have been obtained (40) for $(C_{1e}:O_{2e})$, $(C_{1e}:O_{2a})$, and $(C_{1a}:O_{2e})$, respectively, the nonrigorous nature of the present methods do not merit (22) employing three different values for $(C_1:O_2)$.

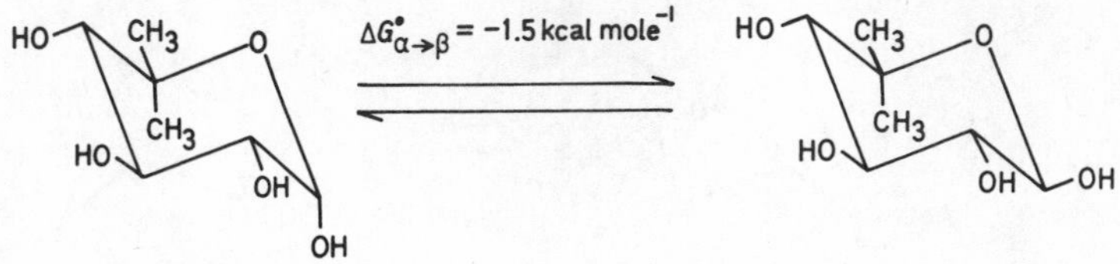

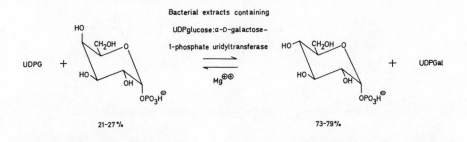

$$\Delta G^{\circ}_{\alpha \to \beta} = -1.5 \, \text{kcal mole}^{-1}$$

8%   (7)   92%   (8)

$(C_a:O_a) + (O_a:H_a)$ $(C_a:H_a) + (O:OH)$

$$\therefore \; \Delta G^{\circ} = (C_a:H_a) + (O:OH) - (C_a:O_a) - (O_a:H_a)$$

$$\therefore -1.5 = 0.9 + 0.55 - (C_a:O_a) - 0.45$$

$$\therefore (C_a:O_a) = 2.5 \, \text{kcal mole}^{-1}$$

Figure 3.14   The determination of the value for $(C_a:O_a)$ from the equilibrium between the α- (7) and β- (8) anomers of 6-deoxy-5C-methyl-D-xylopyranose.

equilibrium (Figure 3.15) established in the enzyme-catalyzed epimerization at C_4 interconverting α-D-glucose-1-phosphate and α-D-galactose-1-phosphate (41), the free energy difference may be estimated to lie somewhere between 0.6 and 0.8 kcal mole^{-1}. Since α-D-galactose-1-phosphate has an additional nonbonded interaction amounting to 0.45 kcal mole^{-1} for $(O_a:H_a)$, this would suggest a small but significant steric interaction in-

Figure 3.15   The enzyme-catalyzed equilibration of α-D-galactose-1-phosphate and α-D-glucose-1-phosphate: UDPG = uridine diphosphate glucose; UDPGal = uridine diphosphate galactose.

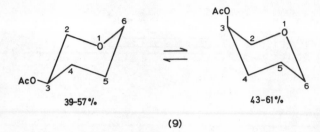

(9)

Figure 3.16 The conformational equilibrium of 3-acetoxy-tetrahydropyran. Note that the numbering of the tetrahydropyran ring differs from that of the pyranoid ring.

volving the axial lone pair. On the other hand, the conformational preference for the acetoxy group in 3-acetoxytetrahydropyran (**9** in Figure 3.16) lies (42) in the region -0.27 to $+0.17$ kcal mole^{-1}, depending on the nature of the solvent, and is much smaller than the estimated value of 0.5 kcal mole^{-1} for its steric preference. In fact, it would appear that an electronic effect is operative (42) and that it favors the axial orientation of the acetoxy group in some solvents, including water. Configurational equilibria in 5-O-substituted 2-isopropyl-1,3-dioxanes have also been found (43–45) to be strongly solvent dependent, and the *cis* isomers with 5-substituents axial predominate in some instances. Figure 3.17 shows that a 5-methoxyl group lacks any significant configurational preference in methanol, whereas a 5-hydroxyl group actually prefers the axial orientation and exists predominantly as the *cis* isomer in isopropyl alcohol.

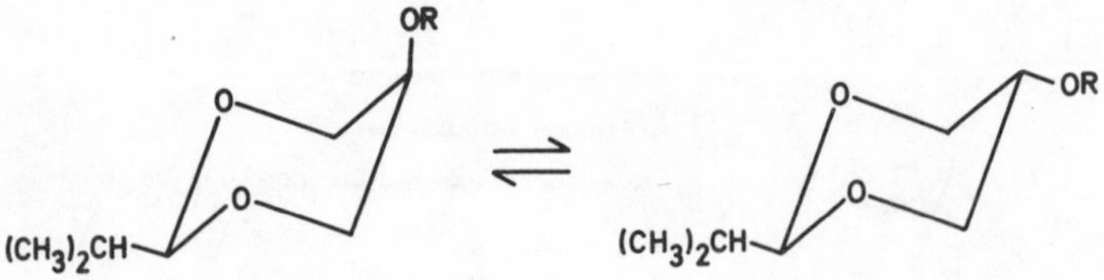

$$R = CH_3, \quad \Delta G^{\circ}_{28} = -0.03 \text{ kcal mole}^{-1} \quad \text{(methanol)}$$

$$R = H, \quad \Delta G^{\circ}_{80} = +0.51 \text{ kcal mole}^{-1} \quad \text{(isopropyl alcohol)}$$

Figure 3.17 The configurational equilibria in 5-methoxy- and 5-hydroxy-2-isopropyl-1,3-dioxanes.

These results may be compared (43–45) with the preferred *gauche* arrangements of the O—CH_2—CH_2—O units in 1,2-dimethoxyethane (46) and polyoxyethylene (47). For the present purpose, it would appear that any *syn*-axial interaction on a pyranose ring between a hydroxyl group on C_2 or C_4 and the lone pair on the ring oxygen atom is small enough in water, either by its intrinsic nature or as a result of an electronic interaction compensating for a steric effect, to be ignored in semiquantitative calculations (*cf.* ref. 22).

The magnitudes of the various steric interactions derived for substituents on cyclitols and pyranoses are summarized in Table 3.1. The values in this

Table 3.1   The Nonbonded Interaction Energies between Substituents on Cyclitol and Pyranose Rings in Aqueous Solution at 22° or 25°.

Interaction	Energy, kcal mole^{-1}
$(C_a:O_a)$	2.5[a]
$(O_a:O_a)$	1.5
$(C_a:H_a)$	0.9
$(O_a:H_a)$	0.45
$(C_1:O_2)$	0.45
$(O_1:O_2)$	0.35

[a] Determined at 40°

table, along with suitable corrections to account for entropy differences, have been used to estimate (*cf.* ref. 21) the relative free energies of the more stable chair conformers of the inositols shown in Figure 2.1 in Section 2.2. These values, which are relative to cyclohexane, are recorded in Table 3.2. Three of the inositols, *allo-*, *muco-*, and *cis-*, have three axial and three equatorial hydroxyl groups and so undergo ring inversion between two equally populated chair conformers. In the case of *allo*-inositol, ring inversion interconverts enantiomers, whereas with *muco-* and *cis*-inositols the interconversion is degenerate. The relative free energies listed in Table 3.2 have been found in some instances to be in good agreement with those obtained (21, 48) on reversible acid-catalyzed epimerization of inositols.

In summing up all the interactions in the chair conformers of pyranoid sugars, electronic, as well as steric, interactions have to be taken into consideration. Although it is becoming evident that several electronic inter-

Table 3.2   The Conformational Free Energies (kcal mole^{-1}) of the Stable Chair Conformers of the Inositols

Inositol	Interaction Energy, kcal mole^{-1}					Relative Free Energy[a]
	$(O_1:O_2)$	$(O_a:H_a)$	$(O_a:O_a)$	$RT \ln \sigma$	$RT \ln 2$ for *dl*-Pair	
myo-	2.10	0.9	...	...	...	3.0
scyllo-	2.10	...	...	1.1	...	3.2
DL-*chiro-*	1.75	1.8	...	0.4	−0.4	3.55
D-*chiro-* or						
L-*chiro-*	1.75	1.8	...	0.4	...	3.95
neo-	2.10	1.8	...	0.4	...	4.3
epi-	2.10	0.9	1.5	...	...	4.5
allo-	1.75	1.8	1.5	...	−0.4	4.65
muco-	1.4	1.8	1.5	...	...	4.7
cis-	2.10	...	4.5	0.65	...	7.25

[a] Relative to the chair conformer of cyclohexane.

actions may be involved in pyranoid sugars, the most important one seems to involve the interaction between an electronegative substituent on the anomeric carbon atom and the ring oxygen atom. As a result of this electronic interaction, which is often discussed in terms of a classical mechanical type of electrostatic interaction, electronegative substituents on the anomeric carbon atom prefer to assume axial rather than equatorial orientations. As shown in Figure 3.18, the orientation (*a*) in which the polar bond is staggered between the lone pairs is destabilized with respect to the orientation (*b*) in which the polar bond is *gauche* to one lone pair and *trans* to the other. This apparently anomolous situation was first discussed by Edward (49) in terms of repulsive electrostatic interactions between the carbon-substituent dipole and the resultant dipole of the lone pair orbitals on the ring oxygen atom[16] and has been termed the *anomeric effect* by Lemieux (50).

The preference of a polar aglycone group X for the axial orientation on the pyranoid ring may be expressed (51, 52) quantitatively as the difference between the conformational free energy $(-\Delta G_X^o)_o$ for the equilibrium shown in Figure 3.19a and the conformational free energy $(-\Delta G_X^o)$ for the corresponding equilibrium, involving an analogously substituted cyclohexane,

[16] When the substituent X is equatorial (*a*), the dipoles are aligned and so experience a repulsive interaction which is relieved when the substituent X becomes axial (*b*).

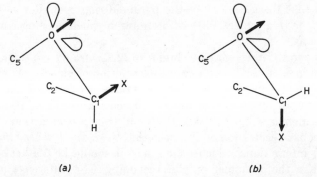

(a)   (b)

Figure 3.18 The relative alignments of the dipoles for equatorial (a) and axial (b) anomeric substituents (X).

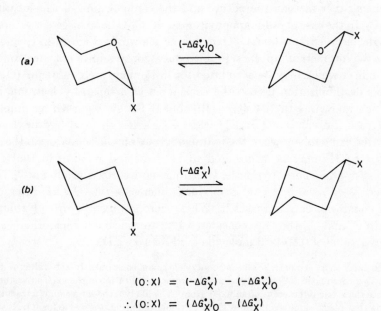

$$(O:X) = (-\Delta G^{\bullet}_X) - (-\Delta G^{\bullet}_X)_O$$

$$\therefore (O:X) = (\Delta G^{\bullet}_X)_O - (\Delta G^{\bullet}_X)$$

Figure 3.19 The quantitative definition of the anomeric effect (O:X) of a polar aglycone group X on a pyranoid ring.

shown in Figure 3.19b; that is, the anomeric effect, which will be designated as (O:X), equals $(-\Delta G_X^\circ) - (\Delta G_X^\circ)_0$ or $(\Delta G_X^\circ)_0 - (\Delta G_X^\circ)$. This definition assumes that the geometry of the pyranoid ring is similar to that of the cyclohexane ring (*cf.* ref. 53), an assumption which is being made in these calculations.[17]

A value for (O:OH) may be obtained (22, 23) from a consideration of the equilibrium composition of an aqueous solution of glucose. At equilibrium, such a solution contains 36% of the α-pyranose and 64% of the β-pyranose (54), corresponding to a free energy difference of 0.35 kcal mole^{-1} in favor of the β-anomer (Figure 3.20a). However, from a comparison of the steric interactions in each anomer, it is seen that the α-anomer has two additional $(O_a:H_a)$ interactions, which means that it should be 0.9 kcal mole^{-1} less stable than the β-anomer on this reckoning. The difference of 0.55 kcal mole^{-1} between the two values corresponds to (O:OH) and represents the electronic stabilization of the axial hydroxyl group of the α-anomer. Similar calculations for the D-mannopyranoses (69% α:31% β) (54) and the 2-deoxy-D-*arabino*hexopyranoses (47.5% α:52.5% β) (22, 23) yield (Figure 3.20b and c) values for (O:OH) of 1.0 and 0.85 kcal mole^{-1}, respectively.

Thus, the magnitude of (O:OH) estimated in this fashion depends on, among other factors, the nature and the configuration of the substituent at C_2. In the case of β-D-mannopyranose, the C_2-O bond bisects the torsional angle between the two C_1-O bonds as shown in Figure 3.21, and this *gauche* interaction appears to introduce some additional electronic instability, which may be accounted for in the increased value for (O:OH). This destabilization used to be considered as a separate electronic interaction known as the $\Delta 2$ *effect* (19), but it is now regarded as simpler to increase the value of (O:OH) when C_2 carries an axial hydroxyl group. By the same token, when the hydroxyl group on C_2 is equatorial, the value for (O:OH) may be considered to be decreased relative to that for 2-deoxy-D-*arabino*hexopyranose, which has no hydroxyl group on C_2. Thus, whereas an axial hydroxyl group on C_2 increases the (O:OH) interaction, an equatorial one decreases it. When there are axial hydroxyl groups on both C_2 and C_3, they are considered (22) to cancel out each other's effect, and a value of 0.85 kcal mole^{-1} is used for (O:OH).

[17] In fact, their geometries are *not* equivalent, and consequently the value of (O:X) does *not* correspond (52) exactly to the electronic stabilization of the axial substituent X. Since the steric interaction of an axial group X is likely to be larger on a pyranoid ring than that of the same axial group X on a cyclohexane ring, the value for (O:X) underestimates the true magnitude of the electronic interaction. However, any errors introduced seem to be small enough to be ignored in the present calculations.

(a)

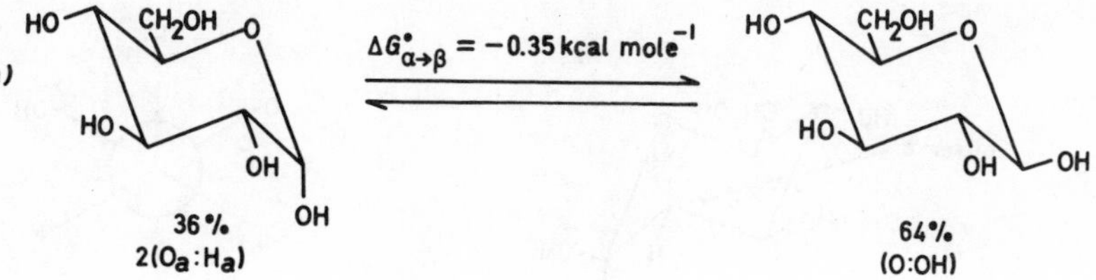

$$\begin{aligned} \therefore\ \Delta G^\circ &= (O{:}OH) - 2(O_a{:}H_a) \\ \therefore\ -0.35 &= (O{:}OH) - 0.9 \\ \therefore\ (O{:}OH) &= 0.55\ \text{kcal mole}^{-1} \end{aligned}$$

(b)

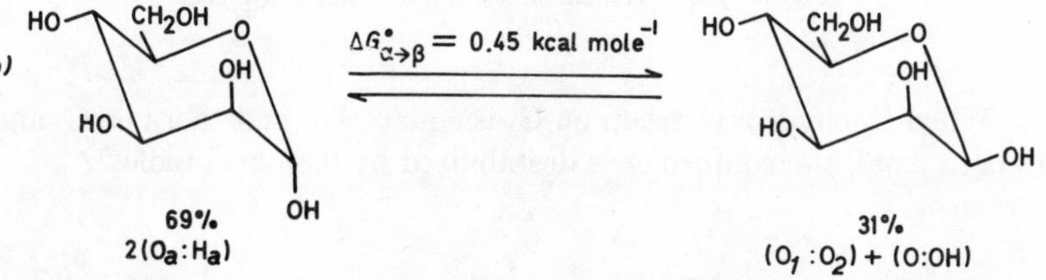

$$\begin{aligned} \therefore\ \Delta G^\circ &= (O_1{:}O_2) + (O{:}OH) - 2(O_a{:}H_a) \\ \therefore\ 0.45 &= 0.35 + (O{:}OH) - 0.9 \\ \therefore\ (O{:}OH) &= 1.00\ \text{kcal mole}^{-1} \end{aligned}$$

(c)

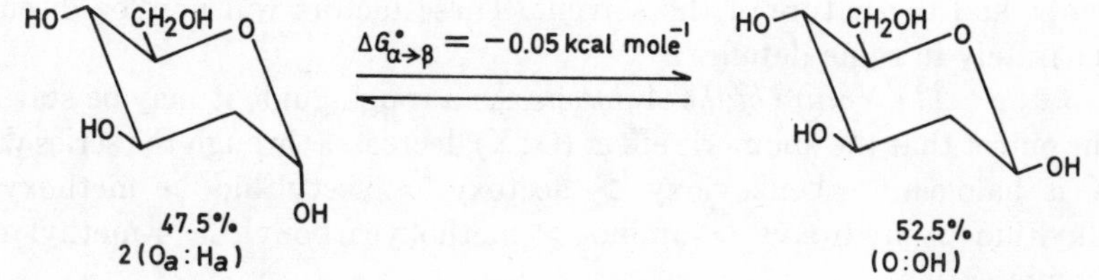

$$\begin{aligned} \therefore\ \Delta G^\circ &= (O{:}OH) - 2(O_a{:}H_a) \\ \therefore\ 0.05 &= (O{:}OH) - 0.9 \\ \therefore\ (O{:}OH) &= 0.85\ \text{kcal mole}^{-1} \end{aligned}$$

Figure 3.20 The calculated values for the anomeric effect (O:OH) associated with (*a*) the D-glucopyranoses, (*b*) the D-mannopyranoses, and (*c*) the 2-deoxy-D-*arabino*-hexopyranoses.

The following rules may be used to assess the magnitude of the anomeric effect for pyranoses in aqueous solution:

1. When the hydroxyl groups on C_1 and C_2 are both equatorial, the conformer is destabilized by 0.55 kcal mole^{-1}.
2. When the hydroxyl group on C_1 is equatorial, and that on C_2 is axial, the conformer is destabilized by 1.00 kcal mole^{-1}.

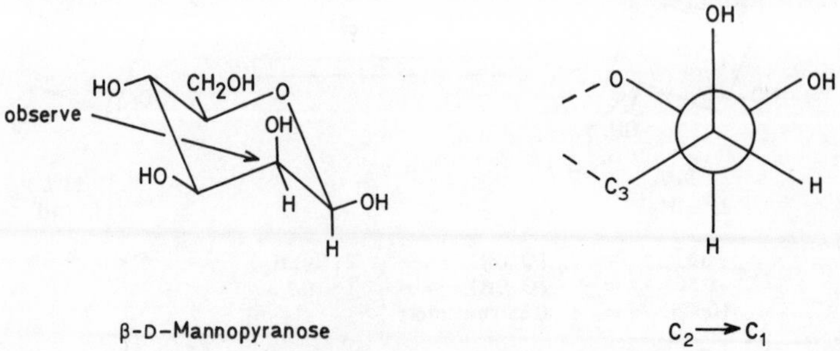

β-D-Mannopyranose $C_2 \longrightarrow C_1$

Figure 3.21   The Δ2 effect in β-D-mannopyranose.

3. When the hydroxyl group on C_1 is equatorial, and those on C_2 and C_3 are both axial, the conformer is destabilized by 0.85 kcal mole^{-1}.

3.2.3   *The Anomeric Effect*

The magnitude of the anomeric effect is dependent on a number of factors, which include the nature of the aglycone, the nature of other substituents, and the nature of the solvent. These factors will now be discussed separately in some detail.

3.2.3a   The Nature of the Aglycone. As a rough guide it may be stated at the outset that the anomeric effect (O:X) decreases through the series where X is halogen > benzoyloxy > acetoxy > acetylthio > methoxyl > alkylthio > hydroxyl > amino > methoxycarbonyl > 4-methyl pyridinium cation.

Acid-catalyzed equilibrations of *cis-* and *trans*-2-halo-4-methyltetrahydropyrans (Figure 3.22) have shown (55) that anomeric effects in favor of

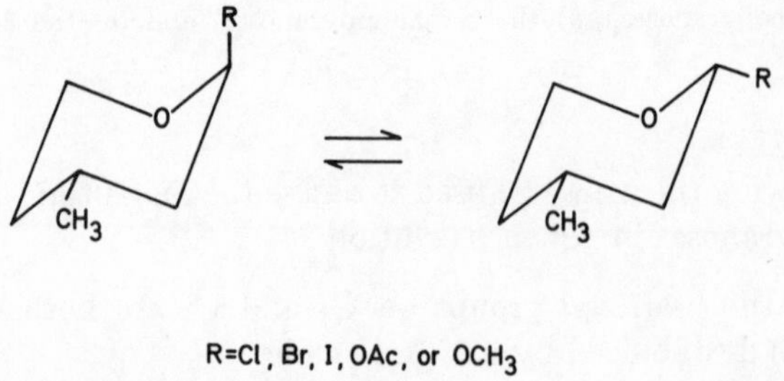

R=Cl, Br, I, OAc, or OCH$_3$

Figure 3.22   The acid-catalyzed equilibrations of *cis-* and *trans*-2-halo, 2-acetoxy-, and 2-methoxy-4-methyltetrahydropyrans.

the axial chloro, bromo, and iodo substituents, respectively, amount to at least 2.65, 3.2, and 3.1 kcal mole^{-1}. The proportion of *cis-* to *trans*-2-chloro-4-methyltetrahydropyran is 3:97, and the only detectable conformer of both 2-chloro- (**10**) and 2-bromo- (**11**) tetrahydropyran is (56) that with the halogen axial. The anomeric effect favoring axial halogen is large enough to cause (57, 58) 2,3,4-tri-*O*-acetyl-β-D-xylopyranosyl chloride (**12**) and fluoride (**13**) to exist predominantly as their all axial $^1C_4$ conformers

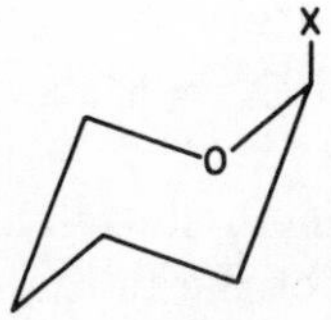

(10) X = Cl

(11) X = Br

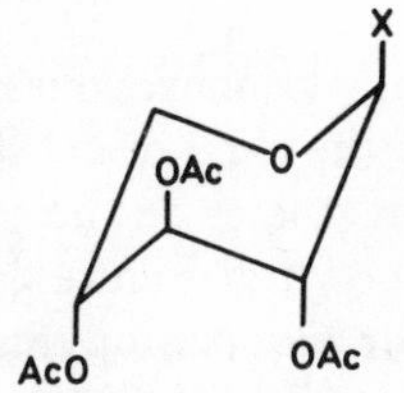

(12) X = Cl

(13) X = F

with four axial substituents and two *syn*-axial interactions. It is also significant that *trans*-2,3-dichlorotetrahydropyran (**14**) (59), as well as *trans*-2,3-dihalogeno- and *trans*-2,5-dihalogenodioxanes (60), dithianes (61), and thioxanes (62), exist as the chair conformers wherein both halogens have axial orientations (e.g., **15–18**). The situation recalls that of the 2-

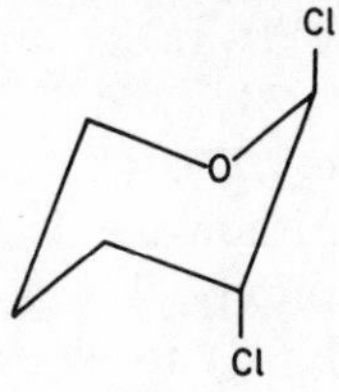

(14)

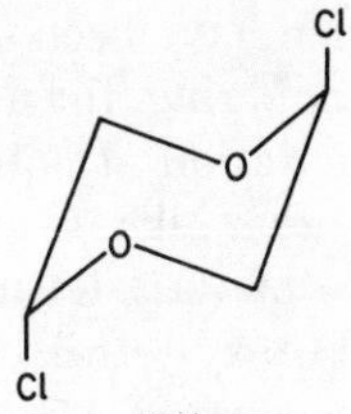

(15)

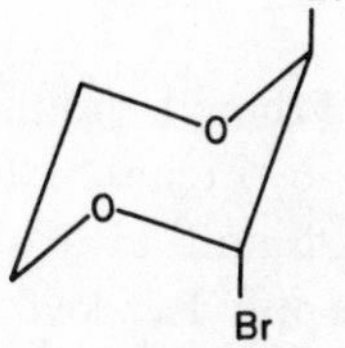

(16)

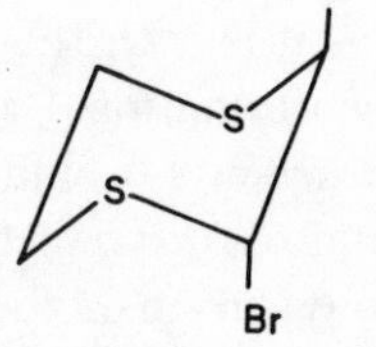

(17)

(18)   (19)

X = Cl, Br

halogenocyclohexanones (**19**), in which the halogen (X = Cl or Br) also prefers the axial orientation (63).

From studies on the equilibration of 2-acetoxy-4-methyltetrahydropyran (51), shown in Figure 3.22, and the anomerization of the tetraacetates of the four aldopentopyranoses (50*c*), a value of 1.3 kcal mole^{-1} has been obtained for (O:OAc). The anomeric effect of a benzoyloxy group is probably larger (64) than that of an acetoxy group, while that of an acetylthio group is probably smaller (65). Whereas the proportion of the *trans* isomer of 2-acetoxy-4-methyltetrahydropyran with an axial acetoxy group was 72–75%, that of the *trans* isomer of 2-methoxy-4-methyltetrahydropyran was (51) only 65% in aqueous methanol. This corresponds to a value of 0.9 kcal mole^{-1} for (O:OCH$_3$) in that mixed solvent.

The preference for an axial methoxyl group is seen also in other situations. In 3-methoxy-4-oxa-5α-cholestane (**20**) and 3-methoxy-4-oxa-5α-estrane (**21**), which have been studied (66) as models for the $^4C_1$ (D) conformer of the pyranoid ring, the methoxyl group is, respectively, 73% and 67% in the axial orientation at equilibrium in methanol (Figure 3.23). The anomeric effect of other alkoxyl groups has also been studied. Although a decrease in the value of (O:OR) in the series 2-methoxy-, 2-ethoxy-, 2-isopropoxy-, and 2-*t*-butoxy-tetrahydropyrans has been ascribed (67) to electrostatic factors because of a correlation with Taft polar constants, an alternative explanation in terms of an increased steric interaction outweighing the anomeric effect is possible (52). Alkylthio groups also show (52) a preference for the axial orientation, but in their case the preference is not as marked as it is with the alkoxyl group.

The conformational preference of the methoxycarbonyl group in 2-methoxycarbonyl-6-*t*-butyltetrahydropyran, shown in Figure 3.24, has been found (53) to be 1.6 kcal mole^{-1}, which is larger than that of a methoxycarbonyl group on the cyclohexane ring, where it is only 1.27 kcal mole^{-1} (32). This difference has been attributed (53) to electronic stabilization of the *equatorial* methoxycarbonyl group, and compared with the effect (68)

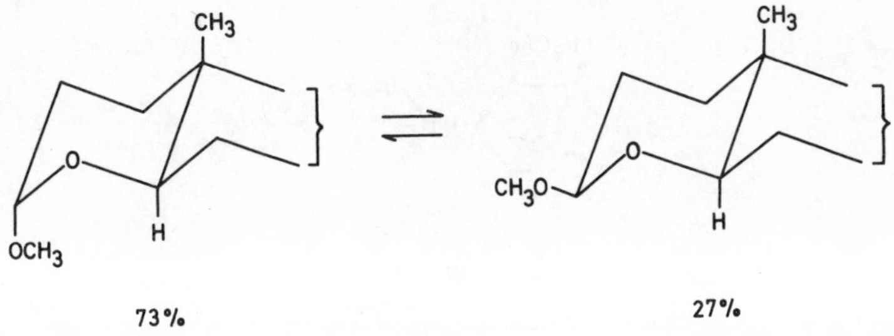

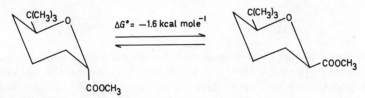

73%   27%

(20)

67%   33%

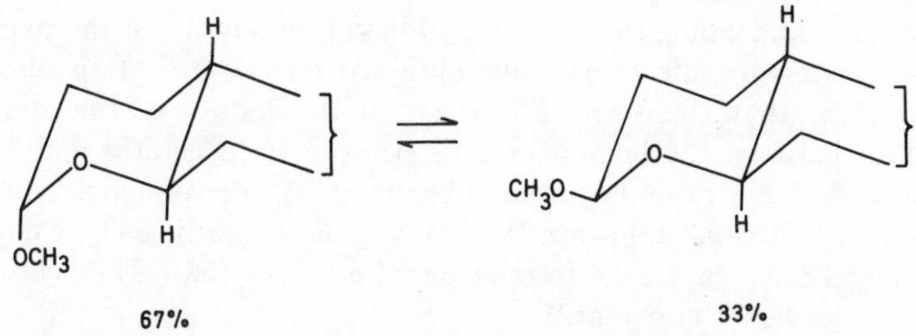

(21)

Figure 3.23   Partial structures, showing the results of acid-catalyzed equilibrations of 3-methoxy-4-oxa-5α-cholestane (**20**) and 3-methoxy-4-oxa-5α-estrane (**21**).

$\Delta G^{\circ} = -1.6$ kcal mole^{-1}

Figure 3.24   The base-catalyzed equilibration of *cis*- and *trans*-2-methoxycarbonyl-6-*t*-butyltetrahydropyrans.

of the positively charged 1-pyridyl substituent in *N*-(tetra-*O*-acetyl-α-D-glucopyranosyl)-4-methyl pyridinium bromide (**22**) in destabilizing the $^{4}C_{1}$ conformer (which would have an axially oriented quaternized nitrogen atom at the anomeric center) and in favoring a "boat-like" conformer where the pyridyl residue is equatorial. For obvious reasons, this electronic effect has been termed (68) the *reverse anomeric effect*.

(22)

It is evident from the few examples which have been mentioned that the magnitude of the anomeric effect (O:X) is fairly closely related to the polarity of the C_1-X bond.

3.2.3b The Nature of Other Substituents. It has already been noted that the presence and configuration of a hydroxyl group on C_2 of the pyranose ring will markedly affect the value obtained for (O:OH). It is also well known (50c) that there are differences in the nature of the anomeric equilibria between the homomorphous pentose tetraacetates and hexose pentaacetates. For example, at equilibrium at 25°, the preference (69) for the α-anomer in 1,2,3,4,6-penta-O-acetyl-D-glucose (23) is 88%, compared with only 78.5% in 1,2,3,4-tetra-O-acetyl-D-xylose (24). The reason for this behavior is not apparent.[18]

(23)

The nature of the substituents at other positions around the pyranoid ring can also have a profound effect on the magnitude of the anomeric effect. It may be seen from Table 3.3 that the equilibrium compositions of D-mannose and some O-methyl derivatives change (23) in favor of the

[18] See, however, refs. 70 and 71. The observation (69) that the preference for the α-anomer in 1,2,3,4,6-penta-O-acetyl-D-galactose is also only 78% has led to the suggestion (70) that a steric interaction between the *trans* diequatorial substituents on C_4 and C_5 of glucose derivatives tends to increase flattening of the pyranoid ring and reduce the steric interaction of the axial group on the anomeric carbon atom. Although this effect may operate with the pentose tetraacetates and hexose pentaacetates, it does not appear to be important in methyl glycosides, where investigations have shown (72) that the percentages of the α-anomers in methyl D-xylopyranoside and methyl D-glucopyranoside at equilibrium are 67% and 69%, respectively (see Table 5.4 in Section 5.3).

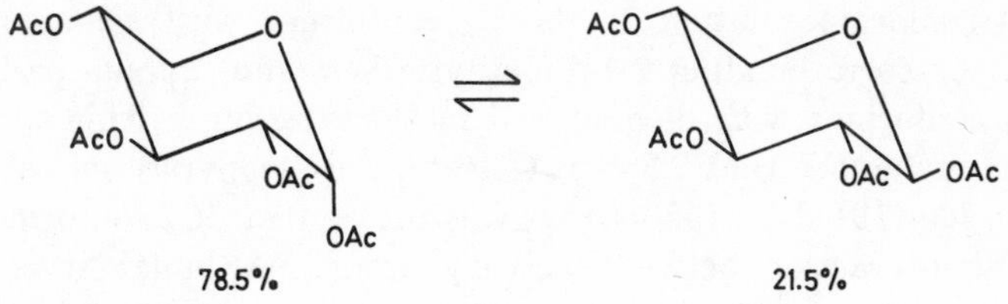

78.5%   21.5%

(24)

α-anomer as the degree of methylation is increased. This trend has been ascribed (23) to changes in the "effective dielectric constant" of the variously substituted molecules altering the magnitude of (O:OH).

Table 3.3   The Equilibrium Compositions of D-Mannose and Some O-Methyl Derivatives

Sugar	α-Pyranose, %
D-Mannose	67
2-O-Methyl-D-mannose	75
2,3-Di-O-methyl-D-mannose	80
2,3,4,6-Tetra-O-methyl-D-mannose	86

Evidence from ^{1}H nuclear magnetic resonance spectroscopy and from optical rotation data indicates (30) that, although methyl 3-deoxy-2,4-di-O-acetyl-β-L-*erythro*-pentopyranoside[19](**25a**) exists predominantly in car-

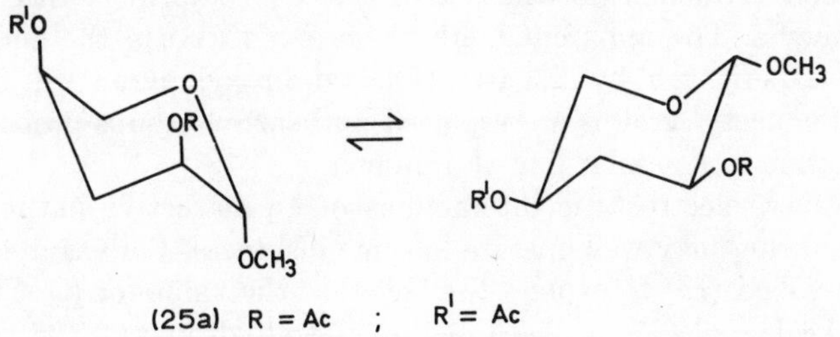

(25a) R = Ac ; R' = Ac

(25b) R = CH₃ ; R' = CH₃

(25c) R = Ac ; R' = CH₃

(25d) R = H   ; R' = H

[19] In the name of this compound, the generic prefix *erythro* refers to the relative configuration at C_2 and C_4, even though these two chiral centers are separated by a nonchiral carbon atom, C_3. The configurational descriptor L defines the absolute configuration at C_4.

bon tetrachloride solution as its $^4C_1$ conformer with *syn*-axial acetoxy groups, the corresponding 2,4-dimethyl ether (**25b**) adopts preferentially the $^1C_4$ conformer with diequatorial methoxyl groups. This situation re-calls the preference that 2,3,4-tri-*O*-acetyl-β-D-xylopyranosyl chloride (**12**) and fluoride (**13**) show (57, 58) for existing as their $^1C_4$ conformers with a *syn*-axial interaction between acetoxy groups. Although it is tempting to suggest (*cf.* ref. 58) that these conformers might be stabilized by an electrostatic attraction between the *syn*-axial acetoxy groups, a more appealing rationalization has been advanced (30) on the assumption that the main interaction between *syn*-axial oxygen atoms is coulombic repulsion between the nonbonded electrons. If this is the case, it is not surprising that the repulsion is minimal when the oxygen atoms carry electron-withdrawing acetyl groups, and much stronger when the oxygen atoms are the electron-rich oxygen atoms of methoxyl groups. Even the derivative (**25c**) of methyl 3-deoxy-β-L-*erythro*-pentopyranoside (**25d**) with 2-acetoxy and 4-methoxy substituents exists predominantly

(26)   (27)

in carbon tetrachloride solution as its $^1C_4$ conformer with diequatorial substituents. The apparent increase observed (58) in the anomeric effect (O:F) experienced by 2,3,4-tri-*O*-acetyl-β-D-xylopyranosyl fluoride (**13**) when the acetyl groups are replaced by benzoyl groups probably finds an explanation in a similar line of argument.

However, electrostatic interactions of an attractive nature across the pyranoid ring may well operate in some instances. For example, they have been invoked (73) to explain the fact that the value for (O:CH$_3$) is larger (1.40 kcal mole^{-1}) in 2,4-dimethoxytetrahydropyran (**26**) than in 2-methoxy-4-methyltetrahydropyran (**27**). The partial positive charge on C$_4$ and C$_6$ of the tetrahydropyran ring may help to stabilize the partial negative charge on the oxygen atom of the anomeric methoxyl group.

3.2.3c The Nature of the Solvent. Generally speaking, the anomeric effect is large in solvents (e.g., carbon tetrachloride) of low dielectric constant and small in solvents (e.g., water) of high dielectric constant. This is exemplified by the acid-catalyzed equilibration of 2-methoxy-6-methyltetrahydropyran

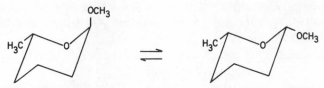

Figure 3.25   The acid-catalyzed equilibration of *cis*- and *trans*-2-methoxy-6-methyl-tetrahydropyrans (see Table 3.4).

(Figure 3.25), which has been studied in several solvents. The results listed in Table 3.4 show that the preference for the axial methoxyl group is lessened in solvents of high dielectric constant.

Table 3.4   Acid-Catalyzed Equilibration of 2-Methoxy-6-Methyl-tetrahydropyran (Figure 3.25) in Different Solvents (33c)

Solvent	Dielectric Constant	ΔG^0_{25} kcal mole^{-1}
Carbon tetrachloride	2.24	0.74
1,4-Dioxane	2.21	0.60
Tetrahydrofuran	8.20	0.60
Nitrobenzene	34.8	0.43
Acetonitrile	37.5	0.35

However, the influence of the dielectric constant on the anomeric effect, and hence on conformational equilibria, is often found to be incidental to other, more important solvation effects involving hydrogen bonding. Thus, methyl 3-deoxy-β-L-*erythro*-pentopyranoside (**25d**) exists predominantly (30) as the $^4C_1$ conformer in solvents such as chlorofrom which do not form strong hydrogen bonds with the hydrogen atoms of the hydroxyl groups. Indeed, under such circumstances, the $^4C_1$ conformer is stabilized by an intramolecular hydrogen bond involving the *syn*-axial hydroxyl groups. However, when these hydroxyl groups are engaged in hydrogen bonding with solvents which are strong proton acceptors, such as pyridine, dimethyl sulfoxide, or water, the $^1C_4$ conformer is favored. The mole fractions (N_{1C_4}) of the $^1C_4$ conformer in different solvents, as estimated from coupling constant and optical rotation data, are shown in Table 3.5. It is also evident from this table that the conformational equilibrium is more sensitive to differences in solvation effects than it is to changes in dielectric constant.

Table 3.5   The Approximate Mole Fractions (N_{1C_4}) of the ${}^1C_4$ Conformer of Methyl 3-deoxy-β-L-erythro-pentopyranoside in Different Solvents (30)

Solvent	J_{H_1,H_2} Hz	$N_{1C_4}{}^a$	$[\alpha]_D^{25}$ deg	$N_{1C_4}{}^b$	Dielectric Constant^c
Chloroform	2.2	0	142	0	4.2
Benzene	2.8	0.16	...	...	2.3
Acetone	3.2	0.26	131	0.23	21
Acetonitrile	3.4	0.32	127	0.31	39
Pyridine	4.35	0.57	113	0.60	12.3
Dimethyl sulfoxide	5.6	0.90	99	0.90	36
Water	6.0	1	94	1	78

^{a} Calculated from the following relationship (see Section 4.5.2):
$$J_{H_1,H_2}^{obs} = N_{1C_4} J_{H_1,H_2}^{D_2O} + (1 - N_{1C_4}) J_{H_1,H_2}^{CDCl_3}$$
^{b} Calculated from the following relationship:
$$[\alpha]_D^{obs} = N_{1C_4} [\alpha]_D^{D_2O} + (1 - N_{1C_4})[\alpha]_D^{CDCl_3}$$
^{c} At 25°.

It has been proposed (30) that hydrogen bonding of hydroxyl groups by proton acceptor solvents (S) causes polarization of the O-H bonds in a manner (R—O←H←S) such that the increase in the R-O bond dipoles is large enough to destabilize the ${}^4C_1$ conformer with *syn*-axial hydroxyl groups and to cause the compound to exist preferentially as its ${}^1C_4$ conformer. In relation to hydrogen-bonding phenomena, another interesting observation has been made (30) concerning the nature of the conformational equilibrium displayed by methyl 3-deoxy-β-L-*erythro*-pentopyranoside (25d). In ethylene dichloride the compound exists predominantly as the ${}^4C_1$ conformer, as expected, but on addition of dimethyl sulfoxide certain very significant changes occur. At very low concentrations of dimethyl sulfoxide (*ca.* 7 moles per mole of diol), the proportion of the ${}^4C_1$ conformer increases to a maximum, as indicated by the increase in the specific rotation of the solution; then, as the concentration of dimethyl sulfoxide is increased, the specific rotation decreases rapidly, indicating that a preference for the ${}^1C_4$ conformer is being felt. This observation has been explained (30) in terms of increased polarization of the O-H bonds, with the movement of electrons toward the oxygen atoms favoring a strong intramolecular hydrogen bond, and therefore stabilization of the ${}^4C_1$ conformer, in the first instance. Subsequently, as more of the proton-acceptor solvent is added, the strong repulsion between the *syn*-axial C-O bonds takes over and forces the equilibrium in the direction of the $^1C_4$ conformer. The strong repulsion between O_2 and O_4 in this case is to be contrasted with the weak repulsion brought about by the electron-withdrawing acetyl groups in the diacetate (**25d**) discussed in Section *3.2.3b*.

3.2.3d   The Origin of the Effect. The factors considered in Sections *3.2.3a–c* show quite clearly that the anomeric effect is polar in origin. The difference in dipole-dipole interaction energies between axial and equatorial orientations of the polar bonds (Figure 3.18) may be calculated (1a, 55, 74) by a classical mechanical approach, which allows estimations of dipole-dipole interaction energies from a knowledge of the magnitudes and relative orientations of the dipoles, of the distance between them, and of the dielectric constant. In this manner, the dipole-dipole interaction energies for 2-chloro- (**10**) and 2-bromo- (**11**) tetrahydropyran have been estimated (55) as 2.7 and 2.4 kcal mole^{-1}, respectively. Comparison of these values with the experimental values of 2.65 and 3.2 kcal mole^{-1} shows that agreement for the bromo derivative is not good. There are several difficulties[20] (10, 74, 75) in making these calculations, and considerable doubt as to how much reliance may be placed on the calculated values always exists.

In view of this situation, semiquantitative approaches for considering dipole-dipole interactions have been developed. In order to assess the importance of dipole-dipole interactions between two oxygen atoms in constitutional fragments of the type —O—CR$_2$—O—, several investigators (27, 43, 44, 50c, 52, 75–77) have found it convenient to consider the interactions between the component dipoles generated along the axes of the lone pairs on the oxygen atoms assumed to be localized tetrahedrally in sp^3 orbitals. As a general rule, the most stable conformer for acyclic and cyclic acetals is the one in which there are a minimum number of *syn*-axial[21] lone pairs on oxygen atoms causing dipolar repulsion.[22] A considera-

[20] The exact location of the dipoles is not always easy to pin-point, and there is often some doubt as to the selection of a reasonable value for the dielectric constant. In addition, it is not justifiable to apply a classical mechanical formula on the molecular scale, particularly when the separation between the dipoles is of the same order of magnitude as the dimensions of the dipoles themselves.

[21] This term is used because, on inspection of molecular models, it is seen that "parallel" lone pairs localized tetrahedrally in sp^3 orbitals have the same relative geometry as *syn*-axial groups on a cyclohexane ring. Although the concept of directed lone pairs has proved useful in semiquantitative arguments, there is some doubt as to its theoretical justification, and it is possible (10, 78) that the nonbonded electrons on oxygen atoms are much more diffuse than is implied by sp^3 hybridization.

[22] In a more general context, Eliel (75, 76) has termed this phenomenon the *rabbit-ear effect*. Whereas Lemieux (77) has recommended that the term *anomeric effect* be retained out of historical interest, Wolfe (78) has suggested that the phenomenon be called the

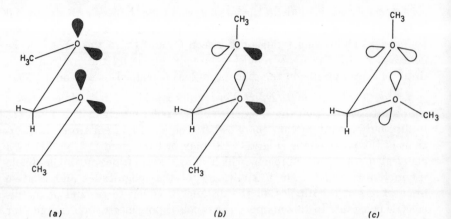

Figure 3.26   The *trans-trans* (a), the *gauche-trans* (b), and the *gauche-gauche* (c) conformers of dimethoxymethane. Lone pairs involved in *syn*-axial interactions are represented by black lobes.

tion of all the possible conformers (Figure 3.26) for dimethoxymethane shows that the *trans-trans* conformer (a) has *two syn*-axial lone pair interactions, the *gauche-trans* conformer (b) has *one syn*-axial lone pair interaction, and the *gauche-gauche* conformer (c) has *none*. Therefore one would predict (*cf.* ref. 50c) that the *gauche-gauche* conformer (c) should be the most favored, and this is indeed the case, as shown by dipole moment measurements (80) and electron diffraction studies (81). *Syn*-axial lone pair interactions are probably responsible for polyoxymethylene (52, 75)—in contrast with polymethylene, which has a planar zigzag conformation—having an *all-gauche* helical conformation (82), wherein such interactions are relieved.

The 2-alkoxytetrahydropyrans are also useful model compounds for studying the anomeric effect. A 2-alkoxytetrahydropyran with an equatorial alkoxyl group (Figure 3.27) has two conformers (*E*1 and *E*2), obtained on torsion around the exocyclic C-O bond, which have a single *syn*-axial lone pair interaction, and a third conformer (*E*3) which has two

Edward-Lemieux effect. Also, the opinion has been expressed (79) that, since the effect is now a generally recognized phenomenon in the much wider field of conformational analysis of heterocyclic compounds, the need for special terms to refer to electronic effects may no longer exist. Nonetheless, in the present context, it will be convenient to use, for electronic interactions associated with the anomeric center, the term *anomeric effect*, while recognizing that it is a particular manifestation of a general phenomenon, which might best be referred to as an *electronic effect*, that is, an effect involving electron distribution.

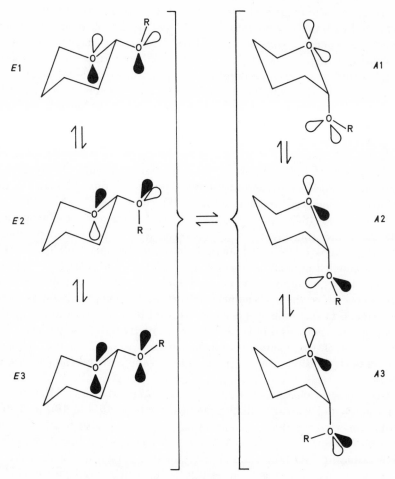

Figure 3.27   The six possible conformers (*E*1, *E*2, *E*3, *A*1, *A*2, and *A*3) of a 2-alkoxy-tetrahydropyran. R = alkyl group.

such interactions. On the other hand, when the alkoxyl group is axial (Figure 3.27) two of the conformers (*A*2 and *A*3) have one interaction, and the third (*A*1) has no *syn*-axial lone pair interactions. Hence, it may be predicted that the axial conformer will be more stable than the equatorial one, a prediction which is in agreement with experimental observations. Moreover, conformer *A*1 should be the most stable of the axial conformers, and conformer *E*1 the most stable of the equatorial conformers, since conformer *E*2 has a destabilizing *syn*-axial interaction between the

R group and the axial hydrogen atom on C_3. These predictions are also consistent with the experimental facts (77, 83, 84). Dipole moment measurements and coupling constant data from ^{1}H nuclear magnetic resonance spectroscopy have revealed (84) that the axial conformers of six 2-alkoxytetrahydropyrans exist predominantly in aprotic solvents as $A1$ conformers, while the equatorial conformers exist preferentially as either $E1$ or $E2$ conformers, these two conformers being indistinguishable from dipole moment measurements. However, there is some evidence (77) from optical rotation studies on (S)-2-methyoxytetrahydropyran that the $A2$ conformer is stabilized in water, possibly by the formation of an H—O—H bridge between the *syn*-axial lone pairs. X-ray crystallographic studies on pyranosides have shown[23] (*cf.* refs. 52 and 84) that *in all cases* the axial anomers exist as $A1$ conformers [e.g., methyl α-D-glucopyranoside (85) and methyl 4,6-dichloro-4,6-dideoxy-α-D-glucopyranoside (86)] and the equatorial anomers as $E1$ conformers (e.g., methyl β-D-xylopyranoside (87) and methyl β-D-maltopyranoside (88)]. In solution, although the axial anomers should exist almost entirely as $A1$ conformers, the equatorial anomers could contain appreciable amounts of $E2$ conformers, since the exo anomeric effect[24] is the same for them as for $E1$ conformers. In fact, this has been shown (83) to be the case in the methyl D-glucopyranosides, and in their 2-deoxy derivatives, by comparison of the magnitudes of the vicinal couplings between the ^{13}C of the aglycone, labeled in the methyl group with ^{13}C, and the anomeric proton (see Section 4.5.2).

The anomeric effect has been interpreted also in other ways. In *trans*-2,5-dihalogeno- and trans-2,3-dihalogenodioxanes (e.g., **15** and **16**), as well as in chloromethoxymethane, attention has been drawn (10) to the fact that axial C-X bonds (where X = halogen) are longer than in chloroalkanes, while adjacent C-O bonds are shorter than in aliphatic ethers. A stereoelectronic explanation has been proposed (10) which may be illustrated by reference to chloromethoxymethane in Figure 3.28a. In either of the two enantiomeric conformers with the chlorine atom *gauche* to the methyl group (but not in the conformer where the chlorine atom is *trans* to the methyl group) the p orbital of the oxygen atom[25] is suitably disposed for mixing with the antibonding σ orbital associated with the C-Cl bond. The

---

[23] In the crystalline state, intermolecular forces are also important in establishing the structure, and hence the conformation, of a molecule, and so it must be appreciated that any correspondence with the solution properties may well be fortuitous.

[24] The preference for axial anomers to exist as $A1$ conformers, and equatorial anomers to exist as either $E1$ or $E2$ conformers, has been termed the *exo anomeric effect* by Lemieux (77, 83).

[25] The oxygen atom is assumed to be sp^2 hybridized since excited states are being mixed.

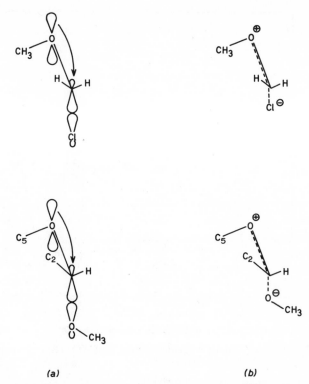

(a)   (b)

Figure 3.28   (a) The stereoelectronic explanation of the anomeric effect in chloromethoxymethane and in α-anomers of methyl-D-glycopyranosides, and (b) the equivalent valence bond representations.

equivalent valence bond representation is shown in Figure 3.28*b*. This kind
of delocalization strengthens the C-O bond and weakens the C-Cl bond.
Indeed, chloromethoxymethane is known (89) to exist predominantly as
the *gauche* conformers with unusually long C-Cl bonds and unusually short
C-O bonds. As shown in Figure 3.28, the situation in α-anomers of methyl
D-glycopyranosides with axial methoxyl groups is analogous to that in
the *gauche* conformers of chloromethoxymethane. This may explain (16)
the relative stability of methyl α-D-glycopyranosides and the relative
shortening of their endocyclic C-O bonds.

Recently, molecular orbital calculations within the Hartree-Fock
framework, based on the suggestion (3) that barrier mechanisms may be
analyzed in terms of attractive-dominant versus repulsive-dominant interactions, have reproduced (78) the expected energy profile for torsion around

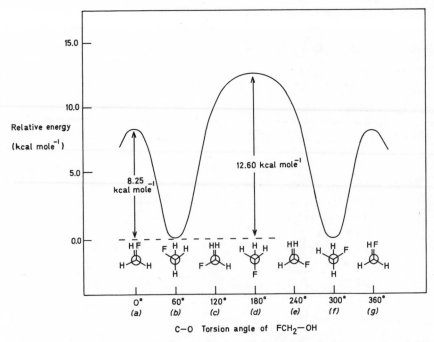

Figure 3.29   The energy profile for torsion around the C-O bond of fluoromethanol (78).

the C-O bond of fluoromethanol, a model compound for studying the anomeric effect. Energy minima correspond (Figure 3.29) to conformers (*b*) and (*f*) with the C-F bonds *syn-clinal* to the O-H bonds. Conformation (*d*), in which the C-F and the O-H bonds are *anti-periplanar*, corresponds to an energy maximum higher than that associated with conformation (*a*) or (*g*), in which the C-F and O-H bonds are *cis-periplanar*. This would suggest that the barrier traversed in the interconversion of the enantiomeric conformers (*b*) and (*f*) is the 0° barrier.

It is also significant that the eclipsed conformations (*c*) and (*e*) associated with the 180° barrier are not much different in energy from conformation (*d*). This means that the interaction of the C-F bond with the lone pairs on the oxygen atom as the C-F bond sweeps through the 120° angle from torsional angles 120° to 240° is virtually constant. Hence the suggestion has been advanced (78) that the lone pairs on the oxygen atom are not directed but are diffuse, as shown in Figure 3.30, and that the anomeric effect exhibited by fluoromethanol has its origin in the interactions between *bonded* electron pairs associated with the polar C-F and O-H bonds.

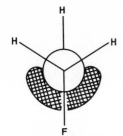

Figure 3.30 Diffuse lone pairs on the oxygen atom of fluoromethanol.

In discussing the origin or origins[26] of the anomeric effect, many questions remain to be answered. Nonetheless, a quantitative estimate of its importance in most pyranoid derivatives can usually be arrived at empirically.

3.2.4 Conformational Free Energies

Now that the nature of the steric and electronic interactions in pyranoid rings has been examined, the results may be used to predict which conformer is preferred in aqueous solution. The conformational free energies of each chair conformer may be calculated by summing all the steric interactions, using the values listed in Table 3.1, and making appropriate allowances for the anomeric effect according to the rules given at the end of Section 3.2.2. Application of this semiquantitative approach to the calculation of conformational free energies is shown in Figure 3.31 for the $^4C_1$ and $^1C_4$ conformers of α- and β-D-allopyranose. On the basis of these results, it may be predicted that both anomers exist predominantly as their $^4C_1$ conformers, and this is indeed the case.

The conformational free energies for the $^4C_1$ and $^1C_4$ conformers of the D-aldohexopyranoses (22), the D-aldopentopyranoses (22), and the D-ketohexopyranoses are shown in Tables 3.6, 3.7, and 3.8, respectively. When the free energy difference between the conformers is less than 0.7 kcal mole^{-1}, which corresponds to a 77:23 mixture at room temperature, both conformers are predicted in the tables (*cf.* ref. 22). Where experimental

[26] It is also a question, for example, of how far one is justified in comparing the properties of chloromethoxymethane and fluoromethanol with those of dimethoxymethane and pyranoid derivatives (*cf.* ref. 10). Also, the quantum mechanical calculations (78) do not explain the solvent dependence of the effect (33c).

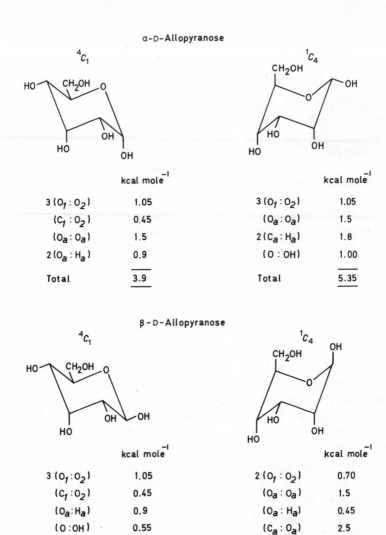

α-D-Allopyranose

$^4C_1$

kcal mole^{-1}

3 (O_1 : O_2)	1.05
(C_1 : O_2)	0.45
(O_a : O_a)	1.5
2 (O_a : H_a)	0.9
Total	3.9

$^1C_4$

kcal mole^{-1}

3 (O_1 : O_2)	1.05
(O_a : O_a)	1.5
2 (C_a : H_a)	1.8
(O : OH)	1.00
Total	5.35

β-D-Allopyranose

$^4C_1$

kcal mole^{-1}

3 (O_1 : O_2)	1.05
(C_1 : O_2)	0.45
(O_a : H_a)	0.9
(O : OH)	0.55
Total	2.95

$^1C_4$

kcal mole^{-1}

2 (O_1 : O_2)	0.70
(O_a : O_a)	1.5
(O_a : H_a)	0.45
(C_a : O_a)	2.5
(C_a : H_a)	0.9
Total	6.05

Figure 3.31 The conformational free energies of the $^4C_1$ and $^1C_4$ conformers of α-D-allopyranose and β-D-allopyranose.

Table 3.6   The Conformational Free Energies (kcal mole⁻¹) of the $^4C_1$ and $^1C_4$ Conformers Calculated (22) for the D-*Aldohexopyranoses in Aqueous Solution*

Aldohexopyranose	$G^{\circ}_{4C_1}{}^a$	$G^{\circ}_{1C_4}{}^a$	Preferred Conformer	
			Predicted	Found[b]
α-D-Allose	3.9	5.35	$^4C_1$	$^4C_1$
β-D-Allose	2.95	6.05	$^4C_1$	$^4C_1$
α-D-Altrose	3.65	3.85	$^4C_1$, $^1C_4$	$^4C_1$, $^1C_4$
β-D-Altrose	3.35	5.35	$^4C_1$	$^4C_1$
α-D-Galactose	2.85	6.3	$^4C_1$	$^4C_1$
β-D-Galactose	2.5	7.75	$^4C_1$	$^4C_1$
α-D-Glucose	2.4	6.55	$^4C_1$	$^4C_1$
β-D-Glucose	2.05	8.0	$^4C_1$	$^4C_1$
α-D-Gulose	4.0	4.75	$^4C_1$	$^4C_1$
β-D-Gulose	3.05	5.45	$^4C_1$	$^4C_1$
α-D-Idose	4.35	3.85	$^4C_1$, $^1C_4$	$^4C_1$, $^1C_4$
β-D-Idose	4.05	5.35	$^4C_1$	
α-D-Mannose	2.5	5.55	$^4C_1$	$^4C_1$
β-D-Mannose	2.95	7.65	$^4C_1$	$^4C_1$
α-D-Talose	3.55	5.9	$^4C_1$	$^4C_1$
β-D-Talose	4.00	8.0	$^4C_1$	

[a] These conformational free energies are relative to a hypothetical pyranoid ring devoid of all nonbonded and electronic interactions.
[b] By ¹H nuclear magnetic resonance spectroscopy (22, 23, 90, 91).

evidence on the basis of ¹H nuclear magnetic resonance spectroscopy (22, 23, 90–92) has been good enough to allow predictions about the conformational equilibria, this fact has been indicated.

In addition, X-ray and neutron diffraction studies have shown (*cf.* ref. 93) that the hexopyranoid derivatives with the *gluco, manno,* and *galecto* configurations which have been investigated so far exist as $^4C_1$ (D) or $^1C_4$ (L) conformers in the crystalline state. Among the crystalline pentopyranoid sugars (*cf.* ref. 73), methyl β-D-xylopyranoside and β-D-lyxose exist as $^4C_1$ conformers, wheras β-D-arabinose and 2-deoxy-β-D-ribose exist as $^1C_4$ conformers. Of the ketohexopyranoid derivatives, α-L-sorbose has been

Table 3.7   The Conformational Free Energies (kcal mole^{-1}) of the $^4C_1$ and $^1C_4$ Conformers Calculated (22) for the D-Aldopento-pyranoses in Aqueous Solution

			Preferred Conformer	
Aldopentopyranose	$G^{\circ}_{4C_1}$[a]	$G^{\circ}_{1C_4}$[a]	Predicted	Found[b]
α-D-Arabinose	3.2	2.05	$^1C_4$	$^1C_4$
β-D-Arabinose	2.9	2.4	$^4C_1$, $^1C_4$	
α-D-Lyxose	2.05	2.6	$^4C_1$, $^1C_4$	$^4C_1$, $^1C_4$
β-D-Lyxose	2.5	3.55	$^4C_1$	$^4C_1$
α-D-Ribose	3.45	3.55	$^4C_1$, $^1C_4$	$^4C_1$, $^1C_4$
β-D-Ribose	2.5	3.1	$^4C_1$, $^1C_4$	$^4C_1$, $^1C_4$
α-D-Xylose	1.95	3.6	$^4C_1$	$^4C_1$
β-D-Xylose	1.6	3.9	$^4C_1$	

[a] These conformational free energies are relative to a hypothetical pyranoid ring devoid of all nonbonded and electronic interactions.

[b] By ^{1}H nuclear magnetic resonance spectroscopy (22, 23, 90, 91).

Table 3.8   The Conformational Free Energies (kcal mole^{-1}) of the $^4C_1$ and $^1C_4$ Conformers Calculated for the D-Ketohexo-pyranoses in Aqueous Solution

			Preferred Conformer	
Ketohexopyranose	$G^{\circ}_{4C_1}$[a]	$G^{\circ}_{1C_4}$[a]	Predicted	Found[b]
α-D-Fructose	3.63	3.85	$^4C_1$, $^1C_4$	
β-D-Fructose	4.95	2.85	$^1C_4$	
α-D-Psicose	3.90	5.35	$^4C_1$	
β-D-Psicose	5.00	3.55	$^1C_4$	
α-D-Sorbose	2.30	6.55	$^4C_1$	$^4C_1$
β-D-Sorbose	3.85	4.35	$^4C_1$, $^1C_4$	
α-D-Tagatose	2.50	6.00	$^4C_1$	$^4C_1$
β-D-Tagatose	4.30	4.00	$^4C_1$, $^1C_4$	$^1C_4$

[a] These conformational free energies are relative to a hypothetical pyranoid ring devoid of all nonbonded and electronic interactions.

[b] By ^{1}H nuclear magnetic resonance spectroscopy (92).

shown (94) to exist as the $^1C_4$ conformer, α-D-tagatose as the $^4C_1$ conformer (95), and β-D-fructose as the $^1C_4$ conformer (95).

When an anomer is a mixture of $^4C_1$ and $^1C_4$ conformers, its free energy is lower than that of *either* conformer by virtue of the entropy of mixing (*cf.* Section 3.1.1 and refs. 21–23). The relative free energy of each anomer, G°_{anomer}, may be calculated by using the expression

$$G^\circ_{\text{anomer}}, = N_{4C_1} G^\circ_{4C_1} + N_{1C_4} G^\circ_{1C_4} + RT(N_{4C_1} \ln N_{4C_1} + N_{1C_4} \ln N_{1C_4}) \quad (9)$$

where N_{4C_1} and N_{1C_4}, the mole fractions of the conformers, may be obtained by solving the equations

$$G^\circ_{4C_1} - G^\circ_{1C_4} = - RT \ln (N_{4C_1}/N_{1C_4}) \quad (10)$$

and

$$N_{4C_1} + N_{1C_4} = 1 \quad (11)$$

for N_{4C_1} and N_{1C_4}. By using the values for G_{4C_1} and G_{1C_4} in Tables 3.6, 3.7, and 3.8, and assuming no contributions from furanose or other forms, G°_α and G°_β for the aldohexopyranoses, the aldopentopyranoses, and the ketohexopyranoses have been calculated (*cf.* refs. 21–23) and are shown in Table 3.9. From the free energy differences between anomers, their proportions at equilibrium may be calculated, and these are expressed as percentages of α-anomers in the table under the heading "Theory." Where available, values which have been obtained for percentages of α-anomers in aqueous solutions at equilibrium by direct integration of ^1H nuclear magnetic resonance spectra are listed in the table under the heading "Experimental." Comparison of the observed and calculated values shows (22, 23) reasonable agreement except in the case of idose. This is not surprising when it is appreciated that idose is the least stable of all the pyranoses and that distortion of chair conformers, or even significant contributions from twist-boat conformers, will seriously invalidate some of the assumptions made at the outset in these calculations.

It is possible to obtain estimates of the relative free energies of the pyranoses, $G^\circ_{\text{pyranose}}$, in aqueous solutions at equilibrium from the expression

$$G^\circ_{\text{pyranose}} = N_\alpha G^\circ_\alpha + N_\beta G^\circ_\beta + RT(N_\alpha \ln N_\alpha + N_\beta \ln N_\beta) \quad (12)$$

where N_α and N_β, the mole fractions of the anomers, may be obtained by solving the equations

$$G^\circ_\alpha - G^\circ_\beta = -RT \ln (N_\alpha/N_\beta) \quad (13)$$

and

$$N_\alpha + N_\beta = 1 \quad (14)$$

Table 3.9   The Relative Free Energies (kcal mole⁻¹) and the Percentage Proportions of the α-Anomer at Equilibrium for the D-Aldohexopyranoses, the D-Aldopentopyranoses, and the D-Ketohexopyranoses in Aqueous Solution (22, 23)

				α-Anomer, %	
Pyranose	G^o_a	G^o_β	$G^o_{pyranose}$	Theory	Experimental[a]
Glucose	2.4	2.05	1.8	36	36
Mannose	2.5	2.95	2.25	68	67
Galactose	2.85	2.5	2.25	36	27
Talose	3.55	4.0	3.3	68	58
Allose	3.85	2.95	2.85	18	20
Altrose	3.35	3.35	2.95	50	40
Gulose	3.85	3.05	2.85	21	22
Idose	3.65	4.0	3.4	64	46
Xylose	1.9	1.6	1.35	37	33
Lyxose	1.85	2.4	1.65	72	71
Arabinose	1.95	2.2	1.65	60	63
Ribose	3.1	2.3	2.15	20.5	26
Sorbose	2.3	3.65	2.25	92	...
Tagatose	2.5	3.7	2.5	89	...
Fructose	3.35	2.85	2.65	28	...
Psicose	3.55	3.15	2.9	33	...

[a] By ¹H nuclear magnetic resonance spectroscopy (22, 23).

for N_α and N_β. The values obtained (22, 23) in this manner for $G^o_{pyranose}$ are listed in Table 3.9. It is perhaps not surprising to find that the pyranoid derivatives most commonly occurring in Nature correspond to the most stable configurational isomers. Thus, glucose, galactose, mannose, xylose, and fructose occur frequently as pyranoid derivatives, whereas the others appear infrequently if at all.

3.2.5   Nonchair Pyranoid Derivatives

Certain anhydro sugars are characterized by pyranoid rings which assume conformations other than chair conformers. Thus, in 1,4-anhydro-2,3,6-tri-O-methyl-β-D-galactopyranose (96), the pyranose ring is forced to exist as its $^{1,4}B$ conformer (**28**), while the glycosidic ring of methyl 2,6-anhydro-3,4-di-*O*-methyl-α-D-mannopyranoside (97) probably prefers to exist as its $^2S_0$ conformer (**29**). In the case of epoxides and unsaturated derivatives, pyranoid rings are forced into half-chair conformers. For example, it has been shown (98) by ^{1}H nuclear magnetic resonance spectroscopy that the α-anomer of 1,2,4,6-tetra-*O*-acetyl-3-deoxy-D-*erythro-*

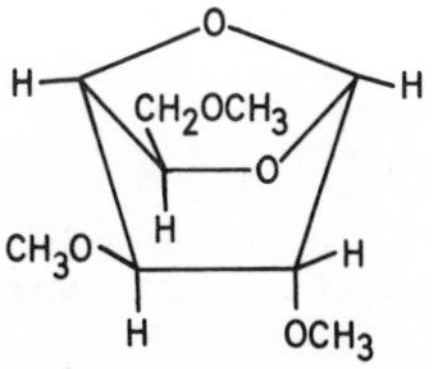

(28)

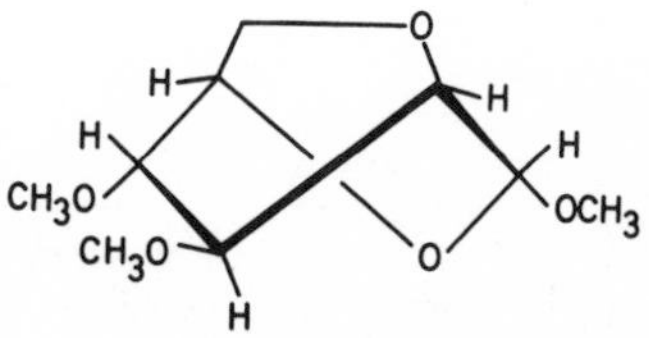

(29)

hex-2-enose exists predominantly as its $^0H_5$ conformer (**30**), while the β-anomer prefers to exist as its $^5H_0$ conformer (**31**). In both these conformers, the anomeric acetoxy group is quasi-axial.

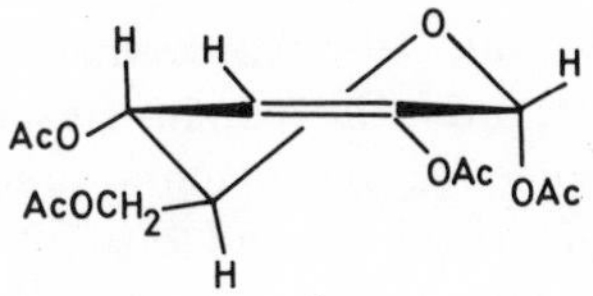

$^0H_5$

(30)

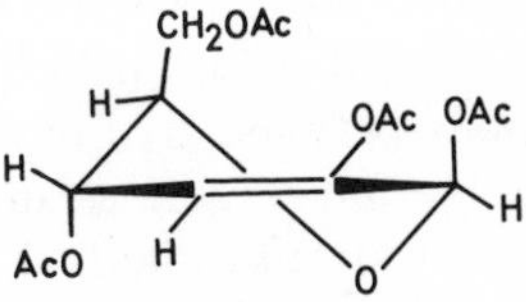

$^5H_0$

(31)

3.3 Acyclic Derivatives

It is well known (1a) that *n*-butane prefers to exist as its *anti* conformer rather than as its *gauche* conformers (*cf.* Section 1.1). At room temperature, the preference is almost 2:1 in favor of the *anti* conformer. Furthermore, polymethylene hydrocarbons tend to adopt planar zigzag conformations wherein all the carbon atoms lie in one plane (*cf.* refs. 82 and 99). On the basis of this knowledge, it will be convenient to begin (*cf.* refs. 93, 100, and 101) by examining the planar zigzag conformers of acyclic carbohydrate derivatives.

The planar zigzag conformers of the three pentitols are shown in Figure 3.32. Close inspection of molecular models shows that there are important

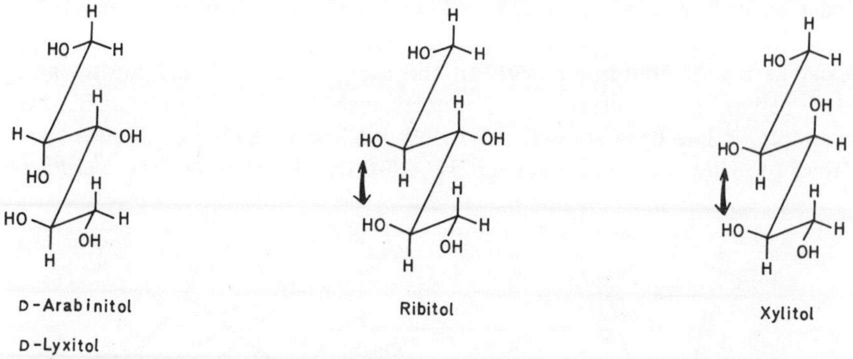

D-Arabinitol   Ribitol   Xylitol

D-Lyxitol

Figure 3.32   The planar zigzag conformers of the three penitols. *Syn*-axial interactions are indicated by the double-headed arrows.

nonbonded interactions between "parallel" hydroxyl groups 1,3 to each other in both xylitol and ribitol. This interaction is analogous (102, 103) to that between 1,3-diaxial hydroxyl groups on a cyclohexane ring, and so we shall refer to it as a *syn*-axial interaction. Of all the interactions in acyclic derivatives, the *syn*-axial ones are the most highly destabilizing and largely determine the relative populations of the different conformers.

From the values listed in Table 3.1, it can be seen that the *syn*-axial interactions between hydroxyl groups in xylitol and ribitol introduce a considerable amount of strain (1.5 kcal mole^{-1}) into the planar zigzag conformers shown in Figure 3.32. This may be relieved by torsion around their C_3-C_4 bonds,[27] as shown in Figure 3.33 for xylitol. Consideration of the magnitude of the *syn*-axial interactions shows that conformer (*b*) should be more highly populated than conformers (*a*) and (*c*). Thus, we may predict that in solution acyclic derivatives with the *xylo* configuration[28] will exist predominantly as conformers of type (*b*). On the other hand, those with the *arabino* or *lyxo* configuration are expected to exist preferentially as planar zigzag conformers.

These predictions are borne out by experimental observations. Examination of a number of acyclic derivatives with the *ribo* and *xylo* configurations by ¹H nuclear magnetic resonance spectroscopy (102–105) has shown that the most stable conformers have 1,2-*gauche* relationships between carbon atoms in their chains; these have been termed (102*b*) *sickle* conformers. For example, tetra-*O*-acetyl-D-ribose diethyl dithioacetal (**32**) probably exists

---

[27] Since the zigzag conformers of both these molecules have a plane of symmetry, torsion around the C_2-C_3 bonds would be isoenergetic.

[28] The same general prediction holds for those with the *ribo* configuration.

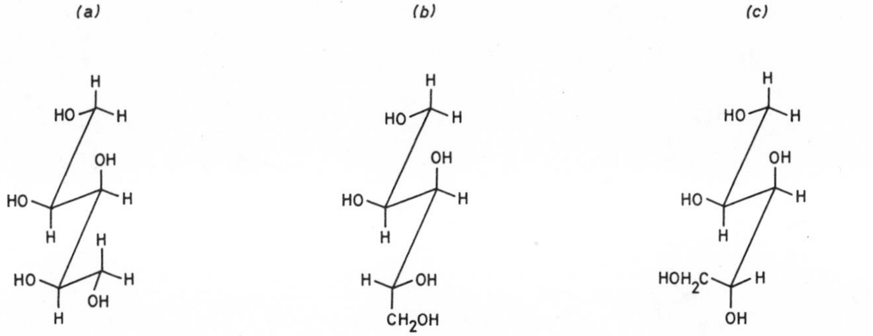

(a)

	kcal mole^{-1}
2(O_a:H_a)	0.9
(O_a:O_a)	1.5
Total	2.4

(b)

	kcal mole^{-1}
2(O_a:H_a)	0.9
(C_a:H_a)	0.9
Total	1.8

(c)

	kcal mole^{-1}
2(O_a:H_a)	0.9
(C_a:O_a)	2.5
Total	3.4

Figure 3.33 The three conformers of xylitol obtained on torsion around the C_3-C_4 bond.

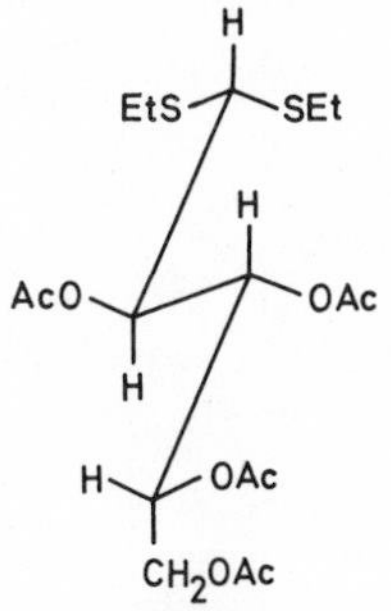

(32)

predominantly as the sickle conformer with a 1,2-*gauche* relationship between C_2 and C_5. In crystalline riboflavin hydrobromide monohydrate, the ribitol chain exists (106) as a sickle conformer with a 1,2-*gauche* relationship between C_1 and C_4. Acyclic derivatives with the *arabino* and *lyxo* configurations exist as planar zigzag conformers in solution (102–105) and in the crystalline state (93, 107).

Figure 3.34 shows the number of *syn*-axial interactions between hydroxyl groups in the planar zigzag conformers of the hexitols: galactitol and mannitol have *none*, glucitol (gulitol) and altritol (talitol) have *one* each, and allitol and iditol have *two* each. Thus, only the acyclic derivatives with the *galacto* and *manno* configurations are expected to exist as planar zigzag

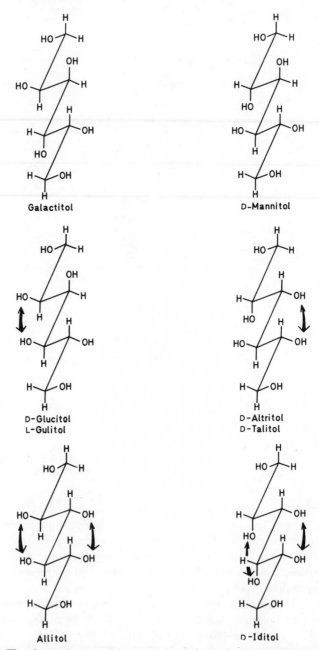

Figure 3.34 The planar zigzag conformers of the six hexitols. *Syn*-axial interactions are indicated by the double-headed arrows.

conformers. The others should contain appreciable amounts of sickle and other bent carbon-chain conformers. So far, it has been shown by ^{1}H nuclear magnetic resonance spectroscopy (102*b*) and by X-ray crystallography (107, 108) that acyclic derivatives with the *galacto* and *manno* configurations exist predominantly as planar zigzag conformers in solution and in the crystalline state. On the other hand, D-glucitol,[29] D-iditol, and allitol all exist (107) as bent carbon-chain conformers in the crystalline state.

Solutions of aldoses contain acyclic *aldehydo* forms in constitutional equilibria with cyclic forms. However, the concentration of the *aldehydo* form—usually partially hydrated—in aqueous solution is generally too low to be detected by ^{1}H nuclear magnetic resonance spectroscopy. Nonetheless, a polarographic determination has indicated (109) that the *aldehydo* content of an aqueous solution of glucose is 0.0026% at a concentration of 0.655 mole liter^{-1}. This corresponds to a free energy difference of about 7 kcal mole^{-1} between the acyclic and the cyclic forms of glucose. It has already been noted in Section 3.2.4 that glucose is the most stable of the aldohexopyranoses and in this section that the *aldehydo* form has one *syn*-axial interaction in its planar zigzag conformer. One might speculate that aqueous solutions of mannose and galactose, which have no *syn*-axial interactions in the planar zigzag conformers of their *aldehydo* forms, and are less stable than glucose in their pyranoid forms, may contain higher proportions of *aldehydo* forms.

3.4 Furanoid Rings

It will be convenient to begin a discussion of furanoid rings by considering the conformational properties of cyclopentane. The three most symmetrical conformations are shown in Figure 3.35. The planar conformation (*a*) has all five carbon atoms in one plane and belongs to point group **D**$_{5h}$. The envelope conformation (*b*),[30] in which one atom is displaced out of a plane defined by the other four, has a σ plane (point group, **C**$_s$) and is often called the **C**$_s$ conformation. The twist conformation[30] has two atoms equally displaced out of the plane defined by the midpoint between these two

---

[29] It should be mentioned that potassium D-gluconate exists as its planar zigzag conformer in the crystalline state (106). Apparently, in this derivative, the *syn*-axial interaction between the hydroxyl groups on C$_2$ and C$_4$ is not as important as intermolecular interactions in the crystal.

[30] There is a whole continuum of envelope and twist conformations corresponding to varying degrees of displacement of one atom and two atoms, respectively, from the reference planes.

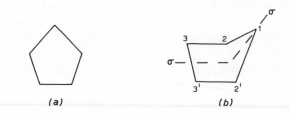

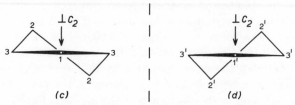

Figure 3.35   The planar (*a*), envelope (*b*), and twist (*c* and *d*) conformations of cyclo-pentane.

atoms and the other three atoms. It exists in two enantiomeric forms (*c* and *d*) and, since each has a C_2 axis of symmetry (point group, $\mathbf{C_2}$), is often called the $\mathbf{C_2}$ conformation. Cyclopentane is flexible, and calculations show (4*a*, 110, 111) that the $\mathbf{C_s}$ and $\mathbf{C_2}$ conformations have approximately the same energy. Since the energy barrier to interconversion of these two forms by pseudorotation is probably less than RT, no discrete energy wells may be identified with certainty, that is, the $\mathbf{C_s}$ and $\mathbf{C_2}$ conformations do *not* qualify as conformers (112).

In the planar conformation all *cis* 1,2 atoms or substituents are eclipsed. Some of these eclipsing interactions are relieved in the $\mathbf{C_s}$ conformation, where only *cis* 1,2 atoms or substituents at positions 3 and 3' are eclipsed. Although all *cis* 1,2 atoms or substituents are partially staggered in the $\mathbf{C_2}$ conformation, there is some increase in the bond-angle-bending strain, compensating for the decrease in nonbonded interactions (110).

In the case of the furanoid ring, there are ten envelope (*E*) and ten twist (*T*) conformations on the envelope-twist pseudorotational itinerary. If the furanoid ring is numbered as described in Section 2.7 and, in addition, the ring oxygen is numbered 0, then *E* and *T* conformations may be designated according to the following set of rules (*cf.* refs. 18*d* and 20):

1. Reference planes are chosen for the E and T conformations corresponding to the ones described for the **C**$_s$ and **C**$_2$ conformations of cyclopentane.

2. Ring atoms which lie above the reference plane (numbering clockwise from above) are written as superscripts and precede the letter, while ring atoms which lie below the reference plane are written as subscripts and follow the letter. 156802

When this convention is employed, the pseudorotational itinerary for a furanoid ring may be represented as shown in Figure 3.36.

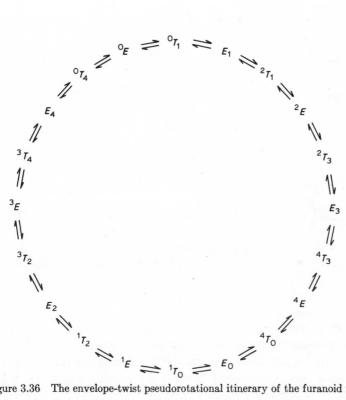

Figure 3.36 The envelope-twist pseudorotational itinerary of the furanoid ring.

Some idea of the stability of the furanoid ring follows from the observation (109) that 4-hydroxybutanal and 5-hydroxypentanal exist in aqueous dioxane at 25° as lactols in equilibrium with 11.4% and 6.2% respectively, of the acyclic hydroxyaldehydes (*cf.* Section 2.7). If it is assumed that the free energies of the two acyclic forms are the same, the difference of 0.4 kcal mole^{-1} between the free energy changes on cyclization calculated from the above percentages corresponds to a measure of the stability of tetrahydropyran-2-ol compared to tetrahydrofuran-2-ol. However, the difference in relative stability is likely to be greater with the sugars, since substituents will tend to destabilize the furanoid ring relative to the pyranoid ring.

Nonbonded interactions between *cis*-1,2 substituents on furanoid rings may be relieved by puckering (23, 50c, 72, 113, 114). Figure 3.37a shows

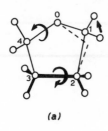

(a)

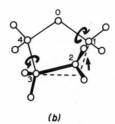

(b)

Figure 3.37   (a) Displacement of C_1 from the plane of the furanoid ring, and (b) displacement of C_2 from the plane of the furanoid ring (113).

that, if C_1 is displaced from the plane of the other four atoms, *cis*-1,2 nonbonded interactions are relieved between substituents on C_1, C_2, and C_3, but not between substituents on C_3 and C_4. Displacement of C_4 or O leads to a similar qualitative result. However, if either C_2 or C_3 is displaced from the plane of the other four atoms (see Figure 3.37b for the effect of C_2 displacement), all *cis*-1,2 nonbonded interactions are relieved. Hence it may be predicted that E conformations with C_2 or C_3 displaced from the plane of the ring (i.e., ^2E, E_2, ^3E, E_3) are more stable than the others. In addition, substituents other than those at C_1 will prefer to take up quasi-equatorial or isoclinal orientations, in which the carbon-substituent bonds have moved toward the plane of the ring. Exception to this rule is made for the orientation of electronegative groups at C_1 because the anomeric effect is also operative (23, 114, 115) in furanoid rings. Thus, a hydroxyl group on C_1 will prefer to assume a quasi-axial orientation in which the C-O bond has moved out of the plane of the ring.

Since *cis*-1,2 interactions are not favorable, it may be predicted (*cf.* ref. 23) that the anomer of a furanose in which the hydroxyl groups on C_1 and C_2 are *trans* will be the more stable. Generally speaking, this is the case (72, 116, 117). However, if an anomer with hydroxyl groups *trans* on C_1 and C_2 also has a *syn*-1,3 interaction, it will be destabilized relative to the other anomer. Thus, 5-O-methyl-β-D-glucose, which exists (23) predominantly in the $^3T_2$ conformation (**33**), has two *syn*-1,3 interactions

(33)

between O_1, and O_3, and between O_1 and C_5, that may be relieved by ano merization to the α-anomer. Indeed, at equilibrium, 5-O-methyl-D-glucose contains (23) approximately equal amounts of each anomer.

Pseudorotation permits $^1T_2 \rightleftharpoons E_2 \rightleftharpoons {}^3T_2 \rightleftharpoons {}^3E \rightleftharpoons {}^3T_4$ and $^2T_1 \rightleftharpoons {}^2E \rightleftharpoons {}^2T_3 \rightleftharpoons E_3 \rightleftharpoons {}^4T_3$ to occur without any 1,2 eclipsing interactions being involved in these interconversions (*cf.* ref. 118). For this reason it is unlikely that any of these E or T conformations could, by themselves, correspond to real energy wells for a furanoid sugar, that is, the energy barriers that separate them are probably less than RT. If this is the situation, these conformations do not correspond to conformers. Consequently, furanoid sugars may be regarded as rapidly interconverting conformations in solution, and nuclear magnetic resonance spectroscopic data should therefore be interpreted in terms of a time-average conformational consensus (*cf.* refs. 23, 118, and 119). All the nuclear magnetic resonance spectroscopic investigations carried out to date indicate (e.g., refs. 115, 118, 120–123) puckering in the C_2/C_3 region of monocyclic furanoid derivatives in solution. This observation is also true of the spiro compound 1′,2-anhydro-[1-(α-D-fructofuranosyl)]-β-D-fructofuranose. Here the average conforma-

(34)

tional picture is best represented (114) by conformation **34**, in which one furanoid ring is shown in the ^2E conformation and the other in the ^3E conformation, that is, C_3 and C_4, respectively, of the fructofuranoid rings are displaced from the reference planes.[31]

Finally, it is significant that, in the large number of X-ray crystallographic studies carried out on furanoid derivatives, including many nucleosides and nucleotides, only puckering at C_2 or C_3 has been observed to date (*cf.* refs. 93 and 124).

3.5   Septanoid Rings

Calculations by Hendrickson (4, 12, 14) aimed at determining the minimum energy conformations of cycloheptane have shown that there are four with similar energy contents. In order of increasing energies, these are (4c) the twist-chair (6.0 kcal mole^{-1}), the chair (7.4 kcal mole^{-1}), the twist-boat (8.4 kcal mole^{-1}), and the boat (8.7 kcal mole^{-1}) conformations.[32] Examination of the symmetry properties (Figure 3.38) of these conformations indicates that, while the chair (C) and the boat (B) conformations each have a σ plane, the twist-chair (TC, TC') and twist-boat (TB, TB') conformations are without reflection symmetry, although they have a C_2 axis of symmetry, and so must exist in two enantiomeric forms. The

[31] It is interesting, in view of electronic effects, that the furanosidic oxygen atoms are axially orientated on the 1,4-dioxane ring (*cf.* **15–18** in Section 3.2.3). Also, the anomeric effect, which favors quasi-axial orientations of the oxygen atoms in the dioxane ring with respect to the furanoid rings, is satisfied in the conformations adopted by both furanoid rings.

[32] These values are relative to the chair conformer of cyclohexane.

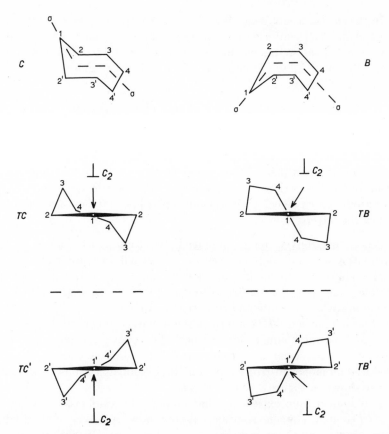

Figure 3.38   The chair (*C*), boat (*B*), twist-chair (*TC*, *TC'*), and twist-boat (*TB*, *TB'*) conformations of cycloheptane.

cycloheptane ring is flexible,[33] and the chair and twist-chair conformations, as well as the boat and twist-boat conformations, are interconvertible (4, 12, 14) via pseudorotation. On the chair/twist-chair pseudorotational itinerary, the twist-chair conformations correspond to energy wells, that is, they are conformers, and the chair conformations correspond to transition states.

[33] Experimental evidence for flexible seven-membered rings comes from the observation that cycloheptane-*trans*-1,2-diol forms (*cf.* ref. 125) an *O*-isopropylidene derivative. In addition, studies (126) on the intramolecular hydrogen-bonding properties of cycloheptane-*cis*-1,2-diol and *trans*-1,2-diol indicate torsional angles between projected C-O bonds of 42° and 51°, respectively.

In the case of a septanoid ring, there are fourteen chair (C) and fourteen twist-chair (TC) conformations on the chair/twist-chair pseudorotational itinerary.[34] If the septanoid ring is numbered from 0 to 6 in the usual manner, different TC and C conformations may be distinguished by using the following set of rules:

1. For a TC conformation, the reference plane is chosen so that positions 1 and 2 (or 1' and 2')[35] and the mid-point between positions 4 (or 4') lie in the same plane. For a C conformation, the reference plane is chosen so that positions 2, 2', 3, and 3' lie in the same plane.[36]

2. Ring atoms which lie above the reference plane (numbering clockwise from above) are written as superscripts and precede the letter(s), while ring atoms which lie below the reference plane are written as subscripts and follow the letter(s).

When this convention is employed, the chair/twist-chair pseudorotational itinerary of the septanoid ring is as shown in Figure 3.39. On the basis of the relative strain energies of the chair and twist-chair conformations of cycloheptane, it will be assumed that the TC conformations are the more stable forms of the septanoid ring, that is, they correspond to conformers. Furthermore, when a TC conformer of a septanoid ring carries substituents, they may be axial, equatorial, or isoclinal, as shown in Figure 3.40 for the twist-chair conformer of cycloheptane. The additional strain energy introduced on monosubstitution by a methyl group at various axial positions is also shown in Figure 3.40 (*cf.* ref. 14).

It is known from experience that none of the aldohexoses exist to any great extent in aqueous solution as septanoses. However, if the hydroxyl groups at C_4 and C_5 are substituted in order to prevent both furanose and pyranose formation, as in 2,3,4,5-tetra-*O*-methyl-D-glucose, for example, then septanose sugars may be formed (127). Examination of the conformers on the chair/twist-chair pseudorotational itinerary of 2,3,4,5-tetra-*O*-methyl-β-D-glucoseptanose (**35**) shows (Figure 3.41) that there are two conformers, $^{1,2}TC_{0,6}$ and $^{0,1}TC_{2,3}$, with *no* axial substituents, and three conformers, $^{5,6}TC_{0,1}$, $^{3,4}TC_{1,2}$, and $^{2,3}TC_{4,5}$, with *one* axial substituent at either position 2a or 3a.[37] Another two possible, contributors, conformers

[34] It is assumed that twist-boat conformations on the boat/twist-boat pseudorotational itinerary are of sufficiently higher energy for their contribution to the conformational equilibria to be minimal.

[35] The numbers refer to the positions on the TC and TC' conformations shown in Figure 3.38.

[36] The numbers refer to the positions on the C conformation shown in Figure 3.38.

[37] These positions correspond to those on the twist-chair conformer of cycloheptane shown in Figure 3.40.

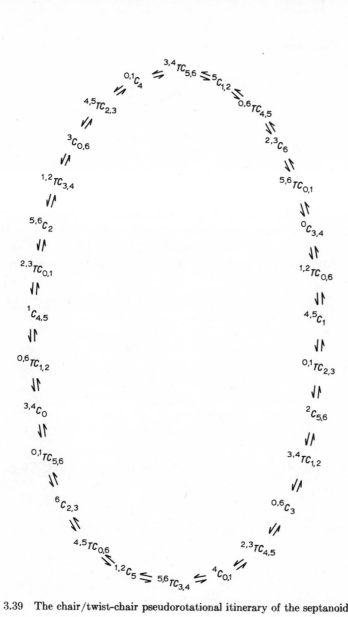

Figure 3.39   The chair/twist-chair pseudorotational itinerary of the septanoid ring.

(35)

$^{5,6}TC_{3,4}$ and $^{4,5}TC_{0,6}$, have, respectively, *one* axial substituent at position $4a$ and *two* axial substituents at positions $2a$ and $4a$[37] but are stabilized relative to the others by anomeric effects. Thus, at least seven conformers could contribute significantly to the conformational equilibrium of the β-anomer.

In contrast, the α-anomer (36) has *no* TC conformers on its chair/

(36)

twist-chair pseudorotational itinerary without at least *one* axial substituent. As shown in Figure 3.42, four conformers, $^{1,2}TC_{0,6}$ $^{0,1}TC_{2,3}$, $^{5,6}TC_{3,4}$, and $^{4,5}TC_{0,6}$. each have *one* axial substituent at position $4a$.[37] The first two are stabilized relative to the other two by anomeric effects. The conclusion

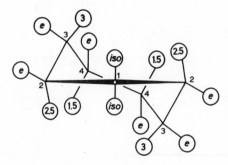

Figure 3.40 The axial, equatorial (*e*), and isoclinal (*iso*) positions on the TC conformer of cycloheptane. The numbers represent the strain energies (kcal mole^{-1}) of a methyl group in the various axial positions.

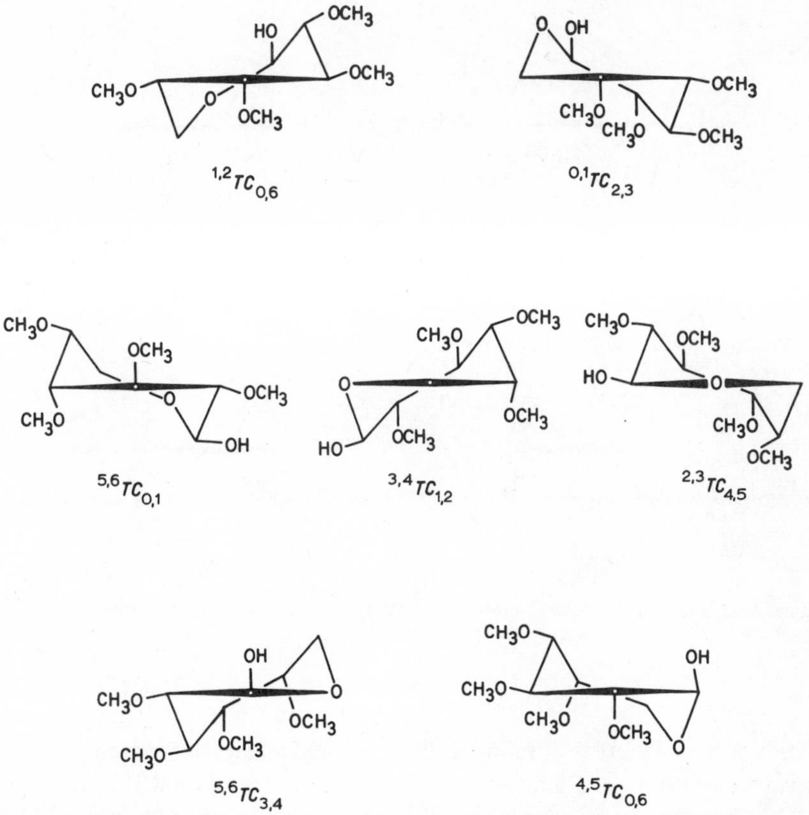

Figure 3.41 The most stable conformers of 2,3,4,5-tetra-O-methyl-β-D-glucoseptanose (**35**).

is that the β-D-septanose should be more stable than the α-D-septanose.[38] Indeed, an equilibrium solution of 2,3,4,5-tetra-O-methyl-D-glucose in chloroform has been shown (127) by ^{1}H nuclear magnetic resonance spectroscopy to contain 60% of the β-septanose and 40% of the acyclic form, that is, no α-septanose was detected. These proportions indicate that the relative free energy of the β-septanose is of the same order of magnitude as that of the acyclic form, which is probably about 7 kcal mole^{-1} less stable than the glucopyranoid ring. Therefore it is not surprising that septanoses cannot be detected in equilibrium mixtures of aldohexoses.

[38] The β-D-septanose will also be favored by an entropy-of-mixing factor, since it may exist as more conformers than the α-anomer.

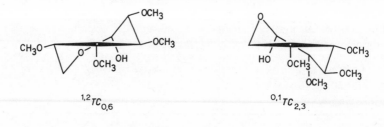

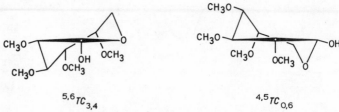

Figure 3.42   The most stable conformers of 2,3,4,5-tetra-*O*-methyl-α-D-glucoseptanose (**36**).

Only a few examples of monocyclic septanoid sugars are recorded in the literature, although 1,6-anhydrohexopyranoses (Section 2.10) and 2,7-anhydroheptulopyranoses contain nominal septanoid rings (*cf*. ref. 127). A thioseptanose ring is present (128) in 6-deoxy-6-mercapto-2,3,4,5-tetra-*O*-methyl-D-galactoseptanose (**37**), and 2,3,4,5-tetra-*O*-acetyl-D-galactose (**38**) and 2,3,4,5-tetra-*O*-methyl-D-galactose (**39**) are known (129, 130) to exist as septanoses.

3.6   Oligosaccharides and Polysaccharides

The conformational properties of oligosaccharides and polysaccharides are determined (16, 131–137) by two factors:

1. The conformations of the individual monosaccharide residues.
2. The relative conformations of respective pairs of monosaccharide residues linked glycosidically to each other.

Since only oligosaccharides and polysaccharides containing pyranose residues have been subjected to detailed conformational analysis to date, this discussion will be limited to situations in which the monosaccharide residues of the carbohydrate polymers are all pyranoid derivatives of one sort or another. It follows that the first requirement in the conformational analysis of these polymers is a knowledge of the conformational properties of the pyranoid monomers (see Section 3.2). The majority of monosaccharides (e.g., D-glucopyranose, D-galactopyranose, D-mannopyranose, and D-xylopyranose) which occur in polysaccharides exist as their $^4C_1$ conformers, and in most instances it is a relatively simple task to derive (131–137) a set of atomic coordinates for each monosaccharide residue, preferably from crystal structure data if available.

If a reasonable value (usually around 117°) is assumed for the bond angle associated with the glycosidic linkage, knowledge of the values of another two variables is all that is required (132, 136) to specify (Figure 3.43) the conformation of the cellobiose residue (*cf.* **46** in Section 2.11), which is the primary structural fragment of *cellulose*, the chief polysaccharide component of the cell walls of higher plants. These variables are the torsional angles defined in Figure 3.43 by the parameters ϕ and ψ,[39] which are related to the torsional angles between C_1—H_1 and $O_{4'}$—$C_{4'}$, and between $C_{4'}$—$H_{4'}$ and $O_{4'}$—C_1, respectively. The D-glucopyranose residues may be designated as **N** or **R**, according to whether they are closer to the nonreducing or the reducing ends, respectively, of the cellulose chain. For each residue, the atomic coordinates are referred to the glycosidic oxygen atom $(O_{4'})$ as origin, with the x axis belonging to the set of axes for residue **N** collinear with the $O_{4'}$—C_1 bond, and with the x axis belonging to the set of axes for residue **R** collinear with the $O_{4'}$—$C_{4'}$ bond. The xz planes are defined by the planes through $O_{4'}$, C_1, and H_1 and through $O_{4'}$, $C_{4'}$, and $H_{4'}$, respectively, and the y axes are perpendicular to these planes.

---

[39] Since the system is so complicated, the parameters ϕ and ψ are best treated as being continuously variable.

The definition of the conformation with $\phi = \psi = 0°$ is an arbitrary one, such as when H_1 and $H_{4'}$ are in the same plane as C_1, $O_{4'}$, and $C_{4'}$, and the geometry around the glycosidic oxygen atom ($O_{4'}$) is the same as that shown in Figure 3.43. Coordinates which refer to any conformation (ϕ, ψ) of the cellobiose residue may be generated by means of standard mathematical expressions for the translation and rotation of sets of axes. New coordinates for **R** which are defined with respect to the axes for **N** may be obtained by rotating the axes of **R** first about the $O_{4'}$-$C_{4'}$ bond through ψ, then about the y axis through the suplement of the angle at the glycosidic oxygen atom ($O_{4'}$) in the plane defined by C_1, $O_{4'}$, and $C_{4'}$, and finally about the $O_{4'}$-C_1 bond through ϕ. Interatomic distances may be calculated from these coordinates, and the extent of nonbonded interactions, as well as the possibility of hydrogen bonding, may be assessed. Electronic computers can be programmed to sample and test an appreciable proportion of the large number of possible conformations.

In one approach (131–136), conformations are said to be "fully allowed" if there are no nonbonded interactions between two atoms over distances less than the sum of their van der Waals radii, and "marginally allowed" if all the nonbonded interactions between two atoms are over distances not greater than the sum of their van der Waals radii and not less than 0.9 times this sum. When all the theoretically possible conformations of the cellobiose residue in Figure 3.43 were sampled (132) at 10° intervals for

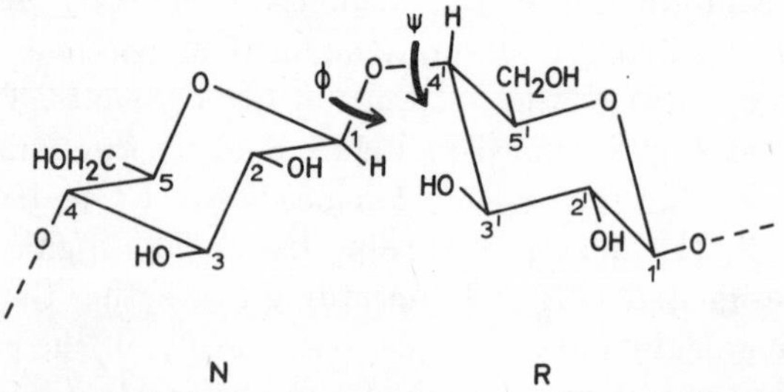

Figure 3.43   The definition of the parameters ϕ and ψ for a cellobiose residue.

both ϕ and ψ, only 24 "fully allowed" and 21 "marginally allowed" conformations out of a total of 36^2 (i.e., 1296)were found. This result is expressed in Figure 3.44 on a "conformational map" that shows (132, 136) which combinations of ϕ and ψ fulfill these conditions. It is significant that the conformer which corresponds to the crystal structure (138, 139) of cellobiose is included within the "marginally allowed" area. When it is

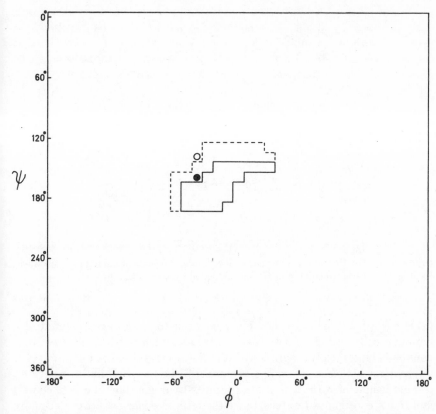

Figure 3.44 The "conformational map" for a cellobiose residue (132, 136). ● corresponds to the crystal structure of cellobiose, and ○ to the Hermans conformation of cellulose.

appreciated that 96% of the relative conformations of β-1,4-linked D-glucopyranose residues are "disallowed" (132, 136), it is not surprising that the cellulose chain is somewhat "stiff" (140). The relative conformations of these residues in the chain are given (131–137) by the parameters (ϕ_1, ψ_1), (ϕ_2, ψ_2), (ϕ_3, ψ_3), ... If these parameters assume the same value at each glycosidic bond, the general conformation is that of a regular helix. Such a helix is characterized by two parameters, n and h, where n is the number of monosaccharide residues per turn of the helix and h is the projected residue height on the axis of the helix.

Systematic exploration of all the possible conformations of cellulose indicates (132, 136) that the "Hermans" or "bent-chain" conformation

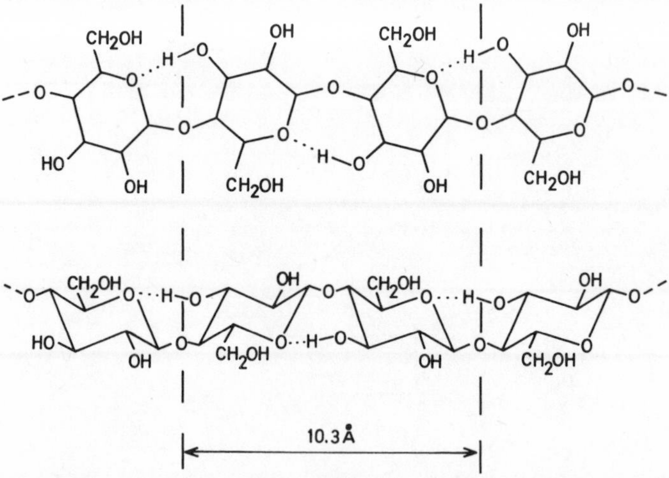

Figure 3.45   The Hermans conformation of cellulose, shown in two different projections. Hydrogen bonds between O_5 and $H_{3'}$ are indicated by the dotted lines.

(141) corresponding to $(-25°, 146°)$ for each (ϕ, ψ) and represented diagrammatically in Figure 3.45 is the only one which is relatively free from nonbonded interactions, agrees with the X-ray crystal structural data (142) in having a *twofold screw axis of symmetry*[40] (i.e., $n = 2$) and a projected residue height of 5.15 Å, and also permits hydrogen bonding between O_5 and $H_{3'}$ of contiguous residues. Since the term *secondary structure* is usually employed to refer to the conformation of a polymer chain of known primary structure, it may be concluded that the "Hermans" conformation $(-25°, 146°)$ represents the most probable secondary structure for cellulose.

More detailed calculations have been carried out (132) on the assumption that the most important contributions to differences in the total intramolecular potential energy (E_T in equation 4) of different secondary structures for cellulose come from nonbonded interactions (E_r) between atoms and groups associated with neighboring D-glucopyranose residues.[41] Contributions from differences in bond-stretching strain (E_d), bond-angle-bending strain (E_θ), torsional strain (E_t), and electronic interactions (E_e),

---

[40] In relation to the regular helix already characterized by the parameters n and h, a twofold screw axis involves rotation about the axis of the helix through 180° followed by a translation of h.

[41] In its nonbonded interactions with other atoms and groups, the hydroxymethyl group has been treated (132) as being equivalent to a methyl group (*cf.* Section 3.2.2).

as well as allowances for differences in hydrogen-bonding energy, solvation energy, and crystal lattice energy, were not taken into account in the calculations, but the significance of some of these factors was assessed qualitatively. On the basis of these computations, the conformation of cellobiose in the crystalline state corresponding to $(-42°, 162°)$ for (ϕ, ψ) was found to be near the energy minimum for nonbonded interactions, with the slight displacement toward higher potential energy favoring the formation of a hydrogen bond between O_5 and $O_{3'}$. There is also some experimental evidence (143) for such a hydrogen bond in dimethyl sulfoxide solution from ^{1}H nuclear magnetic resonance spectroscopy. The minimum energy conformation can also form a fully hydrogen-bonded lattice in the crystal (138, 139).

Although the secondary structure for cellulose represented by the "Hermans" conformation has a slightly higher nonbonded interaction energy than the cellobiose conformation, it still permits hydrogen bonding between O_5 and $O_{3'}$, for which there is some experimental evidence from studies (144) involving infrared dichroism. The somewhat higher nonbonded interaction energy is probably also compensated for by the efficient packing of cellulose chains in the crystal when, and *only* when, the polymer has a simple screw axis of symmetry. Without such a simple screw axis, polymer chains cannot be stacked into a crystal lattice.

One of the most important functions of polysaccharides in Nature is their ability to form *gels*[42] in a wide variety of situations within the bacterial, plant, and animal kingdoms. The opinion that certain polysaccharides can form gels by virtue of intermolecular associations between polysaccharide chains has been vindicated most convincingly by Rees and his associates over the last few years. The manner in which polymer chains of known secondary structure interact defines their *tertiary structure*. The importance of tertiary structure in establishing polysaccharide networks has been demonstrated (133, 135–137, 145) by the results of investigations on a family of related polysaccharides, extractable from red seaweeds and known as carrageenans (see Section 2.12). These polysaccharides have sufficiently regular primary structures to justify the expectation that secondary and tertiary structural features may influence the solid-state and solution properties, and consequently they have been used as models to study gel formation.

It was noted in Section 2.12 that one of the carrageenans, κ-carrageenan, has (136, 146) a primary structure of the masked repeating type, based on the formula shown in Figure 3.46. Some of the 4-O-substituted 3,6-anhydro-

---

[42] A gel displays some properties which resemble the liquid state and others which resemble the solid state.

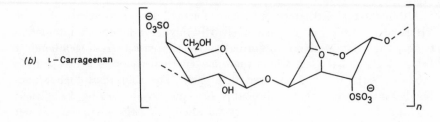

(a) ϰ – Carrageenan

(b) ι – Carrageenan

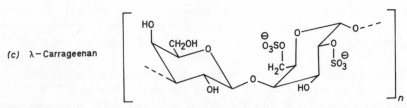

(c) λ – Carrageenan

Figure 3.46 The primary structures of (a) κ-carrageenan, (b) ι-carrageenan, and (c) λ-carrageenan.

D-galactopyranose residues are replaced by D-galactopyranose-6-sulfate residues, and both these residues are partially sulfated at C_2. Another water-soluble component from red seaweed is ι-carrageenan, which also has (136) a masked repeating type of primary structure. In the formula shown in Figure 3.46, about 10% of the 3,6-anhydro-D-galactopyranose-2-sulfate residues are replaced by D-galactopyranose-2,6-disulfate residues. Finally, a third component, λ-carrageenan, has (136, 147) the masked repeating type of primary structure and is represented by the formula in

Figure 3.46, except that occasional 3-O-substituted D-galactopyranose residues are sulfated at C_2. Both κ- and ι-carrageenans may be converted into a more regular type of primary structure by treatment with alkaline borohydride (148), which causes 4-O-substituted residues sulfated at C_6 (A*) to undergo the intramolecular nucleophilic displacement shown in Figure 3.47 to give the corresponding 3,6-anhydride (B).[43] If the position

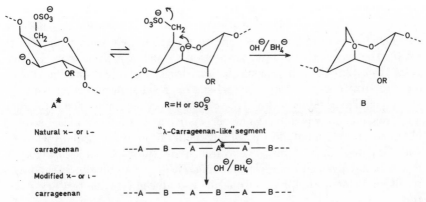

Figure 3.47 Conversion of natural into modified κ- and ι-carrageenans. A = 3-O-substituted D-galactopyranose residue.

of the sulfate group on the 3-O-substituted residues (A) is disregarded (136), it becomes apparent that natural κ- and ι-carrageenans contain "λ-carrageenan-like" segments. It will be seen subsequently that this has important consequences for the secondary, and hence the tertiary, structures of κ- and ι-carrageenans.

X-ray diffraction studies (135) on oriented fibers of salts formed with a series of monovalent cations indicate fiber axis repeat distances of 24.6 Å for κ-carrageenan and 13.0 Å for ι-carrageenan. The X-ray diffraction photographs are capable of the most complete interpretation when it is assumed that both fibers contain polysaccharide chains arranged as *double helices*, so that there are three disaccharide residues in each turn of any single helix. In ι-carrageenan the residues of one helix are located exactly half-way between those of the other helix to give a fiber axis repeat distance

---

[43] Borohydride is present in the reaction mixture to minimize base-catalyzed depolymerization [often referred to (149) as "peeling"] from the reducing end of the polysaccharide. Reducing sugar residues are converted into their corresponding glycitols, and "peeling" from the reducing end is arrested.

of 13.0 Å. The relative orientation of the two helices in κ-carrageenan is unknown at present.

The secondary and tertiary structures of κ-, ι-, and λ-carrageenans can be analyzed (133, 135, 136) by model building in the computer as described previously for cellulose, except that there are four variables, ϕ_{AB}, ψ_{AB}, ϕ_{BA}, and ψ_{BA}, two associated with each distinct glycosidic linkage, to be considered. When this analysis is performed, it transpires that the chains of κ- and ι-carrageenans will form double helices only if each chain has the right-handed screw sense. The representation of the double helix for ι-carrageenan shown in Figure 3.48 was obtained (136) with the aid of a molecular model built to correspond to the calculated coordinates and to satisfy the experimental data. Inspection of such a molecular model suggests (135, 136) that there could be a hydrogen bond between the O_2 of a 3-*O*-substituted D-galactopyranose-4-sulfate residue in one chain and the O_6 of a similar residue in the other chain. Experimental evidence for such a hydrogen bond, which has to be perpendicular to the helix axis, has been obtained (135) from studies involving deuteration and infrared dichroism with oriented fibers. Thus, every free hydroxyl group in ι-carrageenan would be involved in hydrogen bonding within the double helix, and as a result an element of stability would be introduced into the tertiary structure.

Analysis of all the possible arrangements in space for the known primary structure of λ-carrageenan by model building in the computer has revealed (133) a small proportion of left-handed helices, a finding which matches the X-ray diffraction data indicating a helix with threefold screw symmetry and a fiber repeat distance of 25.2Å. Thus, the secondary structure of λ-carrageenan resembles a flat ribbon with some lateral bending.

It follows that natural ι-carrageenan, which contains some "λ-carrageenan-like" segments (Figure 3.46), will be composed of somewhat "kinked" helices. Therefore, in aqueous solution, the polysaccharide chains probably assume secondary structures which librate about potential energy minima in such a way that two chains may readily interact to form segments of double helices as shown in Figure 3.49. This association allows the polysaccharide chains to cross-link in a three-dimensional network and is believed (135, 136, 145, 150) to be responsible for the gel formation on cooling of aqueous solutions of carrageenans. On further cooling, the double helices can associate to form aggregrates reminiscent of the packing in oriented fibers. Support for this theory of gelation comes from the similarities in the cation requirements for gel formation and fiber orientation, as well as from studies (136, 145, 151) on changes in optical rotation with temperature. These changes in optical rotatory power may be attributed to

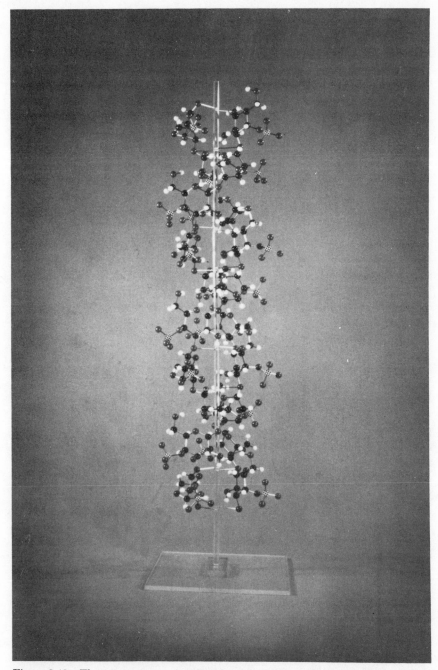

Figure 3.48   The ι-carrageenan double helix. The black balls are carbon atoms; the white ones, hydrogen atoms; the gray ones oxygen atoms; and the speckled ones, sulfur atoms.

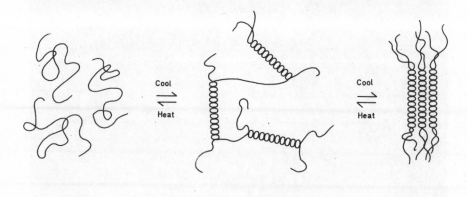

Solution   Gel double helices   Gel aggregates

Figure 3.49   Proposed mechanism (135, 136, 145) for gelation by κ- and ι-carrageenans.

alterations in secondary and tertiary structure associated with the formation of double helices, and subsequently to the aggregation of the helices.

The requirement that only polysaccharide chains with the same senses
can enter into double helix formation (Figure 3.49) means that any intramolecular association must involve loops (136). This realization presents
the possibility that two or more loops may interlock, causing a "catenane-
like" association between polysaccharide chains which will contribute to the
network. Complete double helix formation between two parallel chains is
prohibited by the "kinks" associated with the 6-sulfate residues. An enzyme
has been characterized (136) in red seaweeds that will convert the 6-
sulfate residues into 3,6-anhydride residues. It is tempting to speculate
(136) that such a "de-kinkase" provides the control mechanism for altering
polysaccharide tertiary structure, and hence the composition of polysaccharide networks, in biological situations.

References

1. (a) E. L. Eliel, N. L. Allinger, S. J. Angyal, and G. A. Morrison, *Conformational Analy-sis*, Wiley-Interscience, New York, 1965; (b) M. Hanack, *Conformation Theory*, Acdemic, New York, 1965; (c) J. McKenna, *Conformational Analysis of Organic Compounds*, The Royal Institute of Chemistry Lecture Series, No. 1, London, 1966.
2. J. E. Williams, P. J. Stang, and P. von R. Schleyer, *Ann. Rev. Phys. Chem.*, **19**, 531 (1968).
3. L. C. Allen, *Chem. Phys. Letters*, **2**, 597 (1968).
4. (a) J. B. Hendrickson, *J. Am. Chem. Soc.*, **83**, 4537 (1961); (b) **86**, 4854 (1964); (c) **89**, 7036 (1967).

5. M. Davies and O. Hassel, *Acta Chem. Scand.*, **17**, 1181 (1963).
6. R. Bucourt and D. Hainaut, *Bull. Soc. Chim. France*, p. 2080 (1964).
7. R. A. Wohl, *Chimia*, **18**, 219 (1964).
8. E. L. Eliel and Sr. M. C. Knoeber, *J. Am. Chem. Soc.*, **90**, 3444 (1968).
9. E. W. Garbisch, Jr., and M. G. Griffith, *J. Am. Chem. Soc.*, **90**, 6543 (1968).
10. C. Romers, C. Altona, H. R. Buys, and E. Havinga, in *Topics in Stereochemistry*, Vol. 4, ed. E. L. Eliel and N. L. Allinger, Wiley-Interscience, New York, 1969, p. 39.
11. G. Binsch, in *Topics in Stereochemistry*, Vol. 3, ed. E. L. Eliel and N. L. Allinger, Wiley-Interscience, New York, 1968, p. 97.
12. J. B. Hendrickson, *J. Am. Chem. Soc.*, **89**, 7047 (1967).
13. S. Wolfe and J. R. Campbell, *Chem. Comm.*, p. 874, p. 877 (1967); R. K. Harris and R. A. Spragg, *J. Chem. Soc.*, B, p. 684 (1968).
14. J. B. Hendrickson, *J. Am. Chem. Soc.*, **89**, 7043 (1967).
15. G. A. Jeffrey and R. D. Rosenstein, *Advan. Carbohydrate Chem.*, **19**, 7 (1964).
16. M. Sundaralingam, *Biopolymers*, **6**, 189 (1968).
17. B. Coxon, *Tetrahedron*, **21**, 3481 (1965).
18. (a) R. D. Guthrie, *Chem. Ind.*, p. 1593 (1958); (b) H. S. Isbell and R. S. Tipson, *Science*, **130**, 793 (1959), *J. Res. Natl. Bur. Std.*, **64A**, 171 (1960); (c) R. Bentley, *J. Am. Chem. Soc.*, **82**, 2811 (1960); (d) L. D. Hall, *Chem. Ind.*, p. 950 (1963); (e) D. F. Shaw, *Tetrahedron Letters*, p. 1 (1965).
19. R. E. Reeves, *J. Am. Chem. Soc.*, **71**, 215 (1949); **72**, 1499 (1950); *Advan. Carbohydrate Chem.*, **6**, 107 (1951).
20. J. C. P. Schwarz, Personal communication.
21. Ref. 1a, pp. 351–432.
22. S. J. Angyal, *Aust. J. Chem.*, **21**, 2737 (1968).
23. S. J. Angyal, *Angew. Chem. Intern. Ed.*, **8**, 157 (1969).
24. P. R. Sundarajan and V. S. R. Rao, *Tetrahedron*, **24**, 289 (1968).
25. A. I. Kitaigorodsky, *Tetrahedron*, **14**, 230 (1961).
26. O. Hassel and B. Ottar, *Acta Chem. Scand.*, **1**, 929 (1947).
27. M. A. Kabayama and D. Patterson, *Can. J. Chem.*, **36**, 563 (1958).
28. A. B. Foster, R. Harrison, J. Lehmann, and J. M. Webber, *J. Chem. Soc.*, p. 4471 (1963).
29. R. U. Lemieux and S. Levine, *Can. J. Chem.*, **42**, 1473 (1964).
30. R. U. Lemieux and A. A. Pavia, *Can. J. Chem.*, **47**, 4441 (1969).
31. S. J. Angyal and D. J. McHugh, *Chem. Ind.*, p. 1147 (1956).
32. J. A. Hirsch, in *Topics in Stereochemistry*, Vol. 1, ed. E. L. Eliel and N. L. Allinger, Wiley-Interscience, New York, 1967, p. 199.
33. (a) E. L. Eliel and R. S. Ro, *J. Am. Chem. Soc.*, **79**, 5992 (1957); (b) E. L. Eliel and S. H. Schroeter, *J. Am. Chem. Soc.*, **87**, 5031 (1965); (c) E. L. Eliel and E. C. Gilbert, *J. Am. Chem. Soc.*, **91**, 5487 (1969).
34. S. J. Angyal and V. A. Pickles, *Carbohydrate Res.*, **4**, 269 (1967).
35. G. W. Buchanan and J. B. Stothers, *Chem. Comm.*, p. 1250 (1967).
36. E. L. Eliel, D. C. Neilson, and E. C. Gilbert, *Chem. Comm.*, p. 360 (1968).
37. S. J. Angyal, V. A. Pickles, and R. Ahluwahlia, *Carbohydrate Res.*, **1**, 365 (1966).
38. Ref. 1a, p. 458.
39. Ref. 1a, pp. 439–440.
40. J. Sicher and M. Tichy, *Coll. Czech. Chem. Comm.*, **32**, 3687 (1967).
41. R. G. Hansen and E. M. Craine, *J. Biol. Chem.*, **208**, 293 (1954).
42. C. B. Anderson, D. T. Sepp, M. P. Geis, and A. A. Roberts, *Chem. Ind.*, p. 1805 (1968).

43. E. L. Eliel, *Insights Gained from Conformational Analysis in Heterocyclic Systems*, International Symposium on Conformational Analysis, Brussels, September, 1969.
44. E. L. Eliel, *Accounts Chem. Res.*, **3**, 1 (1970).
45. E. L. Eliel and M. K. Kaloustian, *Chem. Comm.*, p. 290 (1970).
46. R. G. Snyder and G. Zeibi, *Spectrochim. Acta*, **23A**, 391 (1967).
47. J. E. Mark and P. J. Florey, *J. Am. Chem. Soc.*, **87**, 1415 (1965); **88**, 3702 (1966).
48. S. J. Angyal, P. A. J. Gorin, and M. Pitman, *J. Chem. Soc.*, p. 1807 (1965).
49. J. T. Edward, *Chem. Ind.*, p. 1102 (1955).
50. (a) R. U. Lemieux and N. J. Chü, *133rd Meeting Am. Chem. Soc., Abstracts of Papers*, 31N (1958); (b) R. U. Lemieux, *135th Meeting Am. Chem. Soc., Abstracts of Papers*, 5E (1959); (c) *Molecular Rearrangements*, ed. P. de Mayo, Wiley-Interscience, New York, 1963, p. 713.
51. C. B. Anderson and D. T. Sepp, *Chem. Ind.*, p. 2054 (1964).
52. E. L. Eliel and C. A. Giza, *J. Org. Chem.*, **33**, 3754 (1968).
53. C. B. Anderson and D. T. Sepp, *J. Org. Chem.*, **33**, 3272 (1968).
54. H. S. Isbell and W. W. Pigman, *J. Res. Natl. Bur. Std.*, **18**, 141 (1937).
55. C. B. Anderson and D. T. Sepp, *J. Org. Chem.*, **32**, 607 (1967).
56. G. E. Booth and R. J. Ouellette, *J. Org. Chem.*, **31**, 544 (1966).
57. C. V. Holland, D. Horton, and J. S. Jewell, *J. Org. Chem.*, **32**, 1818 (1967).
58. L. D. Hall and J. F. Manville, *Carbohydrate Res.*, **4**, 512 (1967); *Can. J. Chem.*, **47**, 1, 19 (1969).
59. R. U. Lemieux and R. Fraser-Reid, *Can. J. Chem.*, **43**, 1460 (1965).
60. C. Altona, C. Romers, and E. Havinga, *Tetrahedron Letters*, p. 16 (1959); C. Altona and C. Romers, *Rec. Trav. Chim. Pays-Bas*, **82**, 1080 (1963); C. Altona, C. Knobler, and C. Romers, *Rec. Trav. Chim. Pays-Bas*, **82**, 1089 (1963); C. Y. Chen and R. J. W. LeFevre, *J. Chem. Soc.*, B, p. 544 (1966); R. R. Fraser and C. Reyes-Zumora, *Can. J. Chem.*, **43**, 3445 (1965); D. Jung, *Chem. Ber.*, **99**, 566 (1966).
61. H. T. Kalff and C. Romers, *Acta Cryst.*, **18**, 164 (1965); H. T. Kalff and E. Havinga, *Rec. Trav. Chim. Pays-Bas*, **85**, 637 (1966); H. T. Kalff and C. Romers, *Rec. Trav. Chim. Pays-Bas*, **85**, 198 (1966).
62. N. de Wolf, P. W. Henniger, and E. Havinga, *Rec. Trav. Chim. Pays-Bas*, **86**, 1227 (1965); N. de Wolf, C. Romers, and C. Altona, *Acta Cryst.*, **22**, 715 (1967).
63. J. Allinger and N. L. Allinger, *Tetrahedron*, **2**, 64 (1958); N. L. Allinger, J. Allinger, and N. A. LeBel, *J. Am. Chem. Soc.*, **82**, 2926 (1960).
64. P. L. Durette and D. Horton, *158th Meeting Am. Chem. Soc., Abstracts of Papers*, CARB 25 (1969).
65. C. V. Holland, D. Horton, M. J. Miller, and N. S. Bhacca, *J. Org. Chem.*, **32**, 3077 (1967).
66. (a) J. T. Edward, P. F. Morand, and I. Puskas, *Can. J. Chem.*, **39**, 2069 (1961); (b) J. T. Edward and I. Puskas, *Can. J. Chem.*, **40**, 711 (1962); (c) J. T. Edward and J. M. Ferland, *Can. J. Chem.*, **44**, 1299 (1965).
67. G. O. Pierson and O. A. Runquist, *J. Org. Chem.*, **33**, 2572 (1968).
68. R. U. Lemieux and A. R. Morgan, *Can. J. Chem.*, **43**, 2205 (1965); R. U. Lemieux and S. S. Saluja, *Joint ACS/CIC Conference, Abstracts of Papers*, CARB 33 (1970).
69. W. A. Bonner, *J. Am. Chem. Soc.*, **81**, 1450 (1959).
70. D. T. Sepp and C. B. Anderson, *Tetrahedron*, **24**, 6873 (1968).
71. C. B. Anderson and D. T. Sepp, *Tetrahedron*, **24**, 1707 (1968).
72. C. T. Bishop and F. P. Cooper, *Can. J. Chem.*, **41**, 2743 (1963); V. Smirnyagin and C. T. Bishop, *Can. J. Chem.*, **46**, 3085 (1968).
73. F. Sweet and R. K. Brown, *Can. J. Chem.*, **46**, 1543 (1968).
74. F. G. Riddell, *Quart. Rev.*, **21**, 373 (1967).
75. E. L. Eliel, *Kem. Tidskr.*, **81**, 6/7, 22 (1969).

76. R. O. Hutchins, L. D. Kopp, and E. L. Eliel, *J. Am. Chem. Soc.*, **90**, 7174 (1968).
77. R. U. Lemieux, A. A. Pavia, J. C. Martin, and K. A. Watanabe, *Can. J. Chem.*, **47**, 4427 (1969).
78. S. Wolfe, A. Rauk, L. M. Tel, and I. G. Csizmadia, *J. Chem. Soc.*, B, p. 136 (1971).
79. W. D. Ollis and J. H. Ridd, *Ann. Rept. Chem. Soc.*, **63**, 240 (1966).
80. M. Kubo, *Sci. Papers Inst. Phys. Chem. Research (Tokyo)*, **29**, 179 (1936); T. Uchida, Y. Kurita, and M. Kubo, *J. Polymer Sci.*, **19**, 365 (1956).
81. K. Aoki, *J. Chem. Soc. (Japan) Pure Chem. Sect.*, **74**, 110 (1953).
82. P. de Santis, E. Giglio, A. M. Liquori, and A. Ripamonti, *J. Polymer Sci.*, A, 1, 1383 (1963).
83. R. U. Lemieux and J. C. Martin, *Carbohydrate Res.*, **13**, 139 (1970).
84. A. J. de Hoog, H. R. Buys, C. Altona, and E. Havinga, *Tetrahedron*, **25**, 3365 (1969).
85. H. M. Berman and S. H. Kim, *Acta Cryst.*, **B24**, 897 (1968).
86. R. Hoge and J. Trotter, *J. Chem. Soc.*, A, p. 267 (1968).
87. A. McL. Mathieson and B. J. Poppleton, *Acta Cryst.*, **21**, 72 (1966).
88. S. S. C. Chu and G. A. Jeffrey, *Acta Cryst.*, **B24**, 830 (1968).
89. M. C. Planje, L. H. Toneman, and G. Dalinga, *Rec. Trav. Chim. Pays-Bas*, **84**, 232 (1965); M. J. Aroney, R. J. W. LeFevre, and J. D. Saxby, *J. Chem. Soc.*, B, p. 414 (1966).
90. M. Rudrum and D. F. Shaw, *J. Chem. Soc.*, p. 52 (1965).
91. R. U. Lemieux and J. D. Stevens, *Can. J. Chem.*, **44**, 249 (1966).
92. J. C. Jochims, G. Taigel, A. Seegler, P. Lutz, and H. E. Driesen, *Tetrahedron Letters*, p. 4363 (1967).
93. B. Capon, *Chem. Rev.*, **69**, 407 (1969).
94. S. H. Kim and R. D. Rosenstein, *Acta Cryst.*, **22**, 648 (1967).
95. S. Takagi and R. D. Rosenstein, *Carbohydrate Res.*, **11**, 156 (1969).
96. J. Kops and C. Schuerch, *J. Org. Chem.*, **30**, 3951 (1965).
97. E. D. M. Eades, D. H. Ball, and L. Long, Jr., *J. Org. Chem.*, **30**, 3949 (1965).
98. R. J. Ferrier and G. H. Sankey, *J. Chem. Soc.*, C, p. 2345 (1966).
99. J. C. McCoubrey and A. R. Ubbelohde, *Quart. Rev.*, **5**, 364 (1951).
100. R. J. Ferrier and W. G. Overend, *Quart. Rev.*, **13**, 265 (1959).
101. B. Capon and W. G. Overend, *Advan. Carbohydrate Chem.*, **15**, 11 (1960).
102. (a) H. S. El Khadem, D. Horton, and T. F. Page, *J. Org. Chem.*, **33**, 734 (1968); (b) D. Horton and J. D. Wander, *Carbonhydrate Res.*, **10**, 279 (1969); (c) **13**, 33 (1970).
103. J. B. Lee and B. F. Scanlon, *Tetrahedron*, **25**, 3413 (1969); J. M. Williams, *Carbohydrate Res.*, **11**, 437 (1969); S. J. Angyal and K. James, *Aust. J. Chem.*, **23**, 1223 (1970).
104. W. S. Chilton and R. C. Krahn, *J. Am. Chem. Soc.*, **90**, 1318 (1968).
105. G. G. Lyle and M. J. Piazza, *J. Org. Chem.*, **33**, 2478 (1968).
106. C. D. Littleton, *Acta Cryst.*, **6**, 775 (1953).
107. N. Azarnia, G. A. Jeffrey, H. S. Kim, and Y. J. Park, *Joint ACS/CIC Conference, Abstracts of Papers*, CARB 26 (1970).
108. H. M. Berman and R. D. Rosenstein, *Acta Cryst.*, **B24**, 435 (1968); H. M. Berman, G. A. Jeffrey, and R. D. Rosenstein, *Acta Cryst.*, **B24**, 442 (1968); S. H. Kim, G. A. Jeffrey, and R. D. Rosenstein, *Acta Cryst.*, **B24**, 1449 (1968); F. D. Hunter and R. D. Rosenstein, *Acta Cryst.*, **B24**, 1652 (1968).
109. J. M. Los, L. B. Simpson, and K. Wiesner, *J. Am. Chem. Soc.*, **78**, 1564 (1956).
110. K. S. Pitzer and W. E. Donath, *J. Am. Chem. Soc.*, **81**, 3213 (1959).
111. J. B. Hendrickson, *J. Am. Chem. Soc.*, **85**, 4059 (1963).
112. Ref. 1a, p. 200.

113. M. Spencer, *Acta Cryst.*, **12**, 59 (1959).
114. R. U. Lemieux and R. Nagarajan, *Can. J. Chem.*, **42**, 1270 (1964).
115. J. D. Stevens and H. G. Fletcher, Jr., *J. Org. Chem.*, **33**. 1799 (1968).
116. B. Capon, G. W. Loveday, and W. G. Overend, *Chem. Ind.*, p. 1537 (1962).
117. S. J. Angyal and V. A. Pickles, *Carbohydrate Res.*, **4**, 269 (1967).
118. L. D. Hall, P. R. Steiner, and C. Pedersen, *Can. J. Chem.*, **48**, 1155 (1970).
119. R. U. Lemieux and D. R. Lineback, *Ann. Rev. Biochem.*, **32**, 155 (1963).
120. C. D. Jardetzky, *J. Am. Chem. Soc.*, **82**, 229 (1960).
121. R. U. Lemieux, *Can. J. Chem.*, **39**, 116 (1961).
122. R. J. Abraham, L. D. Hall, L. Hough, and K. A. McLauchlan, *J. Chem. Soc.*, p. 3699 (1962).
123. J. F. Stoddart and W. A. Szarek, *Can. J. Chem.*, **46**, 3061 (1968).
124. M. Sundaralingam, *J. Am. Chem. Soc.*, **87**, 599 (1965).
125. W. R. Christian, C. J. Gogek, and C. B. Purves, *Can. J. Chem.*, **29**, 911 (1951).
126. L. P. Kuhn, *J. Am. Chem. Soc.*, **76**, 4323 (1954).
127. E. F. L. J. Anet, *Carbohydrate Res.*, **8**, 164 (1968).
128. J. M. Cox and L. N. Owen, *J. Chem. Soc.*, C, p. 1121 (1967).
129. F. Micheel and F. Suckfüll, *Ann.*, **502**, 85 (1933); **507**, 138 (1933); *Chem. Ber.*, **66**, 1957 (1933); F. Micheel and W. Spruck, *Chem. Ber.*, **67**, 1665 (1934).
130. W. G. Blann, M. Sc. Thesis, Queen's University, Kingston, Canada, 1969.
131. G. N. Ramachandran, C. Ramakrishnan, and V. Sasisekharan, in *Aspects of Protein Structure*, ed. G. N. Ramachandran, Academic, New York, 1963, p. 121; G. N. Ramachandran, in *Structural Chemistry and Molecular Biology*, ed. A. Rich and N. Davidson, Freeman, San Francisco, 1968, p. 77; G. N. Ramachandran and V. Sasisekharan, *Advan. Protein Chem.*, **23**, 284 (1968).
132. D. A. Rees and R. J. Skerrett, *Carbohydrate Res.*, **7**, 334 (1968).
133. D. A. Rees, *J. Chem. Soc.*, B, p. 217 (1969).
134. D. A. Rees and W. E. Scott, *Chem. Comm.*, p. 1037 (1969).
135. N. S. Anderson, J. W. Campbell, M. M. Harding, D. A. Rees, and J. W. B. Samuel, *J. Mol. Biol.*, **45**, 85 (1969).
136. D. A. Rees, *Advan. Carbohydrate Chem. Biochem.*, **24**, 267 (1969).
137. D. A. Rees and R. J. Skerrett, *J. Chem. Soc.*, B, p. 189 (1970).
138. C. J. Brown, *J. Chem. Soc.*, A, p. 927 (1966).
139. S. S. C. Chu and G. A. Jeffrey, *Acta Cryst.*, **24B**, 830 (1968).
140. P. J. Florey, *Proc. Roy. Soc. (London)*, Series A, **234**, 60 (1956); H. Morawetz, *Macromolecules in Solution*, Wiley-Interscience, New York, 1965, p. 111.
141. P. H. Hermans, *Physics and Chemistry of Cellulose Fibers*, Elsevier, New York, 1949.
142. R. H. Marchessault and A. Sarko, *Advan. Carbohydrate Chem.*, **22**, 421 (1967).
143. B. Casu, M. Reggiani, G. G. Gallo, and A. Vigevani, *Tetrahedron*, **22**, 3061 (1966).
144. J. Mann and H. J. Marrman, *J. Polymer Sci.*, **27**, 595 (1958).
145. D. A. Rees, I. W. Steele, and F. B. Williamson, *J. Polymer Sci.*, Part C, **28**, 261 (1969).
146. N. S. Anderson, T. C. S. Dolan, and D. A. Rees, *J. Chem. Soc.*, C, p. 596 (1968).
147. N. S. Anderson, T. C. S. Dolan, C. J. Lawson, A. Penman, and D. A. Rees, *Carbohydrate Res.*, **7**, 468 (1968).
148. D. A. Rees, *J. Chem. Soc.*, p. 5168 (1961).
149. R. L. Whistler and J. N. BeMiller, *Advan. Carbohydrate Chem.*, **13**, 289 (1958).
150. N. S. Anderson, T. C. S. Dolan, A. Penman, D. A. Rees, G. P. Mueller, D. J. Stancioff, and N. F. Stanley, *J. Chem. Soc.*, C, p. 602 (1968).
151. A. A. McKinnon, D. A. Rees, and F. B. Williamson, *Chem. Comm.*, p. 701 (1969).

Physical Methods

4.1 Introduction

In applying physical methods to the investigation of stereochemical problems, it is desirable to employ as many different techniques as possible. Some of the methods which have found wide application in the study of the stereochemical properties of organic compounds in general have been described elsewhere (1). The methods (*cf.* refs. 2–11) which are particularly suited to providing answers to stereochemical problems posed by carbohydrate molecules will now be discussed.

4.2 X-ray Diffraction

In principle, X-ray crystallography is capable of yielding complete information on the structure of any sugar which can be obtained in the crystalline form (5). Even in the case of some polysaccharides (see Section 3.6), natural or man-made fibers contain regions of order called *crystallites*, which are amenable to X-ray diffraction analysis (3). Clearly, intermolecular forces within the crystal lattice will influence the conformation adopted by the molecules in the solid state; and, although it does not necessarily follow that the conformation associated with the structure in the solid state corresponds to the conformer which predominates in the liquid state or in solution, this is often the case. Indeed, a number of instances where such correspondence exists were mentioned in Chapter 3.

Apart from its application as a useful tool in structure determination, X-ray crystallography also supplies useful data on bond lengths and bond angles (5, 7). It will be recalled from Section 3.2 that this information is of vital importance when considering the geometry of the chair conformers of the pyranoid ring, and also when discussing the origins of the anomeric effect.

4.3 Mass Spectrometry

Although mass spectrometry has been found (8, 12) to be not too generally informative about stereochemical differences between configurational isomers, in some instances the technique offers an easy method for the characterization of constitutional isomers. Thus, it has been possible (13) to distinguish between 2,5:3,4-(**1**) and 2,3:4,5-(**2**) di-*O*-methylene-galacti-

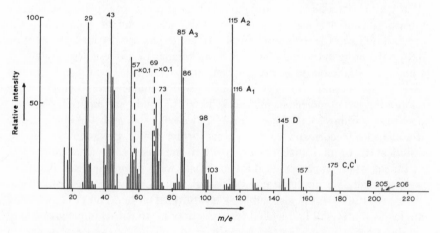

tols by inspection of their mass spectra, which are shown in Figures 4.1 and 4.2, respectively.

In the mass spectrum shown in Figure 4.1, the ion (fragment A_1) with m/e 116 could arise either from a 1,3,6,8-tetraoxacyclo[5.3.0]decane ring system (13) or from a 1,3,6,8-tetraoxacyclo[4.4.0]decane ring system (14), that is, either from the 2,5:3,4-diacetal or from the 2,4:3,5-diacetal.

Figure 4.1 The mass spectrum of 2,5:3,4-di-*O*-methylene-galactitol (**1**).

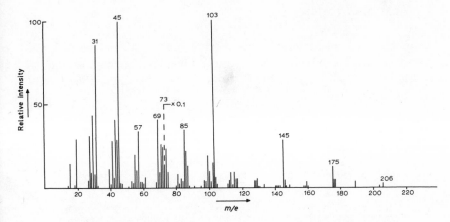

Figure 4.2 The mass spectrum of 2,3:4,5-di-*O*-methylene-galactitol (**2**).

However, the fact that the mass spectrum shows a "half-ion" peak at m/e 103 of *low* relative abundance indicates[1] that the diacetal is *not* 2,4:3,5-di-*O*-methylene-galactitol. The fragmentation process shown in Figure 4.3*a* accounts for the formation of fragment A_1, which may subsequently lose a hydrogen atom to yield fragment A_2 with m/e 115 or a hydromethyl radical to give fragment A_3 with m/e 85.

There are also important peaks in the high mass range to be found at m/e 205 (fragment B), 175 (fragment C), and 145 (fragment D). As shown

[1] The mass spectra of the 2,4:3,5-di-*O*-methylene derivatives of D-glucitol and L-iditol *both* show (15) "half-ion" peaks at m/e 103 of *higher* relative abundance. As shown in Scheme (**A**), electron shifts result (14) in the rupture of three bonds to give a stable "half-radical" and the "half-ion" at m/e 103.

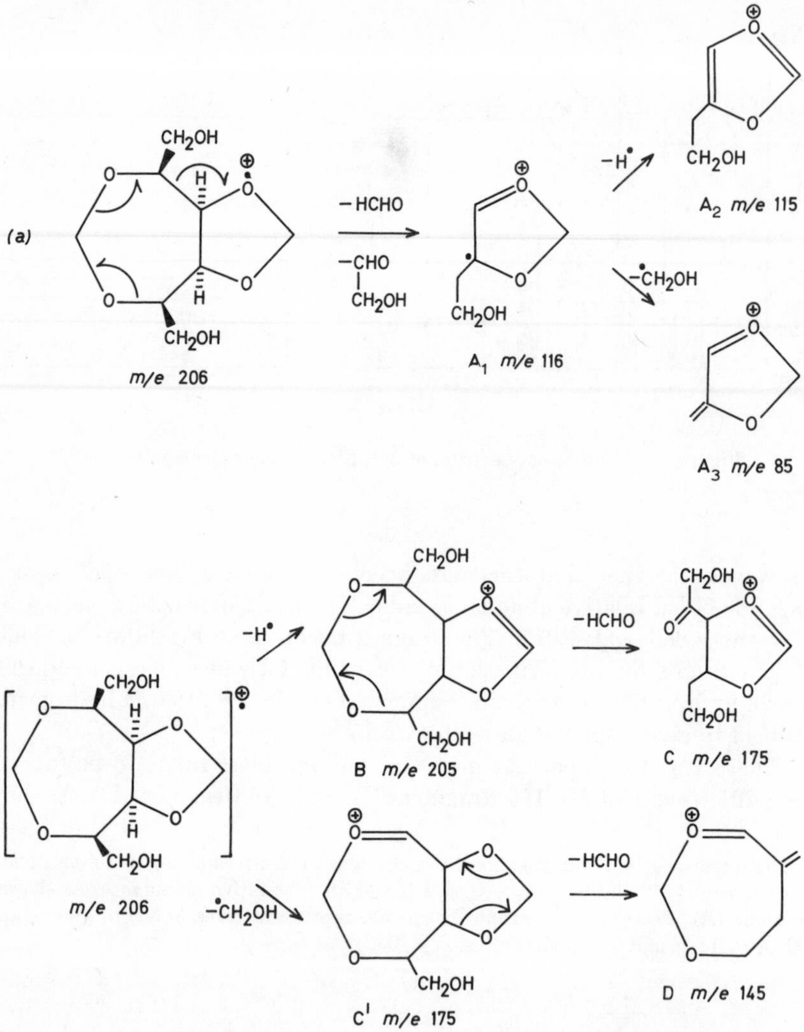

Figure 4.3   The fragmentation processes for 2,5:3,4-di-*O*-methylene-galactitol (**1**).

in Figure 4.3*b*, fragment B results from loss of a hydrogen atom from the molecular ion ($M = 206$). Fragment B may then lose formaldehyde to give fragment C, with the same m/e (i.e., 175) as fragment C′, which is obtained directly from the molecular ion by elimination of a hydroxymethyl radical; fragment C′ may subsequently lose formaldehyde to yield fragment D with m/e 145.

By a fragmentation process similar to that shown in Figure 4.3*b* for the 2,5:3,4-diacetal (**1**), the 2,3:4,5-diacetal (**2**) may eliminate a hydroxymethyl radical followed by formaldehyde to give ions of m/e 175 and 145, respectively (Figure 4.4). However, the mass spectrum of the 2,3:4,5-diacetal (**2**) shown in Figure 4.2 exhibits a "half-ion" peak at m/e 103 of exceptionally high relative abundance on account of cleavage of the C_3-C_4 bond

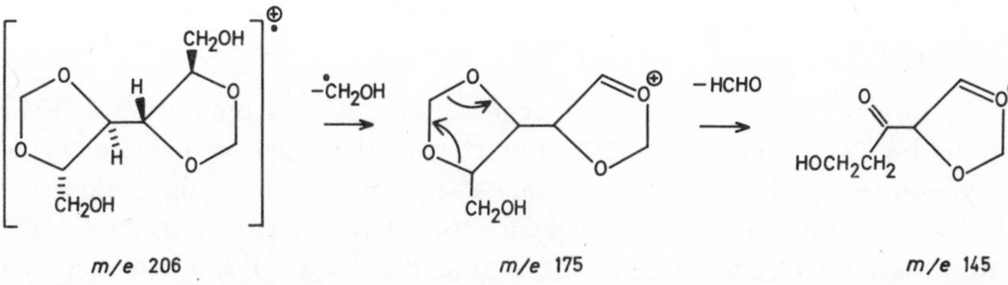

$$m/e\ 206 \qquad m/e\ 175 \qquad m/e\ 145$$

Figure 4.4   The fragmentation process for 2,3:4,5-di-*O*-methylene-galactitol (**2**).

(14, 16). Together with the lack of ions at m/e 115 and 116, this is good evidence that the mass spectrum is characteristic of a 4,4'-bis-1,3-dioxolane.

The constitutional assignments were confirmed (13) by ¹H nuclear magnetic resonance spectroscopy (see Section 4.5.2).

4.4   Infrared Spectroscopy

Although infrared spectroscopy of pyranoid derivatives has facilitated the assignment of configurations at the anomeric carbon atom in the past (9, 17), this problem is now more readily tackled by nuclear magnetic resonance spectroscopy (Section 4.5). However, it is important to realize that, in contrast with the latter technique, infrared spectroscopy offers a means of obtaining data for the solid state of a particular compound, as well as for solutions.

If infrared spectra are recorded at very low dilutions (<0.005 M) in carbon tetrachloride solutions, the intramolecular hydrogen bonding associated with hydroxyl groups in carbohydrate derivatives may yield information about configuration as well as conformation. The method is based on the observation (18) that the O—H stretching frequency, which normally occurs in the region around 3630 cm⁻¹, is shifted to lower frequency when the hydroxyl group is engaged in hydrogen bonding; the lower the frequency, the greater is the strength of the hydrogen bond.

However, recent observations show that care must be exercised when applying this rule. Although the hydroxyl group in the chair conformer of the *trans* isomer (3) of 5-hydroxy-2-isopropyl-1,3-dioxane cannot enter into

HO

O

O

CH(CH₃)₂

(3)

hydrogen bonding with the ring oxygen atoms, the existence of two O—H stretching frequencies, one at 3636 cm⁻¹ and the other at 3605 cm⁻¹, has been confirmed (19). Despite the fact that hydrogen bonding could occur if the chair conformer was converted into a twist-boat conformer (*cf.* ref. 20), the energy of a hydrogen bond is undoubtedly insufficient to overcome the increase of almost 6 kcal mole⁻¹ involved (Section 5.5.2) in transforming the chair conformer into the highly disfavored twist-boat conformer. It has been suggested (19), therefore, that the absorption band at *ca.* 3605 cm⁻¹ may be assigned to one of the conformers associated with a particular torsional orientation of the equatorial hydroxyl group (*cf.* ref. 21). Nonetheless, it has been possible (20) to make configurational assignments to the two diastereomers of 5-hydroxy-2-phenyl-1,3-dioxane (1,3-*O*-benzylidene-glycerol) by comparison of their infrared spectra in carbon tetrachloride solutions. One diastereomer had an absorption band at 3593 cm⁻¹ (ϵ 78) associated with a hydrogen-bonded hydroxyl group and was assigned to the *cis* isomer (4). The other diastereomer had absorption bands at 3633 cm⁻¹ (ϵ 79) and 3601 cm⁻¹ (ϵ 26), both probably associated with free hydroxyl groups, and was assigned to the *trans* isomer (5).

HO

O

O

Ph

(4)

HO

O

O

Ph

(5)

Occasionally, conformational assignments can be made as well. On the basis of an absorption band at 3512 cm⁻¹, which is characteristic of hydrogen bonding between *syn*-axial hydroxyl groups, methyl 2-*C*-methyl-β-L-ribopyranoside is believed (22) to exist as the $^4C_1$ conformer (6) in carbon etrachloride solutions.

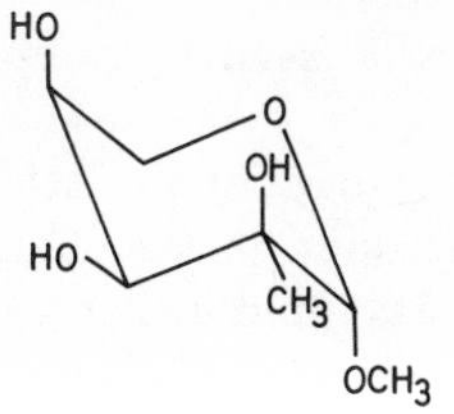

(6)

4.5   Nuclear Magnetic Resonance Spectroscopy

4.5.1   Chemical Shifts

Quite often chemical shift data by themselves turn out to be particularly useful when considering the constitutional, configurational, and conformational properties of carbohydrates and their derivatives. Nonetheless, one usually seeks to corroborate the data by any information that is forthcoming from a consideration of the multiplicity associated with spin-spin coupling.

The observation (23) that, as a general rule in pyranoid rings, equatorial protons resonate at a lower field than constitutionally similar axial protons has led to the formulation of some empirical rules (24, 25). Although a few exceptions have been found, this generalization is of great use in making configurational and conformational assignments.

In fully acetylated pyranoid derivatives, a change in configuration at a chiral carbon atom whereby an equatorial acetoxy group assumes the axial orientation has the effect of deshielding a neighboring axial proton and shielding a neighboring equatorial proton (24). The following empirical rules enable the chemical shifts of H_1 and H_5 in hexopyranose pentaacetates to be predicted relative to the δ values of 5.75 and 3.90 observed for H_1 and H_5, respectively, in β-D-glucopyranose pentaacetate (**7**):

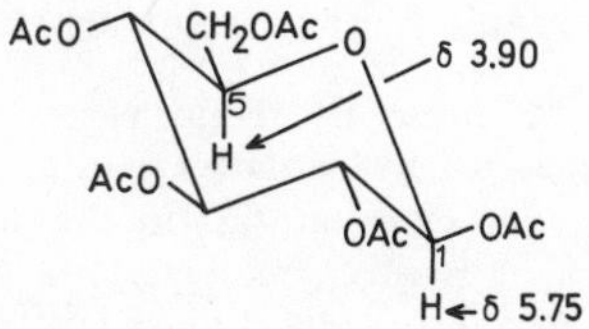

(7)

1. If the proton under consideration has remained axial: (*a*) add 0.2 ppm for each neighboring axial acetoxy group; (*b*) add 0.25 ppm for each *syn*-axial acetoxy group.

2. If the proton under consideration has achieved the equatorial orientation: (*a*) add 0.6 ppm to account for the change of orientation from axial to equatorial; (*b*) subtract 0.20 ppm if there is an axial acetoxy group at a neighboring position.

Table 4.1 shows the measure of agreement between the observed and calculated chemical shifts for a number of hexopyranose pentaacetates.

Table 4.1   Observed and Calculated Chemical Shifts for H_1 and H_5 in a Number of Hexopyranose Pentaacetates (24)

| Hexopyranose Pentaacetate | δ Values, ppm, in Chloroform-d | | | |
| | H_1 | | H_5 | |
	Obs.	Calc.	Obs.	Calc.
α-D-*Altro*-	6.02	5.95	4.5	4.4
α-D-*Galacto*-	6.36	6.35	4.4	4.35
α-D-*Gluco*-	6.34	6.35	4.1	4.15
α-D-*Gulo*-	6.22	6.15	4.6	4.6
α-D-*Manno*-	6.09	6.15	4.1	4.15
β-D-*Allo*-	6.00	6.00	4.2	4.15
β-D-*Galacto*-	5.74	5.75	4.1	4.1
β-D-*Gulo*-	6.00	6.00	4.3	4.35
β-D-*Manno*-	5.93	5.95	3.9	3.9

Comparison of these chemical shifts indicates that H_1 resonates at considerably lower field than does H_5. Indeed, it is a fairly general rule that anomeric protons give rise to signals at lower field than do other ring protons (23). This is a consequence of the fact that the anomeric carbon atom is bonded to *two* oxygen atoms, thus causing the anomeric proton to be somewhat more deshielded than the other ring protons.[2]

[2] The chemical shifts of the ¹⁹F nuclei in ¹⁹F nuclear magnetic resonance spectra of hexopyranosyl and pentopyranosyl fluoride derivatives are also known (26) to be dependent on their orientation, axial or equatorial, at the anomeric center. Just as with anomeric protons in pyranose derivatives, an equatorial fluorine atom is deshielded relative to an axial fluorine atom in pyranosyl fluoride derivatives. Moreover, the ¹⁹F chemical shifts are also subject to some variation that depends on the configuration at the other chiral carbon atoms around the pyranoid ring.

Configurational assignments can often be made on the basis of differences in chemical shift. For example, in both anomers (**8** and **9**) of D-

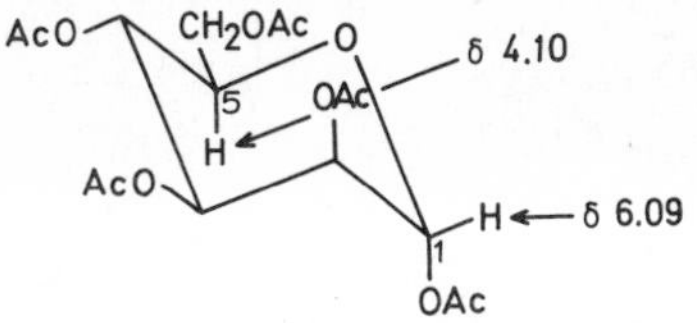

(8)

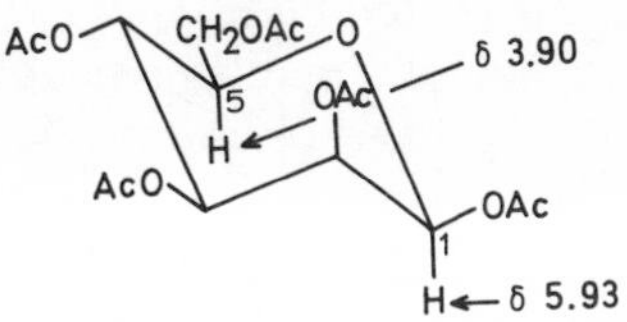

(9)

mannopyranose pentaacetate, H_1 and H_2 bear a *syn-clinal* relationship to each other, and so it is not possible to make configurational assignments at the anomeric center based on spin-spin coupling constant data. However, assignments can be made (24) on the basis of the relative chemical shifts of the anomeric protons. The signal at lower field is assigned to the α-anomer in which H_1 has the equatorial orientation, and the α-anomeric assignment is confirmed by observing the expected deshielding of H_5 by the *syn*-axial acetoxy group on the anomeric carbon atom.

An exception to the rule that equatorial protons resonate at lower field than constitutionally similar axial protons is provided by α-D-altropyranose pentaacetate (**10**), in which the signal for the equatorial proton on C_2

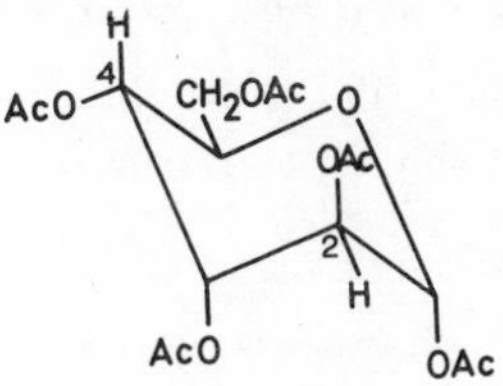

(10)

comes at higher field than does the signal for the axial proton on C_4. This situation arises because H_2 is strongly shielded by the neighboring axial acetoxy groups on C_1 and C_3, whereas H_4 is strongly deshielded by the axial acetoxy groups on C_2 and C_3.

Usually the protons associated with the methyl groups in axial acetoxy groups give rise to signals at lower field than the corresponding protons in equatorial acetoxy groups. The differentiation is not regarded (24) as sufficiently reliable, however, to serve as a basis for making configurational assignments.

Correlations of chemical shifts of ring protons in pentopyranoses with stereochemistry have been expressed (25) in a set of empirical rules based on β-D-xylopyranose (**11**) as standard:

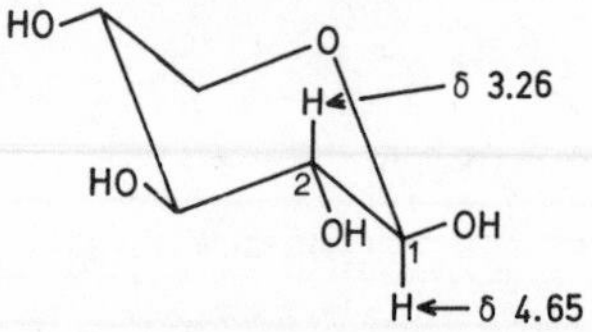

(11)

1. If the proton under consideration has remained axial: (*a*) add 0.3 ppm for each neighboring axial hydroxyl group; (*b*) add 0.35 ppm for each *syn*-axial hydroxyl group.
2. If the proton under consideration has achieved the equatorial orientation: add 0.6 ppm.

The position of the conformational equilibrium of α-D-lyxopyranose (**12**) in aqueous solution has been predicted (25) by comparing the observed chemical shifts (ν_{obs}) of δ 5.08 and δ 3.90 for H_1 and H_2, respectively, with the calculated chemical shifts (ν_{4C_1} and ν_{1C_4}) of these protons, shown in Figure 4.5 for the $^4C_1$ and $^1C_4$ conformers, respectively. From the relationship

$$\nu_{obs} = N_{4C_1}\nu_{4C_1} + N_{1C_4}\nu_{1C_4} \tag{1}$$

the conclusion may be reached that α-D-lyxopyranose (**12**) exists to about equal extents as the $^4C_1$ and the $^1C_4$ conformer.

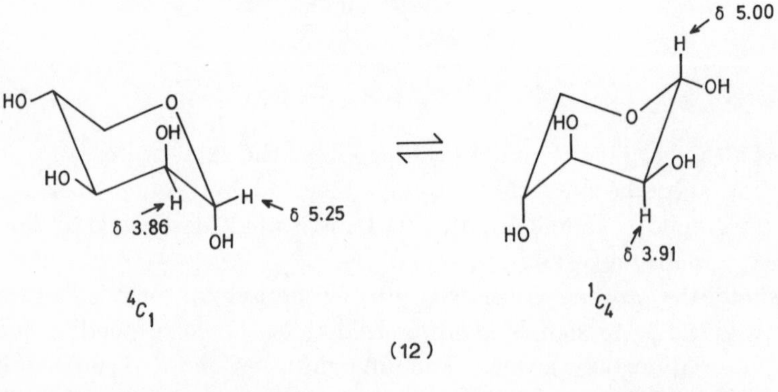

(12)

Figure 4.5   The calculated chemical shifts (25) of H_1 and H_2 in the $^4C_1$ and $^1C_4$ conformers of α-D-lyxopyranose (**12**).

The presence of alkyl substituents on pyranoid rings [*cf.* cyclohexane derivatives (27)] can also influence the chemical shifts of neighboring ring protons. Thus, the H_1 signal of 6-deoxy-5-*C*-methyl-*β*-D-*xylo*hexopyranose (**13**) is shifted (28) to lower field than the H_1 signal of *β*-D-xylopyranose (**11**) on account of deshielding by the *syn*-axial methyl group on C_5.

(13)

In a series of 4-substituted 2-phenyl-1,3-dioxolanes, ^{1}H nuclear magnetic resonance signals for the benzylidene-methine protons of *cis* isomers (**14**) were invariably found (29) at higher field than the corresponding signals of the *trans* isomers (**15**). An analogous situation was found (30) to prevail

$R = CH_3$, CH_2OH , CH_2OAc , $CH(CH_3)_2$, $CH_2CH_2CH_2OH$, $C(CH_3)_3$.

(14)   (15)

for the alkylidene-methine protons in the *syn* and *anti* isomers of some 2,4,5-trisubstituted 1,3-dioxolanes. These observations allow configurational assignments to be made at the acetal carbon atom of 1,3-dioxolane derivatives of carbohydrates.

In many instances, the proportions of *α*-pyranose, *β*-pyranose, *α*-furanose, and *β*-furanose at equilibrium in a solution of an aldopentose or aldohexose in deuterium oxide may be obtained (24, 31, 32) by direct integration of the signals for the anomeric protons. In the identification of furanose forms, the anomer with the *cis* arrangement between the anomeric proton and the oxy substituent on C_2 will normally give rise to a lower field signal for its anomeric proton than the anomer with the *trans* arrangement (33).

A knowledge of the compositions at equilibrium of aqueous solutions of aldohexoses and aldopentoses, as determined by ^{1}H nuclear magnetic resonance spectroscopy, has been extremely useful in identifying ^{13}C signals in proton-decoupled ^{13}C nuclear magnetic resonance spectra (34–37). Tables 4.2, 4.3, and 4.4 record the ^{13}C chemical shifts which have been

Table 4.2 ^{13}C *Chemical Shifts* (*ppm upfield from external carbon disulfide*) *for the Aldopentopyranoses* (*35*)

Pyranose	C_1	$C_2{}^a$	$C_3{}^a$	C_4	C_5
α-D-Xylose	100.0	120.6	119.2	123.1	131.1
β-D-Xylose	95.5	118.0	116.1	122.8	127.2
α-L-Arabinose	95.3	120.1	119.7	123.8	126.1
β-L-Arabinose	95.4	123.6	123.6	123.8	129.9
α-D-Lyxose	98.2	122.1	121.6	124.7	129.4
β-D-Lyxose	98.2	122.1	119.6	125.5	128.3
α-β-Ribose	98.9	123.6	122.0	124.7	129.4
β-D-Ribose	98.4	121.1	121.1	123.7	129.4

^{a} The assignments for C_2 and C_3 are reversed in the paper by Dorman and Roberts (36).

Table 4.3 ^{13}C *Chemical Shifts* (*ppm upfield from external carbon disulfide*) *for Some Aldohexopyranoses* (*35*)

Pyranose	C_1	$C_2{}^a$	$C_3{}^a$	C_4	C_5	C_6
α-D-Glucose	100.4	120.9	119.5	122.8	121.2	131.4
β-D-Glucose	96.5	118.2	116.6	122.8	116.6	131.4
α-D-Galactose	100.0	123.5	123.5	123.8	122.0	131.2
β-D-Galactose	95.8	120.2	119.5	123.1	117.3	131.4
α-D-Mannose	97.6	121.0	121.5	124.9	119.8	130.7
β-D-Mannose	98.2	120.8	118.7	125.2	115.9	130.7
β-D-Allose	99.0	121.2	121.4	125.6	119.0	131.2

^{a} The assignments for C_2 and C_3 are reversed in the paper by Dorman and Roberts (36).

found (35) for some aldopentopyranoses, some aldohexopyranoses, and some methyl aldohexopyranosides, respectively. The electron density associated with a particular carbon atom directly influences its chemical shift. Thus, for example, the anomeric carbon atom, which is attached to two oxygen atoms and has a relatively low electron density associated with it, is shielded and resonates at a relatively low field in the region between 88 and 102 ppm. Other ring carbon atoms resonate at higher field in the region between 116 and 133 ppm. The chemical shift of a particular carbon atom is also dependent on the nature and orientation of the substituent and on

Table 4.4 ^{13}C *Chemical Shifts (ppm upfield from external carbon disulfide) for the Methyl Aldohexopyranosides (35)*

Pyranoside	C_1	$C_2{}^a$	$C_3{}^a$	C_4	C_5	C_6	OCH_3
α-D-*Gluco*-	92.9	120.6	118.9	122.4	120.9	131.3	137.2
β-D-*Gluco*-	89.1	119.1	117.3	122.5	117.3	131.1	135.0
α-D-*Galacto*-	93.0	122.9	122.6	123.9	121.6	131.0	137.2
β-D-*Galacto*-	88.7	121.6	119.5	123.7	117.5	131.4	135.4
α-D-*Manno*-	91.8	122.0	122.7	125.8	120.1	131.6	137.5
β-D-*Manno*-	91.5	122.2	119.5	125.7	116.2	131.4	135.9
α-D-*Altro*-	91.7	122.8	122.8	128.0	122.8	131.5	137.4
α-D-*Ido*-	91.3	121.9	121.0	122.5	122.0	132.6	137.0

^{a} The assignments for C_2 and C_3 are reversed in the paper by Dorman and Roberts (36).

the nature and orientation of neighboring substituents. The dependence on the nature of the substituent is demonstrated by the fact that conversion of an aldopentose or an aldohexose to either of its methyl glycopyranosides (Tables 4.3 and 4.4) causes C_1 to be deshielded by *ca.* 7.0 ppm. The dependence on the orientation of substituents is summarized by the following empirical relationships, which may be deduced (35) by comparing ^{13}C chemical shifts for α-D-glucopyranose and α-D-xylopyranose with those for β-D-glucopyranose and β-D-xylopyranose, respectively:

1. An axial hydroxyl group is associated with increased shielding of the ^{13}C nucleus to which it is attached.

2. A ^{13}C nucleus adjacent to a carbon atom which carries an axial hydroxyl group experiences increased shielding.

3. An axial hydrogen atom in a *syn*-axial relationship with a hydroxyl group is associated with increased shielding of the ^{13}C nucleus to which it is attached.

These observations have the important implication (35) that the introduction of destabilizing interactions around the pyranose ring causes an all-round increase in the shielding of the ^{13}C nuclei.[3] This statement finds quantitative support in Table 4.5, which shows that the sum of the ^{13}C chemical shifts of some pentopyranoses and hexopyranoses is related to their relative free energies (Section 3.2.4).

[3] Similar relationships between destabilizing interactions and ^{13}C chemical shift differences have been found in cyclohexane derivatives (38, 39) and in some inositols and their O-methyl derivatives (40).

Table 4.5   Correlation (35) of the Sum of ^{13}C Chemical Shifts (ppm) with Conformational Free Energies (kcal mole^{-1}) (See Section 3.2.4 and ref. 32)

Pyranose	$\Sigma^{13}C$ Chemical Shifts	Conformational Free Energies
β-D-Glucose	702.1	2.05
β-D-Galactose	707.3	2.5
β-D-Mannose	709.5	2.95
α-D-Glucose	716.2	2.4
α-D-Mannose	715.5	2.5
β-D-Allose	717.4	2.95
α-D-Galactose	724.0	2.85
β-D-Xylose	579.6	1.6
α-L-Arabinose	583.3	1.95
β-D-Lyxose	593.7	2.4
α-D-Xylose	594.0	1.9
β-D-Ribose	594.7	2.3
α-D-Lyxose	596.0	1.85
β-L-Arabinose	598.4	2.2
α-D-Ribose	598.6	3.1

Although anisotropy effects arising from ring currents have been invoked (41) to explain the observation that equatorial protons are usually more deshielded than constitutionally similar axial protons, ^{13}C nuclear magnetic resonance spectroscopic data suggest (35) that the difference may be explained, in part at least, in terms of the relative shielding of the carbon atom to which the proton is attached. It is significant that, when the respective ^{13}C and ^{1}H chemical shifts of α-anomers and β-anomers are compared, a relative shielding of the ^{13}C nucleus of the anomeric carbon atom is accompanied by the relative deshielding of the anomeric proton, and vice versa. This is illustrated in Figure 4.6 for the anomers of D-glucopyranose. Since the anomeric carbon atom is more shielded and hence less positive in the α-anomer, the axial C_1-O_1 bond must be less polarized than the equatorial C_1-O_1 bond in the β-anomer. Therefore a hydroxyl proton associated with an axial C_1-O_1 bond should be more shielded than a hydroxyl proton associated with an equatorial C_1-O_1 bond (35). If this is the case, it would at least partially account for the observation (42) that the hydroxyl proton of the α-anomer with the axial C_1-O_1 bond resonates at higher field than the hydroxyl proton of the β-anomer.

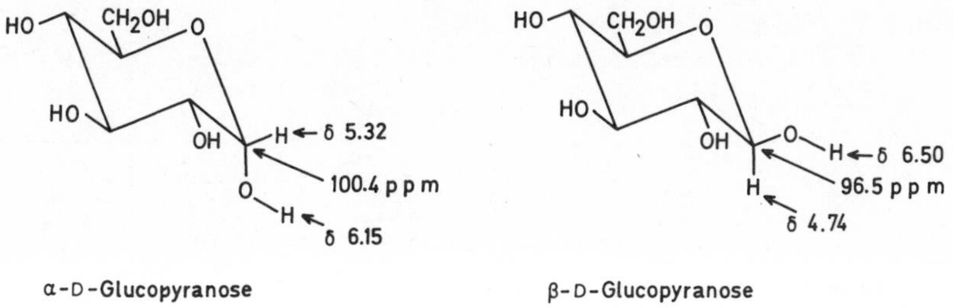

α-D-Glucopyranose   β-D-Glucopyranose

Figure 4.6   A comparison of the ^{13}C and ^{1}H chemical shifts associated with the anomeric centers of α- and β-D-glucopyranoses.

4.5.2   Coupling Constants

The magnitude of the coupling constant between hydrogen atoms on adjacent carbon atoms often yields valuable information about the conformational and configurational properties of carbohydrates. In the system H_1—C_1—C_2—H_2, the main factor which influences the magnitude of J_{H_1,H_2} is the size of the torsional angle ϕ associated with H_1 and H_2 (23). The angular dependence finds quantitative expression in the well-known Karplus (43) relationship:

$$\left. \begin{array}{l} J_{H_1,H_2} = A \cos^2 \phi - C \text{ for } 0° \leq \phi \leq 90° \\ J_{H_1,H_2} = B \cos^2 \phi - C \text{ for } 90° \leq \phi \leq 180° \end{array} \right\} \tag{2}$$

where A, B, and C are constants. The original calculations for an "ethanic"-type fragment yielded (43) values for A, B, and C of 8.5, 9.5, and 0.3 Hz, respectively. Substitution of these values in equation 2 allows the graphical representation shown in Figure 4.7 to be derived for the angular dependence of vicinal coupling constants. In accordance with this graph, protons which are *anti-periplanar* ($\phi \simeq 180°$) on a pyranoid ring usually exhibit a large value for the vicinal coupling constant (7–10 Hz), whereas protons which are *syn-clinal* ($\phi \simeq 60°$) usually exhibit a small value (1–4 Hz).

The importance of the angular dependence of vicinal coupling constants in making configurational assignments is illustrated by considering the ^{1}H nuclear magnetic resonance spectrum of a solution of D-glucose at equilibrium in deuterium oxide, shown in Figure 4.8. On the basis of their relative chemical shifts, the low-field doublet at δ 5.32 may be assigned to the equatorial anomeric proton of α-D-glucopyranose and the high-field doublet at δ 4.74 to the axial anomeric proton of β-D-glucopyranose. This assignment is confirmed by the relative magnitudes of the splittings as-

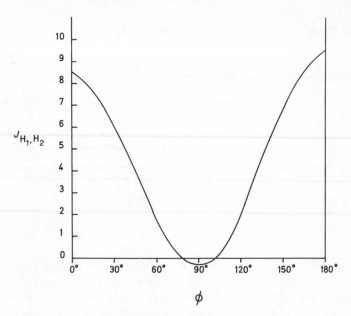

Figure 4.7   A plot of the Karplus relationship between $J_{H1,H2}$ and ϕ.

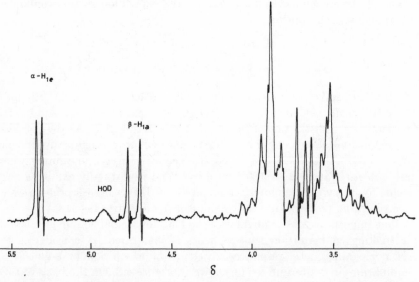

Figure 4.8   A 100 MHz ^{1}H nuclear magnetic resonance spectrum of an equilibrium solution of D-glucose in deuterium oxide. Protons associated with the hydroxyl groups of the sugar were first of all exchanged for deuterons.

sociated with these two signals. In the case of the low-field signal assigned to the anomeric proton of the α-anomer, the value of *ca.* 3.5 Hz for its coupling with H_2 is consistent with the *syn-clinal* relationship which exists between these two protons when α-D-glucopyranose exists as its stable $^4C_1$ conformer. Correspondingly, in the case of the high-field signal assigned to the anomeric proton of the β-anomer, the value of *ca.* 7.5 Hz for its coupling with H_2 is consistent with the *anti*-periplanar relationship which exists between these two protons when β-D-glucopyranose exists as its stable $^4C_1$ conformer.

If, in the system H_1—C_1—C_2—H_2, either C_1 or C_2 carries an electronegative substituent, the magnitude of the vicinal coupling constant for a particular torsional angle is not as large as is predicted by the graph in Figure 4.7 (44–48). The electronegative substituent exerts its maximum effect on the vicinal coupling constant when it is *anti-periplanar* to one of the two protons involved in the vicinal coupling (48, 49). As a result of this electronegativity effect, the magnitude of the coupling constant between *cis* protons on C_1 and C_2 of the pyranose ring falls into two categories:

1. For pyranoses with an axial proton on C_1 and an equatorial proton on C_2, the coupling constant is usually within the range 1.0–1.5 Hz.

2. For pyranoses with an equatorial proton on C_1 and an axial proton on C_2, the coupling constant is usually within the range 2.5–3.5 Hz.

Figure 4.9 shows that for the pyranoses in the first category (A), but not for those in the second (B), H_2 is in an *anti-periplanar* relationship with the

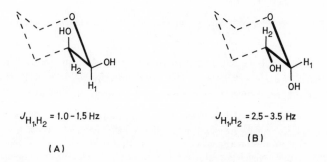

J_{H_1,H_2} = 1.0 - 1.5 Hz

(A)

J_{H_1,H_2} = 2.5 - 3.5 Hz

(B)

Figure 4.9   The steric dependence of the electronegativity effect associated with the ring oxygen atom on $J_{H1,H2}$.

ring oxygen atom. Hence the smaller vicinal coupling constant is to be anticipated.[4]

A more appropriate form of the Karplus relationship has been deduced (50). It gives results so similar numerically (48), however, that its application is hardly justified, especially in view of the uncertainties associated with electronegative substituents.

In the case of some pyranose derivatives it transpires that the observed vicinal coupling constant is intermediate between the ones predicted for the separate chair conformers (25, 31, 32, 51, 52). Since, at room temperature, the free energy of activation associated with the chair-chair interconversion is small enough to ensure rapid conformational interconversion, it follows that, provided the difference in the relative free energies between the $^4C_1$ and $^1C_4$ conformers is also small, the observed coupling constants (J_{4C_1} and J_{1C_4}) associated with the individual conformers are given by the expression

$$J_{obs} = N_{4C_1}J_{4C_1} + N_{1C_4}J_{1C_4} \qquad (3)$$

The equilibrium constants and hence the free energy differences between the $^4C_1$ and $^1C_4$ conformers of the eight D-aldopentopyranose tetraacetates have been deduced (52) from equation 3 with the aid of appropriate coupling constant data and are recorded in Table 4.6. In the case of β-D-ribopyranose tetraacetate (**16**) and β-D-lyxopyranose tetraacetate (**17**) almost

equal amounts of each chair conformer are present in acetone-d_6 at room temperature. Moreover, when the temperature is lowered, the rate of chair-chair interconversion becomes slow enough on the nuclear magnetic

[4] The magnitudes of vicinal ^{19}F—^1H coupling constants also show (26) an angular dependence, and similar electronegativity effects have been observed with pyranosyl fluorides. Also of interest is the observation (34) that in the ^1H nuclear magnetic resonance spectrum of ^{13}C-enriched D-glucose, the signal for the equatorial anomeric proton of the α-anomer exhibits two extra splittings of 5–6 Hz, whereas the signal for the axial anomeric proton of the β-anomer remains as a sharp doublet. It is significant that in the α-anomer H_1 bears *anti-periplanar* relationships with both C_3 and C_5, whereas in the β-anomer H_1 is *syn-clinal* to both C_3 and C_5.

(17)

Table 4.6   The Conformational Equilibria of the Aldopento-pyranose Tetraacetates in Acetone-d_6 at 28° (53)

Aldopentopyranose Tetraacetate	K $^4C_1/^1C_4$	$G°$, kcal mole.[1] $^1C_4 \rightarrow {}^4C_1$
α-D-*Arabino*-	0.23	+0.87 ± 0.36
β-D-*Arabino*-	0.03	+2.1 ± 0.4
α-D-*Lyxo*-	2.9	−0.63 ± 0.28
β-D-*Lyxo*-	0.67	+0.24 ± 0.29
α-D-*Ribo*-	4.0	−0.83 ± 0.36
β-D-*Ribo*-[a]	1.2	−0.11 ± 0.09
α-D-*Xylo*-	50	−2.5
β-D-*Xylo*-[b]	4.0	−0.82 ± 0.14

[a] At 20°.
[b] At 25°.

resonance time scale to permit observation (52–54) of separate signals for the individual conformers. For β-D-ribopyranose tetraacetate (**16**), the observed chemical shift difference ($\nu_{4C_1} - \nu_{1C_4}$) between H_{1a} ($^4C_1$ conformer) and H_{1e} ($^1C_4$ conformer) at −84° was 58.5 Hz. With this information a rate of interconversion k of *ca.* 130 times per second between the $^4C_1$ and $^1C_4$ conformers at −60° (the approximate temperature at which the signals coalesce) has been calculated (52, 54), using the expression

$$k = [\pi(\nu_{4C_1} - \nu_{1C_4})/(2)^{1/2}] \qquad (4)$$

From the Eyring equation (Section 3.1.2), a free energy of activation of *ca.* 10.0 kcal mole^{-1} was obtained (54) for the interconversion. This value compares with a free energy of activation of 9.6 kcal mole^{-1} for the chair-chair interconversion in β-D-lyxopyranose tetraacetate (**17**), as deduced from ^{1}H nuclear magnetic resonance spectra obtained (53) at low temperatures.[5]

In some instances (24, 48, 55–60), the magnitude of long-range spin-spin couplings between protons separated by four (^4J) and five (^5J) single bonds may help to confirm a conformational assignment. Orientational effects associated with couplings across four bonds have been observed (48, 56, 57), and the magnitude of ^4J has been found to attain its maximum value when the bonds assume a planar zigzag conformation, the so-called (60, 61) "W" or "M" conformation.[6] Thus, in the 1,6-anhydro-2,3,4-triacetates of D-glucose (**18**), D-mannose (**19**), and D-galactose (**20**) shown in Figure 4.10,

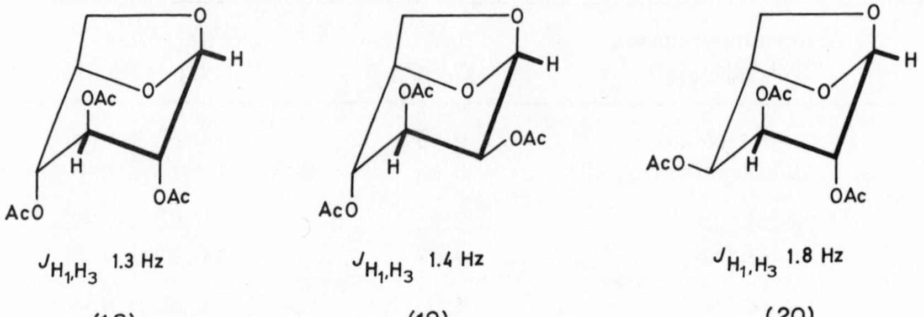

J_{H_1,H_3} 1.3 Hz J_{H_1,H_3} 1.4 Hz J_{H_1,H_3} 1.8 Hz

(18)   (19)   (20)

Figure 4.10   Long-range couplings in the 1,6-anhydro-2,3,4-triacetates of D-glucose (**18**), D-mannose (**19**), and D-galactose (**20**) (55).

long-range couplings of 1–2 Hz between H_1 and H_3 in α-D-gulopyranose pentaacetate (**21**) (24), and between H_2 and H_4, as well as between H_1 and H_3, in α-D-idopyranose pentaacetate (**22**) (59), provide confirmatory evidence that both these derivatives exist predominantly as their $^4C_1$ conformers in solution. Both pentaacetates also exhibit (24, 59) a ^5J coupling between H_1 and H_4. However, it is important to establish that a long-

---

[5] These values must be regarded as approximate, since equation 4—itself an approximate expression—should, strictly speaking, be used only to calculate exchange rates between equally populated sites, a situation which does not prevail for the chair-chair interconversions of β-D-ribopyranose and β-D-lyxopyranose tetraacetates.

[6] The signs of the long-range couplings (^4J) across single bonds in six-membered rings show (62) a stereochemical dependence. Those ($^4J_{ee}$) between two equatorially oriented protons (i.e., the "W" conformation) are *positive*, whereas those ($^4J_{ea}$) between an equatorial and an axial proton are *negative*. It should also be noted that vicinal coupling constants (^3J) are usually *positive*, and geminal coupling constants (^2J) are usually *negative*.

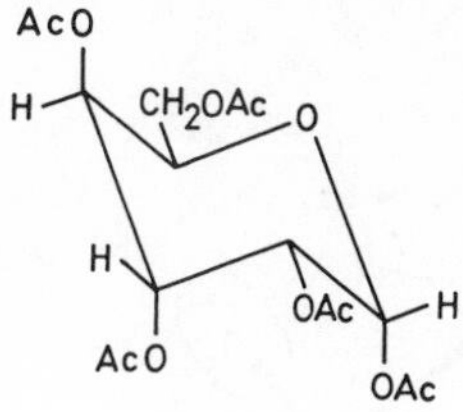

AcO

H — CH$_2$OAc — O

H

OAc — H

AcO

OAc

J_{H_1,H_3} 1.3 Hz

J_{H_1,H_4} 0.7 Hz

(21)

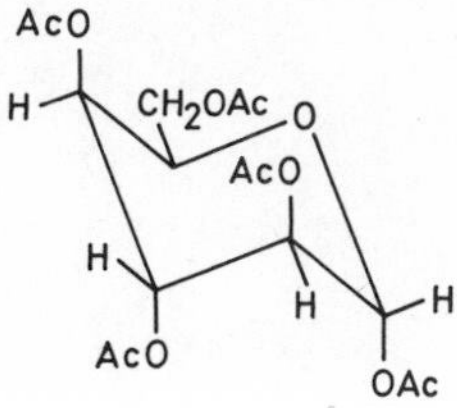

AcO

H — CH$_2$OAc — O

AcO

H

H — H

AcO

OAc

J_{H_1,H_3} 1.0 Hz

J_{H_2,H_4} 0.9 Hz

J_{H_1,H_4} 0.6 Hz

(22)

range coupling is authentic and not attributable to the phenomenon of virtual long-range coupling (63).[7] For example, in β-D-glucopyranose pentaacetate (7), H$_1$ experiences (24) virtual long-range coupling since H$_2$ and H$_3$, which are strongly coupled, have almost the same chemical shift.

In O-methylene derivatives, the magnitude of the coupling constant between the geminal protons is dependent on the orientation of the lone pair orbitals on the oxygen atoms with respect to the protons of the O-methylene group (64–68). This factor can often yield information about the conformation, and hence the constitution, of an acetal. In the absence of oxygen atoms α to methylene groups, geminal coupling constants generally take on values in the region -12 to -18 Hz (48). Positive increments are added to the geminal coupling constant by α oxygen atoms through the inductive removal of electrons from the symmetric bonding orbital of the O-methylene group and through back-donation of lone pair p electrons on the oxygen atoms[8] into the antisymmetric bonding orbital of the O-methylene group.

The positive contribution from the back-donation of a lone pair of p electrons is at a minimum (Figure 4.11a) when the p orbital bisects the H—C—H angle, and at a maximum (Figure 4.11b) when the H—H internuclear axis is perpendicular to the C—O—C plane. The first kind of geometry prevails approximately in 1,3-dioxane derivatives and in some 1,3-dioxepane derivatives; and geminal coupling constants are usually around -6 Hz, that is, by far the most important contribution is from the

---

[7] In an ABC system, a second-order effect on C is observed as a virtual long-range coupling when J_{AB} is large compared with $\Delta\nu_{AB}$, and B is not appreciably coupled to C.
[8] Assumed to be in their excited state and therefore sp^2 hybridized.

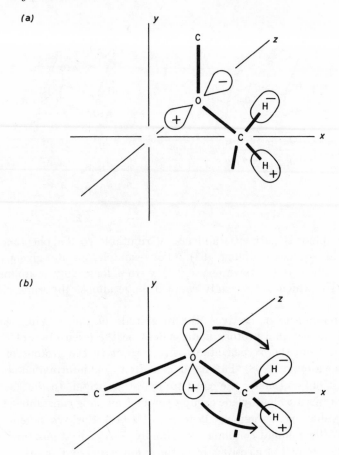

Figure 4.11   (*a*) The geometry for minimum back-donation of lone pair *p* electrons on oxygen atoms into the antisymmetric bonding orbital of an *O*-methylene group. (*b*) The geometry for maximum back-donation of lone pair *p* electrons on oxygen atoms into the antisymmetric bonding orbital of an *O*-methylene group.

inductive effect. To a first approximation, the second kind of geometry occurs in 1,3-dioxolane derivatives and back-donation causes the geminal coupling constant to be close to 0 Hz. Thus, we have a means of distinguishing between constitutionally isomeric *O*-methylene derivatives of carbohydrates. For example, the diacetal which was characterized as 2,5:3,4-di-*O*-methylene-galactitol (**1**) by mass spectrometry in Section 4.3 yielded (13) geminal coupling constants for the *O*-methylene protons in the 1,3-

dioxepane and 1,3-dioxolane rings of -7.3 and *ca.* 0 Hz, respectively. On the other hand, the constitutionally isomeric diacetal, which mass spectrometry had indicated to be 2,3:4,5-di-O-methylene-galactitol (**2**) in Section 4.3, gave (13) a coupling constant of close to 0 Hz for the geminal protons of the enantiotopic O-methylene groups of the 1,3-dioxolane rings.

4.5.3   Nuclear Overhauser Effects

Although this feature of nuclear magnetic resonance spectroscopy has still to be exploited in the carbohydrate field, an elegant confirmation of conformational assignments to the two stereoisomers of 2-O-methyl-4,4,6-trimethyl-1,3-dioxane has been made (69) because it was possible to observe a nuclear Overhauser effect[9] in the case of the *cis* isomer (**24**), but not of the *trans* isomer (**23**). The compound which had been assigned the *cis* configuration on the basis of dipole moment measurements and other ^{1}H nuclear magnetic resonance spectroscopic data showed a 12% enhancement in the integrated area for the proton attached to C_2 when one of the two signals was irradiated. Figure 4.12 shows that in the case of the *cis* isomer

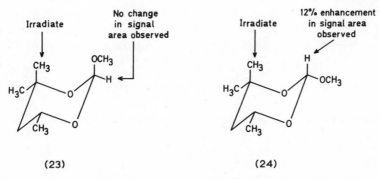

(23)   (24)

Figure 4.12   A nuclear Overhauser effect.

(**24**) the proton attached to C_2 bears a *syn*-axial relationship to one of the two methyl groups on C_4. This brings the proton into sufficiently close proximity with the axial methyl group to exhibit a nuclear Overhauser effect.

[9] For an explanation of this effect see ref. 70.

4.6   Dipole Moment Measurements

In a conformationally mobile system, comparison of the measured dipole moment with the calculated values for the different conformers often allows predictions to be made regarding the nature of the conformational equilibrium. For example, dipole moments of 4.2 D and 1.9 D for μ_O and μ_H, respectively, were calculated (56) for the "O-inside" and "H-inside" conformers of 1,3:2,4-di-*O*-methylene-L-threitol (**25**). The measured

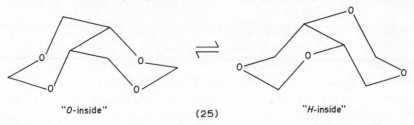

"O-inside"   (25)   "H-inside"

dipole moment μ was 4.00 ± 0.07 D in benzene solution at 25°, and from the equation

$$\mu^2 = N_O\mu_O{}^2 + (1 - N_O)\mu_H{}^2 \tag{5}$$

where N_O is the mole fraction of the "O-inside" conformer, it was estimated that the diacetal (**25**) exists to an extent of 90% as its "O-inside" conformer (see Section 5.5.7).

For the conformational equilibria between the axial and equatorial conformers of a series of 2-alkoxytetrahydropyrans (**26**), a linear relation-

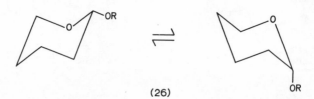

(26)   OR

ship (*cf.* equations 3 and 5) has been found (71) between the squares of the dipole moments and the sum of the vicinal coupling constants of H_X with H_A and H_B, that is $(J_{AX} + J_{BX})$, for which an approximate value may be measured from the separation between the outer peaks of the low-field H_X resonance. From this linear relationship between μ^2 and $(J_{AX} + J_{BX})$ (72), it follows that, of the six possible conformers resulting from torsion around the C-O bond of the C—O—R moiety, one axial conformer and one (or two)[10] equatorial conformer predominate.

---

[10] Two of the three equatorial conformers have the same dipole moment, and so the method is incapable of distinguishing between them (see Section 3.2.3).

4.7 Optical Rotation

The most useful correlations of the configurations and conformations of carbohydrates with optical rotatory power have been achieved by comparisons of *molecular rotations*[11] at single wavelengths, very often measured at the sodium D-line. Empirical approaches have been devised (73–76) for predicting the sign and even the magnitude of the molecular rotation of cyclic carbohydrate derivatives, including cyclitols and pyranoid derivatives. Three (73–75) of these methods assume that separate conformational units in the molecule contribute independently to the molecular rotation and that the total molecular rotation is obtained by summing the contributions.

In one method (74), a center of optical activity is considered to be described by a screw pattern of polarizability of the electrons, with correlations existing (i) between the *handedness* of the screw and the *sign* of the molecular rotation, and (ii) between the *amount* of polarizability and the *magnitude* of the molecular rotation. The most simple conformational unit to consider is the chain of four atoms a—C—C—a'. The Newman projections shown in Figure 4.13 illustrate that the conformational unit exhibits *conformational dissymmetry* caused by the *syn-clinal* and *anti-clinal* conformations in (a), (b), (d), and (e), but not by the *anti-periplanar* conformation in (c). Empirically, it is found that conformations (a) and (b) make dextrorotatory contributions to the molecular rotation which can be expressed mathematically as

$$[M] = +kA \cdot A' \qquad (6)$$

where k is a constant which is the same for conformations (a) and (b), and A and A' are functions of the polarizabilities of atoms a and a', respectively. Conformations (d) and (e) make levorotatory contributions, and conformation (c) does not contribute since it is not dissymmetric. It has been found (74) that these contributions to the molecular rotation may be calculated

---

[11] The molecular rotation $[M]$ is defined by

$$[M] = M[\alpha]/100$$

where M is the molecular weight, and $[\alpha]$ is the *specific rotation*. In some of the early literature of carbohydrate chemistry, the product was not divided by 100. The specific rotation is defined by

$$[\alpha] = 100\alpha/lc$$

where α is the observed rotation, l is the length of the sample cell in decimeters, and c is the concentration in grams per 100 ml. The concentration and the solvent are usually indicated in parentheses after the value; and the temperature in degrees centigrade is expressed by a superscript, and the wavelength of the polarized light by a subscript, both in reference to $[\alpha]$—for example, $[\alpha]_D^{21}$ $-62°$ (c 1.5 in $CHCl_3$).

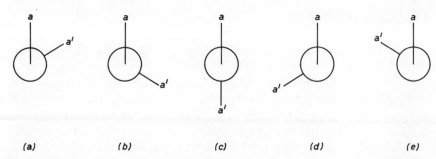

(a)   (b)   (c)   (d)   (e)

Figure 4.13   Newman projections of the conformational unit a—C—C—a' in different conformations.

from the atomic refractions R_a and $R_{a'}$ of atoms a and a', respectively, by the use of the empirical equation

$$[M] = +160°\ R_a^{1/2} \cdot R_{a'}^{1/2} \tag{7}$$

If we consider the conformer of ethylene glycol shown in Figure 4.14, a value for its molecular rotation may be obtained[12] by summing the con-

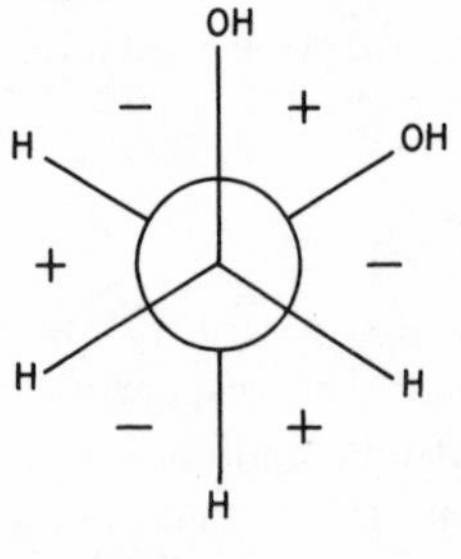

Figure 4.14   The *syn-clinal* conformer of ethylene glycol.

tributions from *all* the dissymmetric conformations to give

$$[M] = k(\text{O}\cdot\text{O} - \text{O}\cdot\text{H} + \text{H}\cdot\text{H} - \text{H}\cdot\text{H} + \text{H}\cdot\text{H} - \text{H}\cdot\text{O})$$

or[13]

$$[M] = k(\text{O}\cdot\text{O} - 2\,\text{O}\cdot\text{H} + \text{H}\cdot\text{H})$$

[12] Ethylene glycol is, of course, achiral. Contributions to optical rotation equal in magnitude but opposite in sign for enantiomeric conformers (which are isoenergetic) cancel each other out.
[13] O.H = H.O.

which is sometimes written symbolically as

$$[M] = k(O - H)^2 \qquad (8)$$

and has been found (74) to have a value of $+45°$ (*cf.* ref. 73). This is an important conformational unit in cyclic carbohydrate derivatives, and the molecular rotations of the cyclitols are readily predicted (77) by adhering to the following simple procedure. Each C-C bond is treated in turn as a conformational fragment of the type shown for ethylene glycol in Figure 4.14. With the hydroxyl group on the nearest carbon atom pointing uppermost, then, if the hydroxyl group on the other carbon atom is *syn-clinal* and to the right a value of $+45°$ is assigned, if it is *syn-clinal* and to the left a value of $-45°$ is assigned, and if it is *anti-periplanar* it makes no contribution to the molecular rotation. The calculated and observed molecular rotations for some cyclitols in their preferred conformers are listed in Table 4.7 and are found to be in reasonably good agreement.

Table 4.7   Observed and Calculated Molecular Rotations for Some Cyclitols (73, 77)

	$[M]_D$	
Compound[a]	Obs.	Calc.
Cyclohexane-		
(−)-1/2-diol	−48°	−45°
(−)-1,2/3-triol	−92°	−90°
(−)-1,2,3/4-tetritol	−49°	−45°
(−)-1,2,4/3-tetritol	−57°	−45°
(−)-1,3/2,4-tetritol	−43°	−45°
(−)-1,2,4/3,5-pentitol	−90°	−90°
(+)-1,3,4/2,5-pentitol	+42°	+45°
(−)-1,2,4/3,5,6-hexitol	−117°	−135°

[a] In this nomenclature scheme, the hydroxyl groups on positions preceding the slash are oriented *above* the plane of the ring and those on positions succeeding the slash are oriented *below* the plane of the ring.

When pyranoid derivatives such as glycosides are considered, additional allowances (*cf.*, however, ref. 75) must be made (74) for the following conformational features:

1. The pyranoid ring has an axis of polarizability difference between O and C_4 when there are different axial substituents on C_1 and C_5 (e.g., *a*),

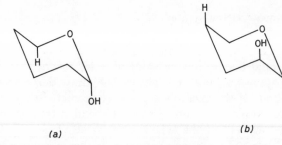

Figure 4.15 Pyranoid rings with an axis of polarizability difference between O and C$_4$.

or on C$_2$ and C$_4$ (e.g., *b*) as shown in Figure 4.15. Conformation (*a*) is considered to contribute +100°, and conformation (*b*) +60°, to the molecular rotation.

2. In hexopyranoid rings, the contribution from the torsional isomers associated with the hydroxymethyl group attached to the chiral center at C$_5$ has been assessed at +25°.

3. In methyl glycopyranosides, the contribution from the torsional isomers associated with the methoxyl group on the anomeric carbon atom has been assessed at +105° for α-anomers, and at −105° for β-anomers.

By means of this empirical approach, the molecular rotations for the $^4C_1$ and $^1C_4$ conformers of the methyl D-aldopentopyranosides have been calculated (74, 77) and are compared in Table 4.8 with the observed values. Although the calculated values obtained by this empirical method are probably insufficiently accurate to allow any unequivocal decisions to be made about conformational properties, nonetheless it is significant that comparison of the observed and calculated molecular rotations in Table 4.8 suggests, for example, that methyl α-D-xylopyranoside (**27**) exists as the $^4C_1$ conformer, whereas methyl β-D-arabinopyranoside (**28**) exists as the $^1C_4$ conformer (*cf.* Section 5.3).

(27)   (28)

Table 4.8 Observed and Calculated Molecular Rotations of the Methyl Pentopyranosides in Water (73, 74, 77)

| | | $[M]_D$ | |
| | | Calc. | |
Methyl Pentopyranoside	Obs.	$^4C_1$	$^1C_4$
α-D-*Arabino*-	−28°	+190°	0°
β-D-*Arabino*-	−403°	−75°	−400°
α-D-*Lyxo*-	+95°	+55°	+135°
β-D-*Lyxo*-	−210°	−210°	−265°
α-D-*Ribo*-	+170°[a]	+250°	+60°
β-D-*Ribo*-	−186°	−150°	−205°
α-D-*Xylo*-	+253°	+250°	+60°
β-D-*Xylo*	−108°	−150°	−205°

[a] In methanol.

The expectation (74) that the nature of the solvent can influence the position of equilibrium between conformers, and hence the molecular rotation of a compound, has been realized (78) for a number of pyranoid derivatives (see Section 3.2.3c). Thus, the ^1H nuclear magnetic resonance spectrum of methyl 3-deoxy-β-L-*erythro*-pentopyranoside (**29**) in deuterium oxide

(29)

indicates (78) that the compound exists almost entirely as the $^1C_4$ conformer, since $J_{H1,H2}$ = 6.0 Hz. The calculated molecular rotation for the $^1C_4$ conformer of +155° is in good agreement with the observed value of +140° in water. On the other hand, the ^1H nuclear magnetic resonance spectrum in chloroform-*d*, showing $J_{H1,H2}$ = 2.2 Hz, requires that the compound exist almost entirely as the $^4C_1$ conformer. Once again, the calculated molecular rotation for the $^4C_1$ conformer of $+205°$ is in excellent agreement with the observed value of $+210°$ in chloroform.

Changes in molecular rotation[14] arising from solvent effects on conformational equilibria are also expected (74) to be sensitive to changes in temperature (*cf.* ref. 54).

Table 4.9 shows a comparison between the observed and the calculated values for the molecular rotations of the $^4C_1$ conformers of the methyl

Table 4.9   Observed and Calculated Molecular Rotations for the $^4C_1$ Conformers of Some Methyl Aldohexopyranosides in Water (77)

Methyl Aldohexopyranoside	$[M]_D$		$[M]_\alpha - [M]_\beta$	
	Obs.	Calc.	Obs.	Calc.
α-D-*Galacto-*	$+380°$	$+375°$	380°	400°
β-D-*Galacto-*	$0°$	$-25°$		
α-D-*Gluco-*	$+309°$	$+325°$	375°	400°
β-D-*Gluco-*	$-66°$	$-75°$		
α-D-*Gulo-*	$+232°$	$+240°$	394°	400°
β-D-*Gulo-*	$-162°$	$-160°$		
α-D-*Manno-*	$+154°$	$+130°$	289°	265°
β-D-*Manno-*	$-135°$	$-135°$		

α- and β-D-glycopyranosides with the *galacto, gluco, gulo,* and *manno* configuratioms (77). The difference in the molecular rotation of the anomeric pairs is seen to be remarkably constant and close to the calculated value of 400° for the glycosides with the *galacto, gluco,* and *gulo* configurations. This observation is a logical expression of Hudson's *rules of isorotation* (79), which attempt to correlate the molecular rotation with the configuration at the anomeric center for a number of pyranoid derivatives. In the case of the methyl D-glycopyranosides (Figure 4.16), the molecular rotation at the anomeric center (A) is considered to contribute to the total molecular rotation independently of the contribution from the remainder of the molecule (B). Thus, in the D-series,

$$[M]_\alpha = B + A$$

and

[14] The term *mutarotation* is often used to refer to a change in optical rotation with time.

$$[M]_\beta = \text{B} - \text{A}$$

and hence

$$[M]_\alpha - [M]_\beta = 2\text{A} \qquad (9)$$

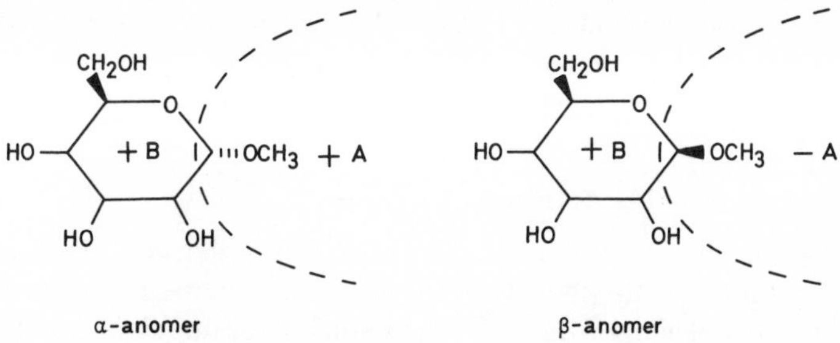

Figure 4.16 Hudson's rules of isorotation as illustrated by the methyl D-glycopyrano-sides. For the sake of generality, the configurations at C_2, C_3, and C_4 have not been specified.

Equation 9 is a quantitative expression of the well-known phenomenon in carbohydrate chemistry that in the D-series of sugars α-anomers are usually more dextrorotatory than β-anomers. The quantitative formulation of the rules of isorotation fails, however, under a number of circumstances. For example, the molecular rotation difference between the α- and β-anomers of methyl D-mannopyranoside is less than the predicted value because of the axial hydroxyl group on C_2 (*cf.* the *galacto*, *gluco*, and *gulo* configurations, which all have equatorial hydroxyl groups on C_2). This reflects the fundamentally unsound nature of the van't Hoff *principle of optical superposition*,[15] of which the rule of isorotation is an example.

The quantum-mechanical theories of optical rotation show (76, 80) that optical activity arises, in fact, not from screw patterns of polarizability of electrons in chiral carbon atoms or dissymmetric conformations,[16] but rather from modifications of such patterns by interactions between pairs of groups. Although the rotatory contribution of a given pair of groups in a

[15] The van't Hoff principle of optical superposition assumes that the molecular rotation is made up of the algebraic sum of the rotatory contributions from all the chiral centers in the molecule. It should be noted that the mannopyranoside anomaly is accommodated by the empirical methods of Whiffen (73), Brewster (74), and Lemieux and Martin (75).

[16] Although the empirical rules proposed by Whiffen (73) and Brewster (74), and modified recently by Lemieux and Martin (75), are theoretically inadequate, they are nonetheless useful because of their very empiricism!

chiral molecule will be influenced by other groups in the molecule, these effects are usually considered to be negligible; and in the *principle of pairwise interactions* the optical rotation is taken as the sum of contributions arising from *all* pairwise interactions in the molecule. Of course, in the ideal situation expressed in the *principle of multiwise interactions*, the optical rotation is taken as the sum of the contributions from pairwise interactions, three-way interactions, four-way interactions, etc. This principle has been used (81) to define a parameter called the *linkage rotation* [Λ] for a disaccharide at a given wavelength as

$$[\Lambda] = [M_{NR}] - [M_{MeN}] + [M_R] \tag{10}$$

where [M_{NR}] is the molecular rotation of the disaccharide, [M_{MeN}] is the molecular rotation of the methyl glycoside of the nonreducing residue **N**, and [M_R] is the molecular rotation of the reducing residue **R** after mutarotation. Thus, the value for [Λ] represents the contribution to the molecular rotation from interactions across the glycosidic linkage minus any contributions to [M_{MeN}] and [M_R] from interactions involving the glycosidic methyl group of **N** and the hydrogen atom of **R**. It has been shown that the linkage rotation may be related to the conformational parameters (ϕ, ψ) defined in Section 3.6 by the relationship

$$[\Lambda]_\alpha = -105° - 120° (\sin \Delta\phi + \sin \Delta\psi) \tag{11}$$

for α-linked disaccharides, and by the relationship

$$[\Lambda]_\beta = 105° - 120° (\sin \Delta\phi + \sin \Delta\psi) \tag{12}$$

for β-linked disaccharides, where $\Delta\phi = \phi - 180°$ and $\Delta\psi = \psi - 180°$. Using values for $\Delta\phi$ and $\Delta\psi$ obtained from crystal structure data, it has been possible, for example, to predict (81) to within a few degrees the linkage rotations of methyl β-cellobioside (**30**) and methyl β-lactoside (**31**).

(30)

(31)

In the case of both κ- and ι-carrageenans, where polysaccharide chains are known to associate (*cf.* Section 3.6), changes in optical rotation brought about by changes in the temperature of aqueous solutions of these polysaccharides have been attributed (82, 83) to the formation of double helices. In such circumstances, the dependence of the optical rotation on the contributions from differing proportions of secondary and tertiary structures is being measured.

Finally, one other empirical correlation of optical rotation with configuration should be mentioned here. This is Hudson's *lactone rule* (84), which in its present-day form (85) states that lactones derived from aldonic acids have a positive rotation if the hydroxyl group involved in lactone formation is on the right of the Fischer projection formula of the aldonic acid. Thus, the δ-lactone of D-galactonic acid (32) has a positive rotation, whereas the γ-lactone has a negative rotation.

$$
\begin{array}{c}
\text{COOH} \\
|\\
\text{H—C—OH} \\
|\\
\text{HO—C—H} \\
|\\
\text{HO—C—H} \\
|\\
\text{H—C—OH} \\
|\\
\text{CH}_2\text{OH}
\end{array}
$$

(32)

References

1. (a) E. L. Eliel, *Stereochemistry of Carbon Compounds*, McGraw-Hill, New York, 1962, p. 126; (b) E. L. Eliel, N. L. Allinger, S. J. Angyal, and G.A. Morrison, *Conformational Analysis*, Wiley-Interscience, New York, 1965, p. 129.
2. Ref. 1b, p. 381.
3. L. Hough and A. C. Richardson, in *Rodd's Chemistry of Carbon Compounds*, Vol. 1F, Ch. 23, ed. S. Coffey, Elsevier, Amsterdam, 1967, p. 124.
4. R. J. Ferrier, *Chem. Britain*, p. 15 (1969); in *Progress in Stereochemistry*, Vol. 4, ed. B. J. Aylett and M. M. Harris, Butterworths, London, 1969, p. 43.
5. G. A. Jeffrey and R. D. Rosenstein, Advan. Carbohydrate Chem., **19**, 7 (1964).
6. R. H. Marchessault and A. Sarko, *Advan. Carbohydrate Chem.*, **22**, 421 (1967).
7. M. Sundaralingam, *Biopolymers*, **6**, 189 (1968); **7**, 821 (1969).
8. N. K. Kochetkov and O. S. Chizov, *Advan. Carbohydrate Chem.*, **21**, 39 (1966).
9. H. Spedding, *Advan. Carbohydrate Chem.*, **19**, 23 (1964).
10. L. D. Hall, *Advan. Carbohydrate Chem.*, **19**, 51 (1964).
11. T. D. Inch, in *Annual Review of NMR Spectroscopy*, Vol. 2, ed. E. F. Mooney, Academic, London, 1969, p. 35.

12. See however, K. Heynes and H. Scharmann, *Tetrahedron*, **21**, 507 (1965).

13. J. F. Stoddart, Unpublished results.

14. O. S. Chizov, L. S. Golovkina, and N. S. Wulfson, *Carbohydrate Res.*, **6**, 138, 143 (1968).

15. D. M. Kilburn, M. Sc. Thesis, Queen's University, Kingston, Canada, 1969.

16. N. S. Wulfson, O. S. Chizov, and L. S. Golovkina, *Z. Organ. Zhim.*, **4**, 744 (1968).

17. Ref. 1*b*, p. 394.

18. L. P. Kuhn, *J. Am. Chem. Soc.*, **74**, 2492 (1952); **76**, 4323 (1954).

19. E. L. Eliel, *Accounts Chem. Res.*, **3**, 1 (1970).

20. N. Baggett, M. A. Bukhari, A. B. Foster, J. Lehmann, and J. M. Webber, *J. Chem. Soc.*, p. 4157 (1963).

21. L. Joris, P. von R. Schleyer, and E. Osawa, *Tetrahedron*, **24**, 4759 (1968).

22. R. J. Ferrier, W. G. Overend, G. A. Rafferty, H. M. Wall, and N. R. Williams, *Proc. Chem. Soc.*, p. 133 (1963).

23. R. U. Lemieux, R. K. Kullnig, H. J. Bernstein, and W. G. Schneider, *J. Am. Chem. Soc.*, **80**, 6098 (1958).

24. R. U. Lemieux and J. D. Stevens, *Can. J. Chem.*, **43**, 2059 (1965).

25. R. U. Lemieux and J. D. Stevens, *Can. J. Chem.*, **44**, 249 (1966).

26. L. D. Hall, J. F. Manville, and N. S. Bhacca, *Can. J. Chem.*, **47**, 1 (1969); L. D. Hall and J. F. Manville, *Can. J. Chem.*, **47**, 19 (1969).

27. H. Booth, *Tetrahedron*, **22**, 615 (1966).

28. S. J. Angyal, V. A. Pickles, and R. Ahluwahlia, *Carbohydrate Res.*, **1**, 365 (1966).

29. N. Baggett, K. W. Buck, A. B. Foster, M. H. Randall, and J. M. Webber, *J. Chem. Soc.*, p. 3394 (1965).

30. E. L. Eliel and W. E. Willy, *Tetrahedron Letters*, p. 1775 (1969); W. E. Willy, G. Binsch, and E. L. Eliel, *J. Am. Chem. Soc.*, **92**, 5394 (1970).

31. M. Rudrum and D. F. Shaw, *J. Chem. Soc.*, p. 52 (1965).

32. S. J. Angyal, *Aust. J. Chem.*, **21**, 2737 (1968); *Angew. Chem. Intern. Ed.*, **8**, 157 (1969).

33. H. J. Fletcher, Jr., and J. D. Stevens, *J. Org. Chem.*, **33**, 1799 (1968).

34. A. S. Perlin and B. Casu, *Tetrahedron Letters*, p. 2921 (1969).

35. A. S. Perlin, B. Casu, and H. J. Koch, *Can. J. Chem.*, **48**, 2596 (1970).

36. D. E. Dorman and J. D. Roberts, *J. Am. Chem. Soc.*, **92**, 1355 (1970).

37. L. D. Hall and L. F. Johnson, *Chem. Comm.*, p. 509 (1969).

38. J. D. Roberts, F. J. Weigert, J. I. Kroschwitz, and H. J. Reich, *J. Am. Chem. Soc.*, **92**, 1338 (1970).

39. A. S. Perlin and H. J. Koch, *Can. J. Chem.*, **48**, 2639 (1970).

40. D. E. Dorman, S. J. Angyal, and J. D. Roberts, *Proc. Natl. Acad. Sci.*, **63**, 612 (1969); *J. Am. Chem. Soc.*, **92**, 1351 (1970).

41. J. A. Pople, W. G. Schneider, and H. J. Bernstein, *High Resolution Nuclear Magnetic Resonance*, McGraw-Hill, New York, 1959, p. 183.

42. B. Casu, M. Reggiani, G. G. Gallo, and A. Vigevani, *Tetrahedron*, **22**, 3061 (1966).

43. M. Karplus, *J. Chem. Phys.*, **30**, 11 (1959).

44. K. L. Williamson, *J. Am. Chem. Soc.*, **85**, 516 (1963).

45. D. H. Williams and N. S. Bhacca, *J. Am. Chem. Soc.*, **86**, 2742 (1964).

46. P. Laszlo and P. von R. Schleyer, *J. Am. Chem. Soc.*, **85**, 2709 (1963).

47. R. U. Lemieux, J. D. Stevens, and R. R. Fraser, *Can. J. Chem.*, **40**, 1955 (1962).

48. S. Sternhell, *Quart. Rev.*, **23**, 236 (1969).

49. H. Booth, *Tetrahedron Letters*, p. 411 (1965).

50. M. Karplus, *J. Am. Chem. Soc.*, **85**, 2870 (1963).

51. B. Coxon, *Tetrahedron*, **22**, 2281 (1966).
52. N. S. Bhacca and D. Horton, *J. Am. Chem. Soc.*, **89**, 5993 (1967).
53. P. L. Durette and D. Horton, *Chem. Comm.*, p. 516 (1969).
54. P. L. Durette and D. Horton, *Carbohydrate* Res., **10**, 565 (1969).
55. L. D. Hall and L. Hough, *Proc. Chem. Soc.*, p. 382 (1962).
56. R. U. Lemieux and J. Howard, *Can. J. Chem.*, **41**, 393 (1963).
57. S. Sternhell, *Rev. Pure Appl. Chem.*, **14**, 15 (1964).
58. B. Coxon, *Carbohydrate Res.*, **1**, 357 (1966).
59. N. S. Bhacca, D. Horton, and H. Paulsen, *J. Org. Chem.*, **33**, 2484 (1968).
60. J. Feeney, M. Anteunis, and G. Swaelens, *Bull. Soc. Chim. Belges*, **77**, 121 (1968).
61. A. Rassat, C. W. Jefford, J. M. Lehn, and B. Waegell, *Tetrahedron Letters*, p. 233 (1964).
62. L. D. Hall and J. F. Manville, *Carbohydrate Res.*, **8**, 295 (1968).
63. J. I. Musher and E. J. Corey, *Tetrahedron*, **18**, 791 (1962).
64. J. A. Pople and A. A. Bothner-By, *J. Chem. Phys.*, **42**, 1339 (1965).
65. A. A. Bothner-By, *Advan. Mag. Res.*, **1**, 195 (1965).
66. R. C. Cookson and T. A. Crabb, *Tetrahedron Letters*, p. 679 (1964); *Tetrahedron*, **24**, 2385 (1968).
67. R. C. Cookson, T. A. Crabb, J. J. Frenkel, and J. Hudec, *Tetrahedron Suppl.*, No. 7, p. 355 (1966).
68. R. Cahill, R. C. Cookson, and T. A. Crabb, *Tetrahedron*, **25**, 4681 (1969).
69. E. L. Eliel and F. Nader, *J. Am. Chem. Soc.*, **91**, 536 (1969); **92**, 584 (1970).
70. F. A. L. Anet and A. J. R. Bourn, *J. Am. Chem. Soc.*, **87**, 5250 (1965).
71. A. J. de Hoog, H. R. Buys, C. Altona, and E. Havinga, *Tetrahedron*, **25**, 3365 (1969).
72. C. Romers, C. Altona, H. R. Buys, and E. Havinga, in *Topics in Stereochemistry*, Vol. 4, ed. E. L. Eliel and N. L. Allinger, Wiley-Interscience, New York, 1969, p. 39.
73. D. H. Whiffen, *Chem. Ind.*, p. 964 (1956).
74. J. H. Brewster, *J. Am. Chem. Soc.*, **81**, 5475, 5483 (1959); in *Topics in Stereochemistry*, Vol. 2, ed. E. L. Eliel and N. L. Allinger, Wiley-Interscience, New York, 1967, p. 1.
75. R. U. Lemieux and J. C. Martin, *Carbohydrate Res.*, **13**, 139 (1970).
76. W. Kauzmann, F. B. Clough, and I. Tobias, *Tetrahedron*, **13**, 57 (1961).
77. Ref. 1*b*, p. 381.
78. R. U. Lemieux and A. A. Pavia, *Can. J. Chem.*, **46**, 1453 (1968); **47**, 4441 (1969).
79. C. S. Hudson, *J. Am. Chem. Soc.*, **31**, 66 (1909).
80. W. Kauzmann, *Quantum Chemistry*, Academic, New York, 1957.
81. D. A. Rees, *J. Chem. Soc.*, B, p. 877 (1970).
82. D. A. Rees, I. W. Steele, and F. B. Williamson, *J. Polymer Sci.*, Part C, **28**, 261 (1969).
83. A. A. McKinnon, D. A. Rees, and F. B. Williamson, *Chem. Comm.*, p. 701 (1969).
84. C. S. Hudson, *J. Am. Chem. Soc.*, **32**, 338 (1910).
85. W. Klyne, *Chem. Ind.*, p. 1198 (1954).

Isomerism

5.1 Introduction

Much of the chemistry of carbohydrates is characterized by isomerisms, and many of the important interconversions and reactions of carbohydrates involving isomerisms eventually lead to the establishment of dynamic equilibria. A number of these isomerisms, such as the conformational isomerism between $^4C_1$ and $^1C_4$ conformers of pyranoid derivatives and the configurational isomerism between α- and β-anomers of furanoid and pyranoid derivatives, were discussed in Chapters 3 and 4. However, many of the thermodynamically controlled processes encountered in carbohydrate chemistry display a remarkable stereochemical versatility which can rarely, if ever, be discussed in terms of a dynamic equilibrium between two states. Indeed, conformational, configurational, and constitutional isomerisms may all occur together in the same system. This chapter will be concerned with a discussion of the interplay among these three kinds of isomerism in a few of the important isomerizations exhibited by carbohydrates.

5.2 Lactol Ring Isomerization

When a crystalline aldose or ketose is dissolved in a solvent, isomerizations take place and an equilibrium is eventually established. The anomerization of an aldopyranose or a ketopyranose may occur by a mechanism involving a cyclic intermediate, or it may proceed via an acyclic *aldehydo* or *keto* intermediate. In fact, the mechanism involving an acyclic intermediate, as shown in Figure 5.1 for the anomerization of the D-glucopyranoses, is (1–4) the generally accepted one.[1] However, when a crystalline α-

---

[1] For more detailed mechanistic discussions, see refs. 3 and 4.

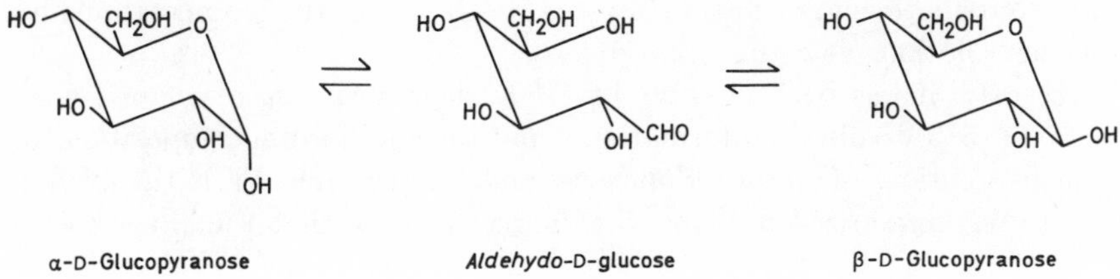

α-D-Glucopyranose   *Aldehydo*-D-glucose   β-D-Glucopyranose

Figure 5.1   The anomerization of the D-glucopyranoses.

pyranose is dissolved in a solvent, it may not only anomerize to the β-pyranose but may also isomerize to the furanose or septanose[2] anomers by virtue of the constitutional isomerisms summarized in Figure 5.2. This

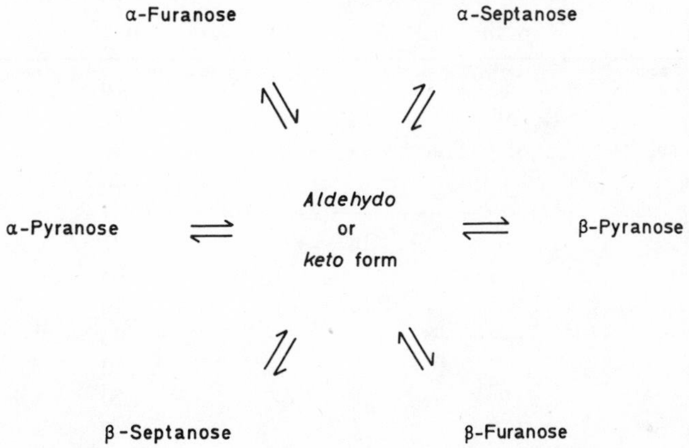

Figure 5.2   Constitutional isomerism among the aldohexoses and the ketoheptoses.

type of constitutional isomerization between different ring sizes of cyclic hemiacetals may be referred to as *lactol ring isomerization*.

When equilibrium has been established in solution by lactol ring isomerization and by anomerization, the proportions of the various constitutional and configurational isomers will be determined by their relative free energies. It will be recalled from Chapter 3 that, for monocyclic aldoses dissolved in water, the populations of the *aldehydo* forms and of septanose anomers at equilibrium are both very small—probably much less than 1%—and are not detectable (5) by ^{1}H nuclear magnetic resonance spectroscopy in deuterium oxide. However, in the case of some aldoses, furanose anomers

---

[2] In the case of the aldopentoses and ketohexoses, the septanose anomers do not come into play.

may contribute significantly (up to 30–40%) to the compositions in aqueous solutions at equilibrium.

Recently, it has been possible by ^{1}H nuclear magnetic resonance spectroscopy (5–9) to obtain information about the equilibrium compositions of aqueous solutions of all the aldohexoses and aldopentoses. From the results, which are summarized in Table 5.1, it may be seen that the aldoses with

Table 5.1   The Compositions of Aqueous Solutions of the Aldohexoses and Aldopentoses at Equilibrium, as Determined by [1]H Nuclear Magnetic Resonance Spectroscopy (5–9)

Aldose	Furanose		Pyranose	
	α, %	β, %	α, %	β, %
D-Allose	5	7	18	70
D-Altrose	20	13	27	40
D-Galactose	←——Trace[a]——→		36	64
D-Glucose	...	...	36	64
D-Gulose[b]	←——————————22——————————→			78
D-Idose	16	16	31	37
D-Mannose	...	...	68	32
D-Talose	20	11	40	29
D-Arabinose	←———3———→		63	34
D-Lyxose	...	...	72	28
D-Ribose	6	18	20	56
D-Xylose	...	...	37	63

[a] See refs. 8 and 9.
[b] The homomorphous D-*glycero*-D-guloheptose contains (5) furanose anomers (2%), α-pyranose (10%), and β-pyranose (88%).

the lowest relative free energies as their pyranoses (see Table 3.9 in Section 3.2.4) contain very small amounts of furanoses. Thus, no furanose anomers have been detected in the ^{1}H nuclear magnetic resonance spectra of glucose, mannose, lyxose, and xylose after equilibration in deuterium oxide. This means that the positions of the pyranose-furanose equilibria shown in Figure 5.3 lie almost completely in favor of the pyranose anomers. Hence, when a crystalline α-pyranose or β-pyranose anomer of one of the aldoses in Figure 5.3 is dissolved in water, anomerization occurs and ultimately an equilibrium is established between the two pyranose anomers. The change in optical rotation which accompanies this anomerization obeys the rate

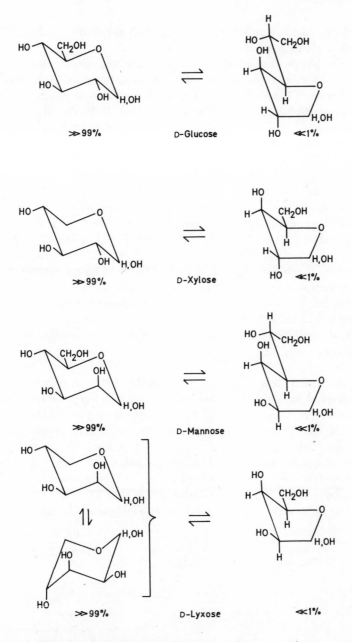

Figure 5.3 The pyranose-furanose equilibria for D-glucose, D-xylose, D-mannose, and D-lyxose. Furanose rings are represented in ^3E or E_3 conformations, although, of course, other conformations are undoubtedly involved.

law for a first-order reversible reaction and is often called (*cf.* refs. 3, 4, and 5) a *simple mutarotation.*

The other aldoses, that is, allose, altrose, galactose, gulose, idose, talose, arabinose, and ribose, for which the pyranose-furanose equilibria are shown in Figure 5.4, all contain sufficient of the furanose anomers (Table 5.1) in aqueous solution at equilibrium for them to be detectable by ^{1}H nuclear magnetic resonance spectroscopy (5-9) in deuterium oxide. These aldoses have high relative free energies as their pyranoses (see Table 3.9 in Section 3.2.4), and freshly prepared aqueous solutions exhibit the phenomenon known as (*cf.* refs. 3, 4, and 5) *complex mutarotation.* This is characterized by an initial fast mutarotation associated with pyranose-furanose isomerization and subsequently by a slow mutarotation which may be attributed to pyranose anomerization. The fast and the slow components need not necessarily be in the same direction, and consequently aqueous solutions of some aldoses, such as ribose, which exhibit complex mutarotation, show reversals in the directions of mutarotation before their optical rotatory powers attain constant values.

Although the relative stabilities of the pyranoses would appear to be the determining factor in deciding the compositions of aqueous solutions of aldoses at equilibrium, it cannot be denied that the relative stabilities of the furanoses may also play a minor role. As yet, it has not been possible to calculate the relative free energies of the various furanoses in Figures 5.3 and 5.4. Nonetheless, a qualitative estimate of their relative stabilities may be derived by assuming that *cis* interactions between neighboring substituents on furanose rings will have a destabilizing influence (5). The number and the nature of the 1,2-*cis* interactions may be classified in terms of the four groups of homomorphous furanoses (see Figure 2.24). If *cis* interactions between O_1 and O_2 are ignored, for they may be relieved by anomerization, the number and nature of the 1,2-*cis* interactions in the homomorphous furanoses are as tabulated in Table 5.2.

From the observation (6) that 3-deoxy-D-*ribo*hexose (**1**) contains 32%

68%   32%

(1)

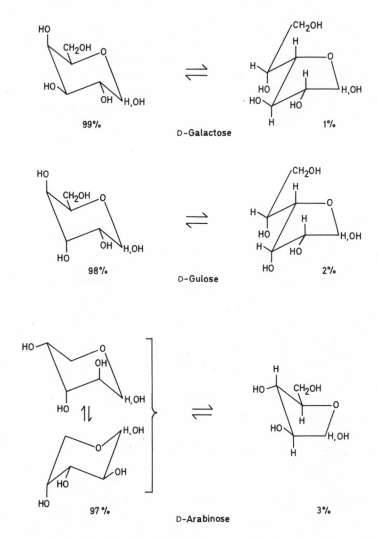

Figure 5.4 The pyranose-furanose equilibria for D-galactose, D-gulose, D-arabinose, D-allose, D-ribose, D-talose, D-idose, and D-altrose. Furanose rings are represented in ^3E or E_3 conformations, although, of course, other conformations are undoubtedly involved.

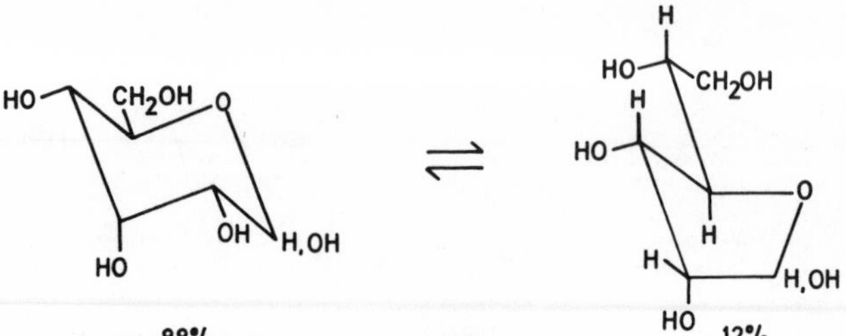

88% D-Allose 12%

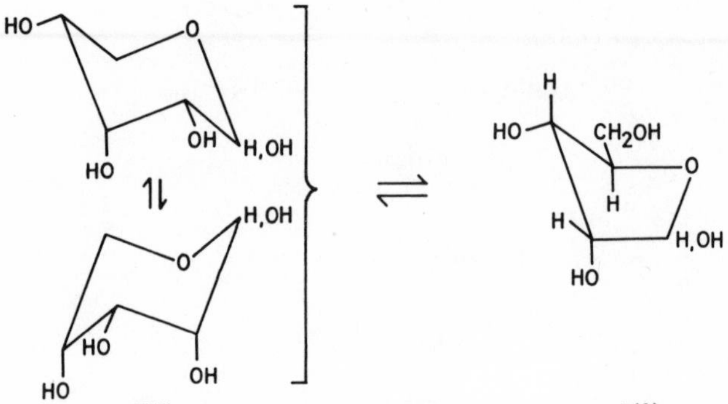

76% D-Ribose 24%

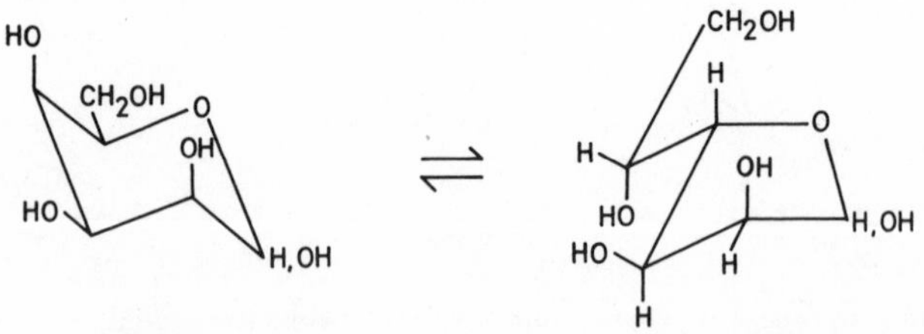

69% D-Talose 31%

Figure 5.4 (continued)

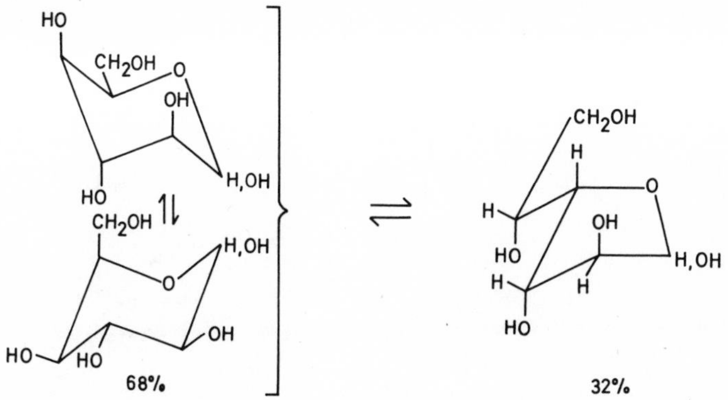

Figure 5.4 (continued)

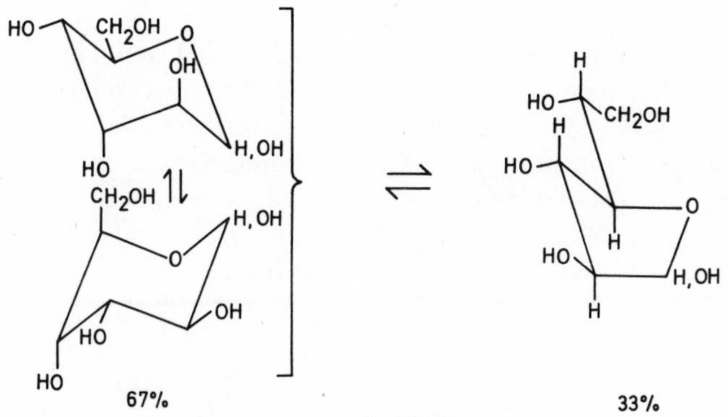

Table 5.2   The Number and the Nature of the 1,2-cis Interactions in the Four Groups of Homomorphous Furanoses

Aldose	Number of 1,2-*cis* Interactions	Nature of 1,2-*cis* Interactions
Gulose Mannose Lyxose	2	O_2/O_3; O_3/C_5
Glucose Idose Xylose	1	O_3/C_5
Allose Talose Ribose	1	O_2/O_3
Altrose Galactose Arabinose	0[a]	. . .

[a] That is, all *trans*.

of furanose anomers at equilibrium in aqueous solution, it would appear that a *cis* interaction between O_3 and C_5 is particularly unfavorable.[3] The *cis* interaction between O_2 and O_3 is probably not so unfavorable, as indicated by the fact (5) that no furanose anomers were detected at equilibrium in the ^1H nuclear magnetic resonance spectrum of 2-deoxy-D-*arabino*hexose (**2**) in deuterium oxide. Hence, of all the aldohexoses and aldopentoses which have an O_3/C_5 *cis* interaction in their furanose rings (i.e., gulose,

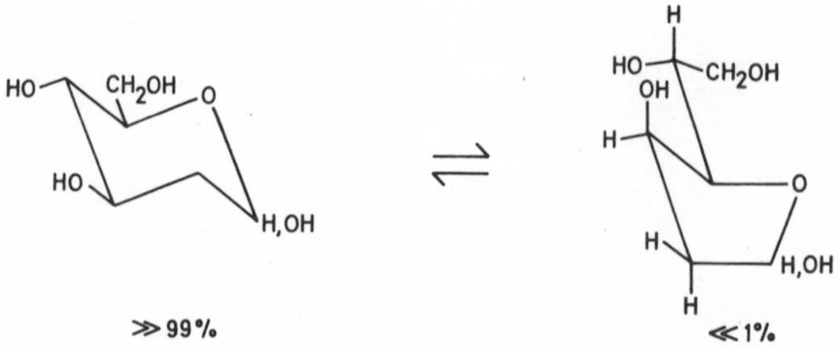

$\gg 99\%$ $\ll 1\%$

(2)

[3] This situation should be compared with that of D-glucose, which does not give rise to any significant proportions of furanose anomers at equilibrium in aqueous solution.

mannose, lyxose, glucose, idose, and xylose), only idose contains appreciable amounts, and gulose small amounts, of furanose anomers. However, the pyranose anomers of idose and gulose are relatively unstable, and this undoubtedly explains the presence of furanose anomers in their aqueous solutions at equilibrium. The pyranose anomers of allose, talose, and ribose are not particularly stable either, and so even with an O_2/O_3 *cis* interaction in their furanose rings, it is not surprising to find appreciable amounts of furanose anomers in their aqueous solutions at equilibrium.

It might be expected that, at equilibrium, aqueous solutions of altrose, galactose, and arabinose, each with an all-*trans* arrangement of neighboring substituents on their furanose rings, would contain large amounts of furanose anomers. Indeed, altrose contains 33% of furanose anomers at equilibrium in aqueous solution, the relative stabilities of the furanose anomers undoubtedly combining with the relative instabilities of the pyranose anomers to give the highest proportion of furanose anomers among all of the aldohexoses and aldopentoses. However, unlike the pyranose anomers of altrose, those of galactose and arabinose are relatively stable, and consequently the proportions of furanose anomers in their aqueous solutions at equilibrium are small, although they are detectable by ^{1}H nuclear magnetic resonance spectroscopy in deuterium oxide.

The positions of pyranose-furanose equilibria can be markedly altered by changes in temperature or in the solvent. When arabinose, galactose, or altrose is dissolved in dimethyl sulfoxide (9, 10), dimethylformamide (11), or pyridine (12, 13), substantial proportions of furanose anomers are found to be present at equilibrium. Thus, it has been shown (9) by ^{1}H nuclear magnetic resonance spectroscopy in dimethyl sulfoxide-d_6 that an arabinose solution contains 33% (*cf.* 3% in water), a galactose solution 15% (*cf.* a trace in water), and an altrose solution 44% (*cf.* 33% in water) of furanose anomers at equilibrium. These changes can be explained if it is assumed (*cf.* ref. 14) that solvents (S) such as dimethyl sulfoxide, which are excellent proton acceptors, cause polarizations of O-H bonds in a manner (R—O←H←S) that increases the negative charges on the oxygen atoms involved in hydrogen bonding with the solvent. Thus, through increased coulombic repulsions between lone pairs associated with oxygen atoms in 1,2-*gauche* relationships on the pyranose rings, a proton-accepting solvent has the effect of destabilizing the pyranose anomers. In contrast, the corresponding furanose anomers with oxygen atoms in mainly 1,2-*trans* relationships, are not destabilized to any great extent. Although water is also an excellent proton-accepting solvent, it is possible that repulsions between lone pairs on oxygen atoms are not as great as in dimethyl sulfoxide, because of the fact that water, unlike dimethyl sulfoxide, may also donate protons to oxygen atoms to form hydrogen bonds. Moreover, when water solvates a sugar molecule, the structure of the water suffers very little disorientation when, and *only* when, a pyranose chair conformer occurs (9, 10, 15). Hence, water tends to stabilize pyranose anomers in a manner that is not possible for dimethyl sulfoxide. That, for a particular sugar, the proportion of furanose anomers in dimethylform-amide is also greater than that in water is shown (11, 16) by the results of methylations carried out in dimethylformamide as solvent. For example, when 3-*O*-β-L-arabinopyranosyl-L-arabinose (**3**) is methylated with methyl

(3)

iodide and silver oxide in dimethylformamide,the products obtained after hydrolysis of the *O*-methyl derivative include (16) appreciable amounts of 2,5-di-*O*-methyl-L-arabinose, indicating[4] that the reducing arabinose residue exists partially as its furanose anomers at equilibrium in dimethyl-formamide. It has also been shown (12) that trimethylsilylation of galac-tose, previously equilibrated in refluxing dry pyridine, with hexamethyl-disilazane and trimethylchlorosilane yields appreciable amounts of fur-

---

[4] Such conclusions are justified only if the rate of mixing of the reactants, and the rate of product formation, are both very fast compared with the rates of lactol ring isomeriza-tion. If this qualification does not hold, the Curtin-Hammett principle (17, 18) will begin to operate and, in the limit where the principle is obeyed, the ratio of the products will be characteristic of the relative free energy levels of the transition states and in-dependent of the relative free energy levels of the pyranose and furanose anomers. In actuality, the reaction rates for methylation and trimethylsilylation are probably both much faster than the rates of lactol ring isomerization, and so, to a first approximation, product ratios may be assumed to reflect the pyranose/furanose ratios in the reaction solvents at equilibrium.

anoid derivatives, indicating[4] that galactose exists to some extent as its furanose anomers at equilibrium in pyridine.[5]

The introduction of substituents may also have a profound effect on the pyranose/furanose ratio. As shown in Table 5.3, the 2,3-dimethyl ethers of

Table 5.3   The Pyranose/Furanose Ratios, Expressed as Percentage Furanose Forms for D-*Arabinose,* D-*Galactose, and* D-*Altrose, and Their 2,3-Di-O-Methyl Derivatives in Deuterium Oxide and in Dimethyl Sulfoxide-d₆ (9)*

Aldose	Deuterium Oxide	Dimethyl Sulfoxide-d_6
D-Arabinose	3	33
2,3-Di-O-methyl-D-arabinose	17	65
D-Galactose	Trace	*ca.* 15
2,3-Di-O-methyl-D-galactose	10	38
D-Altrose	33	44
2,3-Di-O-methyl-D-altrose	45	*ca.* 80

arabinose, galactose, and altrose show (9) an even greater tendency than the unsubstituted sugars to isomerize to the furanose anomers in both water and dimethyl sulfoxide. There is little doubt that the electron-rich oxygen atoms associated with the methyl ether groupings of the dimethyl ethers will experience larger repulsive interactions (*cf.* ref. 14) than those associated with the oxygen atoms of hydroxyl groups on the unsubstituted sugars. These stronger repulsive interactions will increase the magnitude of the 1,2-*gauche* interactions on the pyranose rings, and consequently the pyranose anomers of the 2,3-dimethyl ethers will be destabilized relative to the pyranose anomers of the unsubstituted sugars. This argument provides a possible explanation for the differences in composition of the 2,3-dimethyl ethers and the unsubstituted sugars in dimethyl sulfoxide. In water, the tendency to form furanose anomers is not so great, and this probably finds some explanation, at least, in the ability of water to stabilize (9, 10, 15) pyranose anomers preferentially.

Furanose anomers are often stabilized (19–23) when other rings are fused to aldoses. Thus, 6-deoxy-2,3-O-isopropylidene-L-mannose (**4**) has

[5] Very recently, it has been demonstrated [S. J. Angyal and K. D. Davies, Private Communication] by ^{1}H nuclear magnetic resonance spectroscopy that pyranoses with the axial-equatorial-axial sequence of hydroxyl groups, and furanoses with three *cis* hydroxyl group, form complexes with metal ions in aqueous solutions which are strong enough to affect the positions of configurational and conformational equilibria.

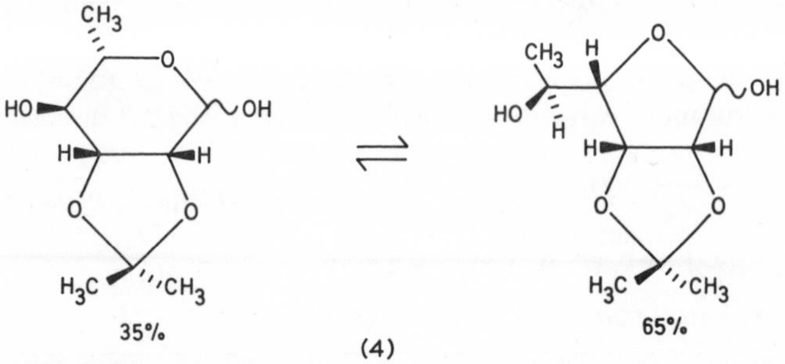

(4)

been shown (20, 23) to contain 65% of furanose anomers at equilibrium in aqueous solution. In the case of D-mannose 2,3-carbonate (**5**) (10, 20)

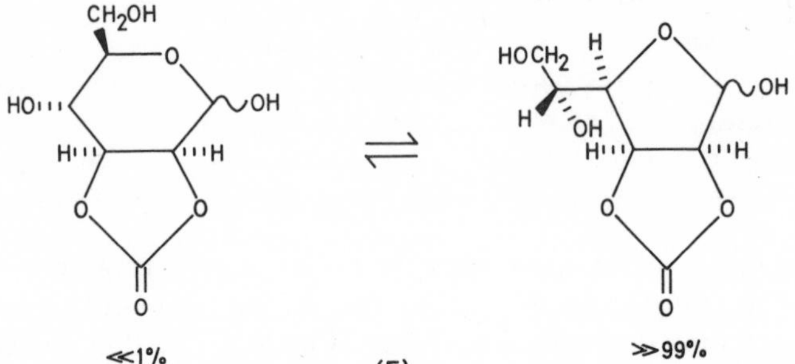

(5)

and 3,6-anhydro-D-glucose (**6**) (5), the equilibria are displaced, albeit entirely in favor of the furanose anomers. These observations indicate that in the *cis*-fused forms of the dioxabicyclooctane ring systems, the [3.3.0] system is more stable (*cf.* ref. 24) than either the [4.3.0] system (see **4** or **5**) or the [3.2.1] system (see **6**). However, *cis*-fused [3.3.0] ring systems are not

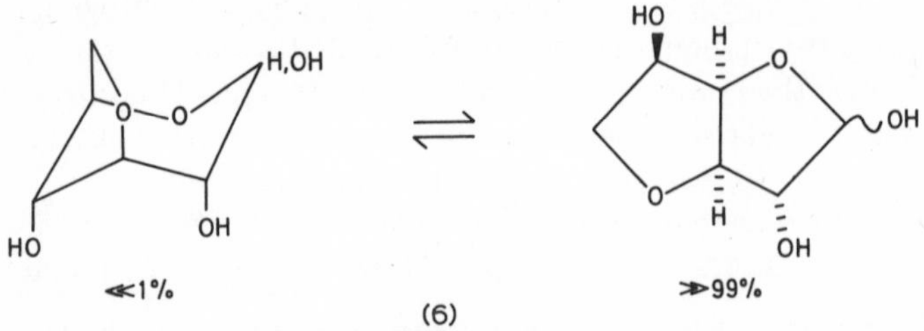

(6)

possible in all situations. Thus, 3,6-anhydro-2-deoxy-D-galactose (**7**) (25) may exist to some extent in aqueous solution at equilibrium in the *aldehydo*

(7)

form,[6] since the *trans*-fused [3.3.0] ring system derived from **7** for the potential furanose anomers is sterically impossible.

5.3   Glycoside Ring Isomerization

In the presence of an acid catalyst, aldoses and ketoses will react (see Section 2.10) with alcohols to form glycosides. Although, initially, aldohexoses and aldopentoses form furanosides preferentially under kinetic control, at equilibrium the thermodynamically more stable pyranosides predominate. Under conditions which permit equilibrium control, the proportions of α- to β-pyranosides are determined by their relative free energies. The percentages of methyl α-pyranosides formed by some of the aldohexoses and aldopentoses which contain only trace amounts of furanosides in acidic methanol at equilibrium (27, 28) are listed in Table 5.4, together with the percentages of the corresponding α-pyranoses present in aqueous solution at equilibrium.

From a comparison of these values, it is evident immediately that the equilibria in the case of the pyranosides have been shifted in favor of the α-anomers. It may be predicted from the conclusions drawn in Section 3.2.2 that the greater preference for the α-pyranosides is chiefly a result of the anomeric effect of a methoxyl group being somewhat larger than that of a hydroxyl group in water. Interaction energies of 0.45 and 0.35 kcal

---

[6] This anhydro sugar gives a positive Schiff test, that is, it restores a pink coloration to an aqueous solution of rosaniline hydrochloride saturated with sulfur dioxide, indicating that it has the properties of an aldehyde. This does not necessarily mean that the *aldehydo* form is present in high concentration at equilibrium; the Curtin-Hammett principle may be operating. For example, 3,6-anhydro-D-glucose gives a positive Schiff test (26), but shows (5) only signals for the furanose anomers in its ¹H nuclear magnetic resonance spectrum, that is, the concentration of the *aldehydo* form is too low to be detected by ¹H nuclear magnetic resonance spectroscopy.

mole^{-1} have been used for $(O_a:H_a)$ and $(O_1:O_2)$, respectively (see Table 3.1 in Section 3.2.2), to calculate approximate values[7] for $(O:OCH_3)$, which are recorded in Table 5.4. The relatively large anomeric effect associated

Table 5.4   A Comparison of the Anomeric Effect of a Hydroxyl Group in Water (O:OH) and a Methoxyl Group in Methanol (O:CH$_3$)

Pyranose or Pyranoside	α, %	(O:OH), kcal mole^{-1}	(O:OCH$_3$), kcal mole^{-1}
D-Glucopyranose	36[a]	0.55	. . .
Methyl D-glucopyranoside	67[b]	. . .	1.31
D-Xylopyranose	37[a]	0.55	. . .
Methyl D-xylopyranoside	69[b]	. . .	1.37
D-Mannopyranose	68[a]	1.00	. . .
Methyl D-mannopyranoside	94[b]	. . .	2.15

[a] See Table 3.9 in Section 3.2.4.
[b] Values from refs. 27 and 28, expressed as a percentage of the pyranosides, and not as a percentage of all glycosides.

with the methyl D-mannopyranosides no doubt has the same explanation as that discussed in Section 3.2.2 for the relatively large anomeric effect associated with the D-mannopyranoses. The following rules may be applied when assessing the magnitude of the anomeric effect of a methoxyl group in methanol:

1. When the anomeric methoxyl group and the C_2 hydroxyl (or methoxyl) group are both equatorial, the conformer is destabilized by 1.4 kcal mole^{-1}.

2. When the anomeric methoxyl group is equatorial and the C_2 hydroxyl (or methoxyl) group is axial, the conformer is destabilized by 2.2 kcal mole^{-1}.

It is significant that in ether or chloroform solutions in the presence of traces of acid, methyl 3,6-anhydro-2,4-di-*O*-methyl-α-D-galactopyranoside (8) undergoes anomerization (29) almost entirely to the β-anomer (9). Although the suggestion (30) that the β-anomer (9) assumes a $B_{1,4}$ con-

[7] These values are only approximate, since the interaction energies used for $(O_a:H_a)$ and $(O_1:O_2)$ were determined in aqueous solution and may not apply directly in methanol.

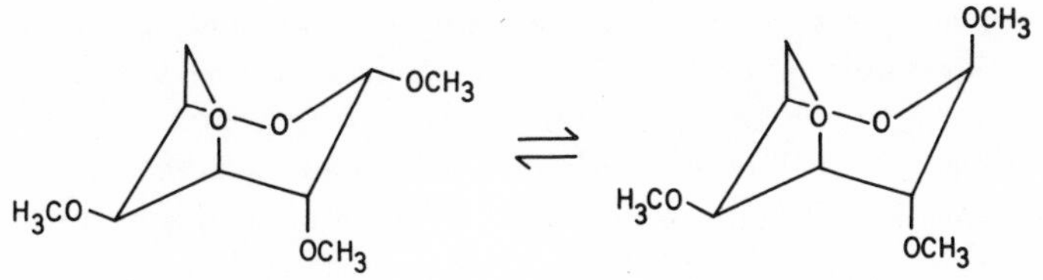

(8)   (9)

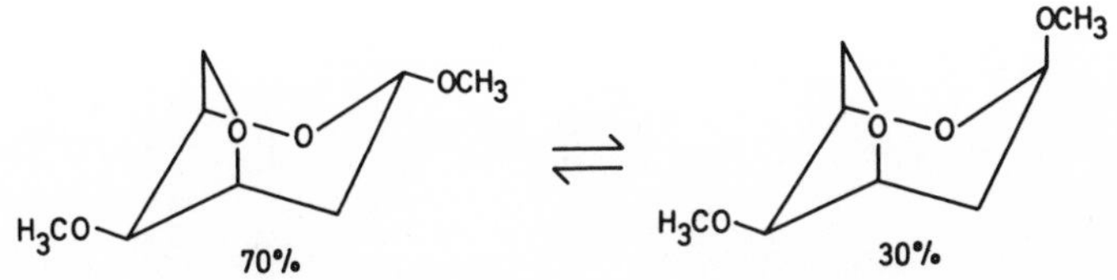

70%   30%

(10)   (11)

formation as shown in Figure 5.5 seems to have gained some acceptance (31, 32), a boat conformation would appear to be improbable (*cf.* ref. 33) since it would be about 6 kcal mole^{-1} less stable than its chair conformer (9) on steric grounds, in addition to having to accommodate a strongly destabilizing anomeric effect. The $^1C_4$ conformer of the α-anomer (8) is also destabilized by a large anomeric effect (2.2 kcal mole^{-1}). However, it may be relieved by anomerization to the β-anomer (9), which probably exists as its $^1C_4$ conformer, albeit slightly distorted by the 3,6-anhydro ring. Such a

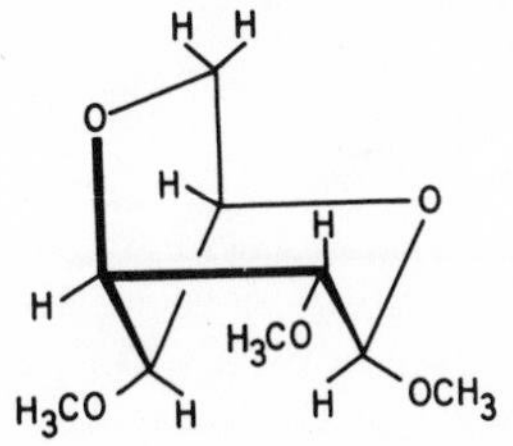

Figure 5.5   The $B_{1,4}$ conformation of the pyranoid ring of methyl 3,6-anhydro-2,4-di-*O*-methyl-β-D-galactopyranoside (9).

distortion probably reduces the magnitude of the steric interaction between the axial methoxyl group on the anomeric carbon atom and the anhydro bridge.

It is noteworthy that, in contrast with the situation in methyl 3,6-anhydro-2,4-di-*O*-methyl-D-galactopyranoside, the α-anomer (10) of the 2-deoxy derivative predominates over the β-anomer (11) when it is equili-

brated in acidic ether solution. Presumably the explanation for this observation is the smaller anomeric effect destabilizing the α-anomer (**10**) when
there is no axial methoxyl group on C_2. This point is amplified by the following observations. The proportions of the anomeric glycosides of methyl
3,6-anhydro-2,4-di-*O*-methyl-D-glucopyranoside at equilibrium in acidic
ether solution may be deduced (25) from specific rotation data (26) to be
32% of the α-anomer (**12**) and 68% of the β-anomer (**13**). In the 2-deoxy de-

rivative, the equilibrium mixture contains (25) 55% of the α-anomer (**14**)
and 45% of the β-anomer (**15**). If it is assumed that the magnitudes of
the steric interactions associated with the anhydro bridges are the same in
both **13** and **15**, the anomeric effect of the methoxyl group in **14** must be
smaller than that in **12** to account for the higher proportion of **14** at equilibrium,[8] that is, the anomeric effect is smaller when there is no axial methoxyl group on C_2.

The compositions of some methyl glycoside mixtures have been determined (27, 28) after equilibration in 1% methanolic hydrogen chloride at
35°; the results are recorded in Table 5.5. It is evident that, compared with
the behavior of the aldopyranoses in aqueous solutions, the stronger
anomeric effect associated with a methoxyl group causes an increase in the
proportion of the anomer with an axial methoxyl group on the more stable
conformer of a methyl pyranoside. Thus, as already pointed out in this

---

[8] Differences of a similar nature were noted in Section 3.2.2 for the hexoses and the 2-
deoxyhexoses in water.

Table 5.5   Methyl Glycoside Compositions at Equilibrium[a]
(27, 28)

Aldose	Furanoside		Pyranoside	
	α, %	β, %	α, %	β, %
D-Galactose	6.2	16.3	57.8	19.7
D-Glucose	0.6	0.9	65.8	32.7
D-Mannose	0.7	0.0	93.9	5.4
D-Arabinose	21.5	6.8	24.5	47.2
2-*O*-Methyl-D-arabinose	←——66.7——→		←——33.3——→	
3-*O*-Methyl-D-arabinose	←——50.7——→		←——49.3——→	
2,3-Di-*O*-methyl-D-arabinose	←——75.4——→		←——24.6——→	
D-Lyxose	1.4	0.0	88.3	10.3
D-Ribose	5.2	17.4	11.6	65.8
D-Xylose	1.9	3.2	65.1	29.8
2-*O*-Methyl-D-xylose	←——12.8——→		←——87.2——→	
3-*O*-Methyl-D-xylose	←—— 9.0——→		←——91.0——→	
2,3-Di-*O*-methyl-D-xylose	←——16.4——→		←——83.6——→	

[a] For aldoses (2%) equilibrated in 1% methanolic hydrogen chloride at 35°.

section, there is an increase in the proportions of the α-anomers in methyl-pyranosides with the *galacto, gluco, manno, lyxo,* and *xylo* configurations which exist as $^4C_1$ (D) conformers, and in the proportion of the β-anomer of methyl arabinopyranoside which exists as the $^1C_4$ (D) conformer. Since both anomers of ribopyranose are conformationally mobile in aqueous solution, the change in the anomeric ratio on conversion into its methyl pyranosides in methanol is not so pronounced (5).

When it is recalled from Section 5.2 that aqueous solutions of galactose and arabinose contain only very small amounts of furanose anomers at equilibrium, the fact that these two aldoses form significant proportions of methyl furanosides, that is, they exhibit *glycoside ring isomerization,* is noteworthy. The propensity for methyl furanoside formation is strikingly reminiscent of the greater tendency for the 2,3-dimethyl ethers of galactose and arabinose, than for the unsubstituted sugars, to isomerize to their furanose anomers. Undoubtedly, methyl pyranosides are destabilized relative to their isomeric methyl furanosides because of increases in the magnitudes of the 1,2-*gauche* interactions associated with the anomeric methoxyl groups on the pyranoid rings. Destabilization of the pyranoid rings by strong 1,2-*gauche* interactions between methoxyl groups would also account for the large amounts of methyl furanosides formed by the mono- and di-methyl ethers of arabinose and xylose (Table 5.5). It is also significant that the percentages of methyl furanosides are much greater in the case of the arabinofuranosides than in the xylofuranosides. However, it may be recalled from Table 5.2 that furanoid derivatives with the *arabino* con-figuration may adopt an all-*trans* arrangement between neighboring sub-stituents, whereas those with the *xylo* configuration must accommodate a destabilizing O_3/C_5 *cis* interaction. Finally, it should be noted that among the methyl pentofuranosides, as would be predicted, the more stable anomer is the one with a *trans* disposition of substituents on C_1 and C_2, that is, the α-anomers in the case of the *arabino* and *lyxo* configurations, and the β-anomers in the *ribo* and *xylo* configurations.

Furanosides are also stabilized by *cis* fusion of five-membered rings in [3.3.0] systems. Thus, one of the major products obtained (34) on reaction of a mixture of methyl D-ribopyranosides with acetone and an acid catalyst is a mixture of methyl 2,3-*O*-isopropylidene-D-ribofuranosides, as shown in Figure 5.6. The reaction presumably proceeds via the methyl 2,3-*O*-

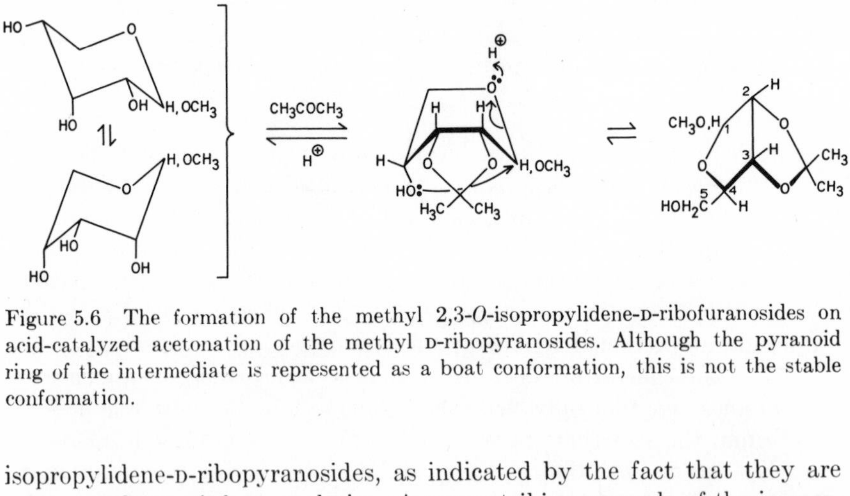

Figure 5.6   The formation of the methyl 2,3-*O*-isopropylidene-D-ribofuranosides on acid-catalyzed acetonation of the methyl D-ribopyranosides. Although the pyranoid ring of the intermediate is represented as a boat conformation, this is not the stable conformation.

isopropylidene-D-ribopyranosides, as indicated by the fact that they are minor products of the acetalation. A more striking example of the isomer-ization of pyranosides to furanosides with *cis*-fused [3.3.0] systems is given in Figure 5.7. Both anomers of methyl 3,6-anhydro-D-glucopyrano-side isomerize (26) in ether solution in the presence of trace amounts of acid to the corresponding furanosides with retention of the anomeric configurations.[9] When *cis*-fused [3.3.0] ring systems are excluded as possi-

[9] Kinetic control probably operates during glycoside ring isomerization to ensure retention of configuration. It is possible that both anomers exist at equilibrium and that this state was not attained in the experiments described in ref. 26.

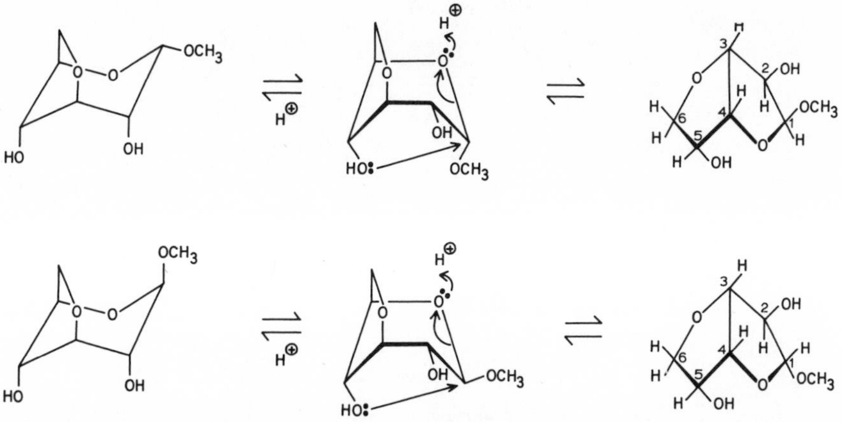

Figure 5.7   Acid-catalyzed isomerization of the α- and β-anomers of methyl 3,6-anhydro-D-glucopyranoside to the corresponding α and β-anomers of the furanosides. Although the pyranoid rings of the intermediates are represented as boat conformations, this is not the stable conformation.

bilities, dimethyl acetals are often found (25, 26) to be more stable than methyl pyranosides. Thus, 3,6-anhydro-D-galactose forms (29) a dimethyl acetal (**16**) on refluxing with methanolic hydrogen chloride.

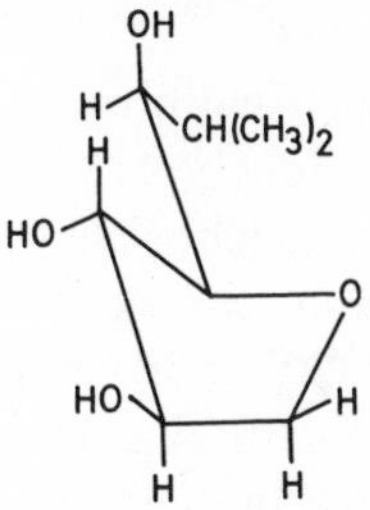

(16)

5.4   Lactone Ring Formation

In aqueous solution, γ-hydroxybutyric acid (**17**) and δ-hydroxyvaleric acid (**19**) exist (*cf.* ref. 31) in equilibrium with their respective lactones, namely, γ-butyrolactone (**18**) and δ-valerolactone (**20**). As is shown in Figure 5.8, the position of the equilibrium (acid $\rightleftharpoons$ lactone + water) at 25° favors the γ-lactone appreciably more than the δ-lactone. It is a well-established fact (35) that a sp^2 hybridized carbon atom is incorporated

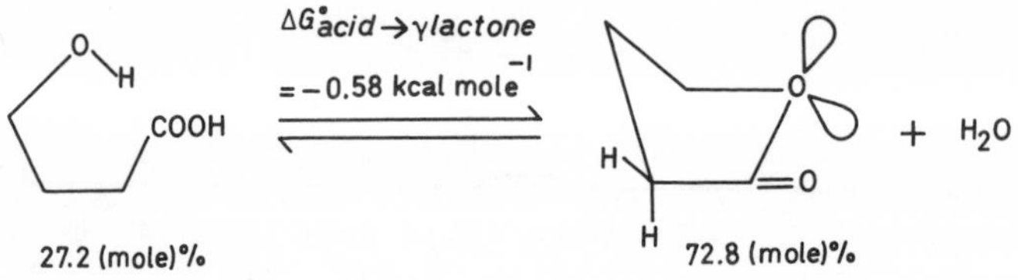

(17)   (18)

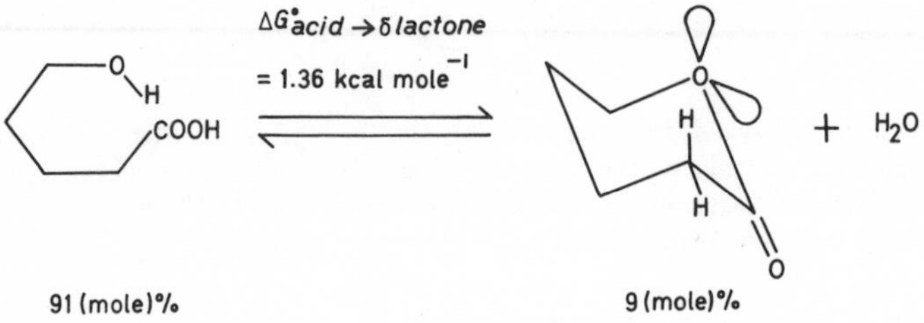

(19)   (20)

Figure 5.8   The lactonization of γ-hydroxybutyric acid (17) and δ-hydroxyvaleric acid (19) at 25°.

into a five-membered ring much more readily than into a six-membered ring. In the case of γ-butyrolactone[10] (18), the carbonyl group is approximately staggered between the neighboring C-H bonds and between the neighboring lone pair orbitals on the oxygen atom, whereas in the chair conformer of δ-valerolactone (20) it is eclipsed with a neighboring C-H bond and with one of the neighboring lone pair orbitals. Accordingly, δ-lactones should be destabilized by both steric and electronic interactions relative to γ-lactones, and so it is not surprising that lactonization occurs more readily for γ-hydroxybutyric acid (17) than for δ-hydroxyvaleric acid (19). The difference of about 2 kcal mole^{-1} between $\Delta G^{\circ}_{\text{acid} \to \gamma-\text{lactone}}$ and $\Delta G^{\circ}_{\text{acid} \to \delta-\text{lactone}}$ in Figure 5.8 may be considered as an estimate of the relative stabilities of γ-butyrolactone (18) and δ-valerolactone (20).

In view of this situation it is not surprising to find that aldonic acids

[10] Although γ-butyrolactone (18) is shown to be in one particular envelope conformation in Figure 5.8, it must be considered to be undergoing pseudorotation in the liquid state.

usually form γ-lactones much more readily than they form δ-lactones. However, in the lactonization of aldonic acids, differences in nonbonded interactions in the acyclic acids and in their lactones will also affect the positions of equilibria. This is illustrated in Figure 5.9 with some partially methylated aldonic acids, for which the degrees of δ-lactonization have been determined (36) at 18°.[11] In the case of *O*-methyl derivatives with the *arabino, galacto,* and *manno* configurations, the acyclic aldonic acids have *no syn*-axial interactions in their planar zigzag conformers and so must be relatively stable.[12] Figure 5.9 shows that in fact the acyclic aldonic acids predominate considerably over their δ-lactones at equilibrium. Of these three δ-lactones, the comparatively higher proportion of 2,3,4,6-tetra-*O*-methyl-D-mannonolactone is probably a result of its having an axial C_2 methoxyl group, thus allowing the eclipsing interaction of the C_2-O bond with the carbonyl group experienced in the other two lactones to be relieved (*cf.* ref. 39 and also the relatively lower proportion of the C_2 epimeric 2,3,4, 6-tetra-*O*-methyl-D-gluconolactone in equilibrium with its hydroxy acid). The *O*-methyl derivatives of the acyclic aldonic acids with the *xylo* and *gluco* configurations have *one syn*-axial interaction in their planar zigzag conformers, whereas the chair conformers of their δ-lactones carry only equatorial substituents. It might be predicted that the δ-lactones will not be too unfavorable, and this is indeed the case (Figure 5.9), especially with 2,3,4-tri-*O*-methyl-D-xylonolactone.

The degrees of γ-lactonization of the corresponding partially methylated aldonic acids have also been determined (36) at 18°. Figure 5.10 shows that

[11] Although the δ-lactones in Figure 5.9 have been drawn as chair conformers, their actual conformers are probably somewhat distorted in order to relieve the eclipsing interaction of the carbonyl group with the equatorial bond on C_2. Indeed, it has been shown recently (37) by X-ray crystallography that the conformation of 1,5-D-glucono-lactone is a distorted chair (**A**)—not a half-chair, as claimed by the authors—in the solid state.

(A)

[12] The relative instability of 2,3,4-tri-*O*-methyl-L-arabinonolactone is well illustrated by its facile conversion in an atmosphere of hydrogen chloride to a cyclic polyester (38), wherein the proposed macrocyclic ring contains ten 2,3,4-tri-*O*-methyl-L-arabinonic acid residues esterified head-to-tail.

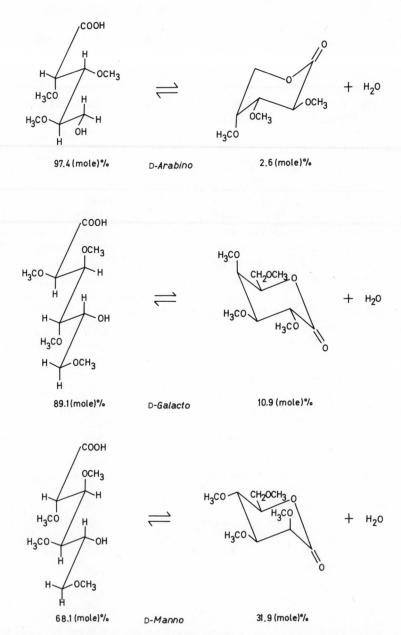

Figure 5.9 The degrees of δ-lactonization at 18° of the partially methylated aldonic acids with the D-*arabino*, D-*galacto*, D-*manno*, D-*xylo*, and D-*gluco* configurations.

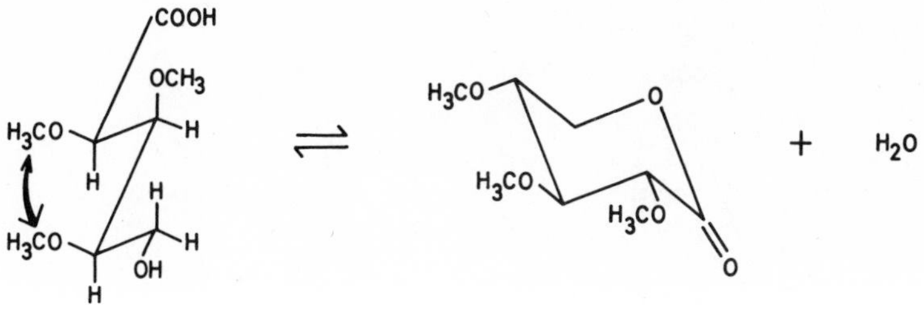

53.3 (mole)%.   46.7 (mole)%.

D-*Xylo*

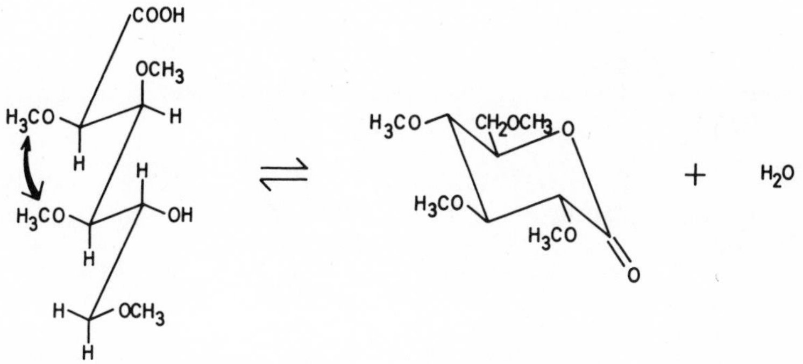

78.4 (mole)%.   21.6 (mole)%.

D-*Gluco*

Figure 5.9 (continued)

in the case of the γ-lactones[13] the extents of lactonization are greater than for the corresponding δ-lactones. If it is assumed that the free energy change on formation of γ- and δ-lactones from 4-hydroxy and 5-hydroxy aldonic acids with identical configurations is the same,[14] then the differences between the free energy changes on lactonization, that is, $\Delta(\Delta G^\circ)_{\gamma \to \delta}$, indicate the relative stabilities of the γ- and δ-lactones. From Table 5.6 it

[13] Envelope conformations have been selected for diagrammatic representation of the γ-lactones in Figure 5.10, although it is recognized that they are almost certainly undergoing pseudorotation in aqueous solution. However, there is some precedent for γ-lactones assuming envelope conformations in the solid state. Thus, 1,4-D-galactonolactone has been shown (40) by crystal structure analysis to exist in the E_3 conformation.
[14] In the formation of lactones from substituted cis-3-hydroxycyclohexanecarboxylic acids, this assumption has been justified (41).

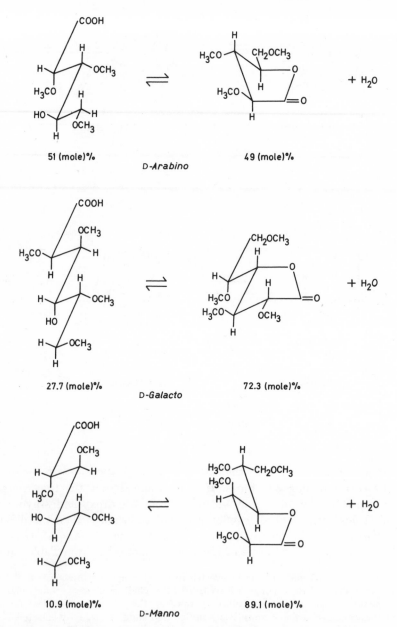

Figure 5.10   The degrees of γ-lactonization at 18° of the partially methylated aldonic acids with the D-*arabino*, D-*galacto*, D-*manno*, D-*xylo*, and D-*gluco* configurations.

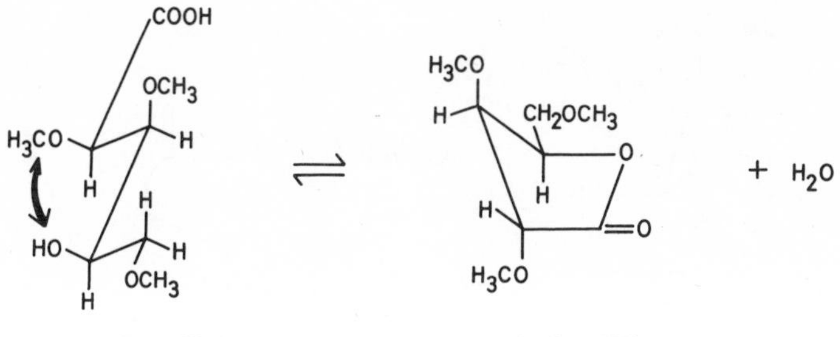

61.5 (mole)%   D-*Xylo*   38.5 (mole)%

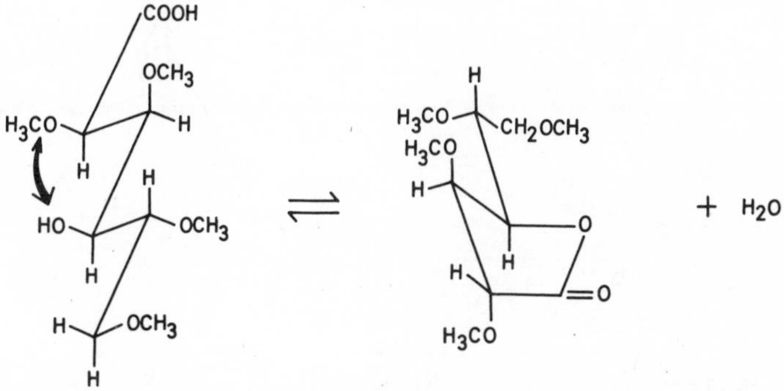

75.7 (mole)%   D-*Gluco*   24.3 (mole)%

Figure 5.10 (continued)

is evident that, apart from the lactones with the *xylo* configuration, the γ-lactones are more stable than their configurationally related δ-lactones.

Table 5.6   The Difference between the Free Energies of Lactonization, $\Delta(\Delta G^\circ)_{\gamma \to \delta}$ *(kcal mole*$^{-1}$*), of Some γ-Lactones and δ-Lactones*

Lactone	$\Delta G^\circ_{\text{acid} \to \gamma\text{-lactone}}$	$\Delta G^\circ_{\text{acid} \to \delta\text{-lactone}}$	$\Delta(\Delta G^\circ)_{\gamma \to \delta}$
Tri-*O*-methylarabinono-	0.02	3.41	3.39
Tetra-*O*-methylgalactono-	−0.55	1.23	1.78
Tetra-*O*-methylmannono-	−1.21	0.44	1.65
Tetra-*O*-methylglucono-	0.65	0.74	0.09
Tri-*O*-methylxylono-	0.27	0.08	−0.19

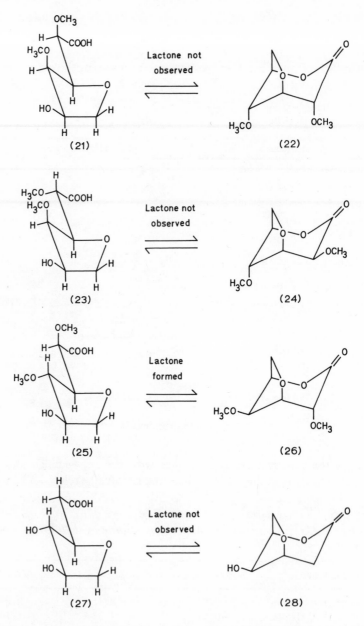

Figure 5.11 The attempted δ-lactonization of some 3,6-anhydro-2,4-di-O-methyl-D-hexonic acids and a 2-deoxy derivative.

It is significant that attempts to lactonize the 3,6-anhydro-2,4-di-*O*-methyl-D-hexonic acids with the *gluco* (**21**) (26), *manno* (**23**) (25), and *galacto* (**25**) (29) configurations shown in Figure 5.11 have not met with much success. Only in the case of 3,6-anhydro-2,4-di-*O*-methyl-D-galactonic acid (**25**) was any lactonization achieved (29), and this occurred only under the forcing conditions of heating the acid above its melting point and distilling. In the derivatives with the *gluco* (**21**) and *manno* (**23**) configurations, the lactones would experience unfavorable interactions, namely, a *syn*-axial interaction between methoxyl groups on C_2 and C_4 in D-glucono-lactone (**22**), and an unfavorable steric and electronic interaction between the C_2-O bond and the carbonyl group, in addition to an axial methoxyl group on C_4, in D-mannonolactone (**24**). Finally, it should be noted that, although 3,6-anhydro-2,4-di-*O*-methyl-D-galactonic acid (**25**) forms a lactone (**26**), 3,6-anhydro-2-deoxy-D-galactonic acid (**27**) does not lactonize to the 2-deoxy lactone (**28**). At first sight this seems somewhat surprising. It would appear to suggest that the axial methoxyl group on C_2 of D-galactonlactone (**26**) exerts a stabilizing influence, perhaps as a result of attractive electronic interactions involving the carbonyl group. However, it must be conceded that this suggestion is based on a minimum of experimental evidence and that 3,6-anhydro-2-deoxy-D-galactonic acid (**27**) may simply have undergone degradation before it had the opportunity to lactonize.

It is noteworthy that some of the uronic acids also exist in aqueous solution in equilibrium with their γ-lactones in which two five-membered rings are *cis*-fused in a [3.3.0] system—a particularly stable arrangement (*cf.* Sections 5.2 and 5.3) which is possible only in uronic acids with the *gluco, gulo, manno,* and *ido* configurations. Thus, D-glucuronic acid and D-mannuronic acid are usually obtained (42, 43) in crystalline form as their respective 6→3 lactones (**29** and **30**).[15] In aqueous solution, the equilibrium

(29)   (30)

[15] It is also of interest that D-glucosaccharic acid and D-mannosaccharic acid crystallize (44) as their 1→4−6→3-dilactones.

(Figure 5.12) between D-glucopyranosyluronic acid (**31**) and D-glucofurano-sylurono-6→3-lactone (**32**) is highly temperature dependent (45), with higher temperatures favoring the lactone, probably on account of a favorable entropy factor for the flexible *cis*-fused five-membered rings.

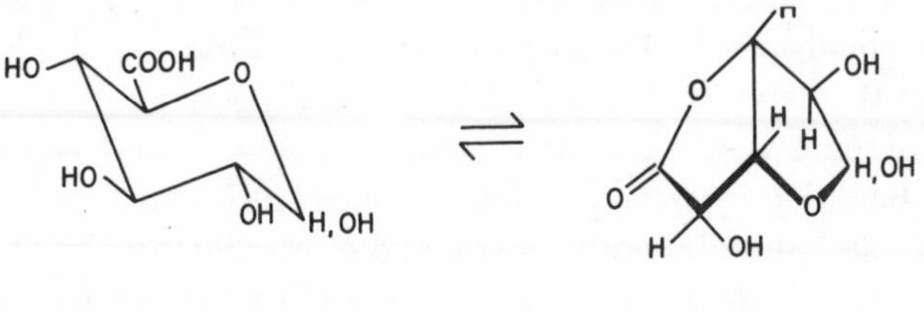

(31)   (32)

Figure 5.12   The equilibrium between D-glucopyranosyluronic acid (**31**) and D-gluco-furanosylurono-6→3-lactone (**32**).

5.5   Cyclic Acetal Formation

5.5.1   Introduction

Cyclic and acyclic carbohydrate derivatives react readily with aldehydes and ketones in the presence of acid catalysts to form cyclic acetals. After prolonged reaction times, an equilibrium is eventually established in which the composition of the reaction mixture is determined by the relative free energies of the different cyclic acetals. From the stereochemical point of view, the equilibria are often complex. Thus, when an equilibrium exists between cyclic acetals of different ring sizes, *acetal ring isomerization* has to be considered, often in conjunction with configurational and/or conformational isomerizations. This point is illustrated in Figure 5.13 by the equilibrium which results on acid-catalyzed condensation of glycerol with acetaldehyde. Condensation of the two primary hydroxyl groups of glycerol with acetaldehyde gives two diastereomeric cyclic acetals with 1,3-dioxane ring systems. On the other hand, since the primary hydroxyl groups of glycerol are enantiotopic, four stereoisomeric cyclic acetals with 1,3-dioxolane ring systems are produced when acetaldehyde condenses with vicinal hydroxyl groups on glycerol.

The first part of this section will be concerned with a short review of the configurational and conformational properties of some monocyclic acetals. In the light of this introduction, acetal ring isomerizations of the kind shown in Figure 5.13 will then be considered. In the last part of the section,

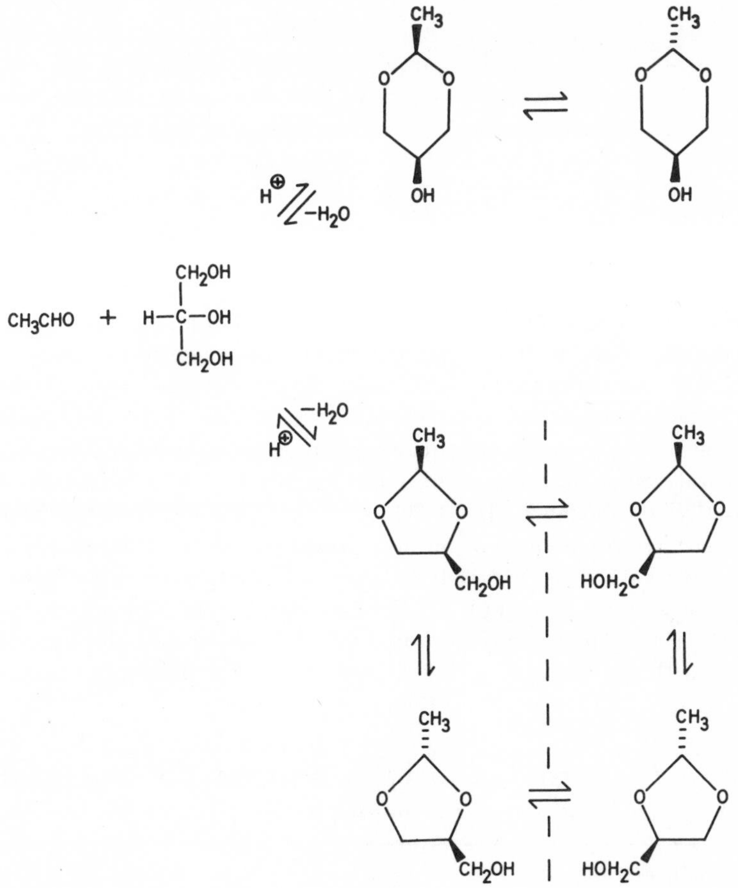

Figure 5.13   Acetal ring isomerization—the acid-catalyzed condensation of glycerol with acetaldehyde.

the stereochemical properties of some bicyclic and tricyclic acetals formed by carbohydrate derivatives will be discussed.

5.5.2   Monocyclic Acetals with 1,3-Dioxane Ring Systems

There is good evidence (46–58) believing that 1,3-dioxane (**33**) and most of its derivatives exist as chair conformers. However, chiefly because C-O bonds are about 10% shorter than C-C bonds, the chair conformer of 1,3-dioxane is puckered in the O_1—C_2—O_3 region and flattened in the C_4—C_5—C_6 region. This is evident immediately from an examination

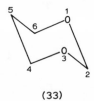

(33)

(52, 54) of molecular models and has been substantiated experimentally by ^{1}H nuclear magnetic resonance spectroscopy (54, 58, 59). Recently, an X-ray crystallographic investigation of 2-*p*-chlorophenyl-1,3-dioxane has shown (60) that, while the torsional CO—CO angle in the puckered region is 63°, the torsional OC—CC angle in the flattened region is 55°. As might be expected, the stereochemical properties of 1,3-dioxane derivatives are often a direct consequence of these geometrical features.

Acid-catalyzed equilibrations of some conformationally biased 2-, 4-, and 5-methyl-1,3-dioxanes (52–54, 56, 57) have yielded information about the orientational preferences of methyl groups on the three different positions of the 1,3-dioxane ring system. The conformational free energies of methyl groups on C_2, C_4, and C_5 of the 1,3-dioxane ring, which have been obtained in this manner, are shown in Table 5.7, and these values may be compared with the value of 1.70 kcal mole^{-1} (61) for the conformational free energy of a methyl group on the cyclohexane ring.

Table 5.7 *The Conformational Free Energies of Methyl Groups on* C_2, C_4, *and* C_5 *of the 1,3-Dioxane Ring*

Position on the 1,3-Dioxane Ring	$-\Delta G^\circ_{CH_3}$ kcal mole^{-1}	Refs.
C_2	3.97	57
C_4	2.9	54, 56, 57
C_5	0.8	54, 56, 57

When the geometry of the 1,3-dioxane ring system is considered, it is not surprising that the conformational free energy of a methyl group on C_2 is as large as 3.97 kcal mole^{-1}. On the assumption of bond distances for C-C, C-O, and C-H bonds of 1.537 Å, 1.417 Å, and 1.096 Å, respectively, and bond angles for C—C—C, C—O—C, and H—C—H angles of 111.5°, 111.5°, and 109.5°, respectively, calculations have afforded (52) the internuclear distances between the nonbonded hydrogen atoms shown in Figure 5.14 for the chair conformers of 2-methyl-1,3-dioxane and methyl-

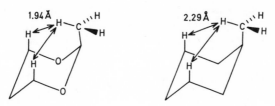

Figure 5.14   Calculated internuclear distances between nonbonded hydrogen atoms in the chair conformers of 2-methyl-1,3-dioxane and methylcyclohexane with axial methyl groups.

cyclohexane with axial methyl groups. The crowding of the axial methyl group in 2-methyl-1,3-dioxane is not only a consequence of the shortness of the C-O bonds as compared to the C-C bonds in methylcyclohexane, but also an outcome of the fact that the puckering in the O_1—C_2—O_3 region causes an axial substituent on C_2 to "lean toward" the *syn*-axial hydrogen atoms on C_4 and C_6. Since an axial methyl group on C_4 is involved in a "normal" interaction with the *syn*-axial hydrogen atom on C_6, as well as in a "severe" interaction with the *syn*-axial hydrogen atom on C_2, its smaller conformational free energy of 2.9 kcal mole^{-1}, compared with that of a methyl group on C_2, is to be expected.[16] Finally, with a value of 0.8 kcal mole^{-1}, the conformational free energy of a methyl group on C_5 is substantially lower than that of a methyl group on cyclohexane. Presumably the reason is that, whereas an axial methyl group on cyclohexane interacts with *syn*-axial hydrogen atoms, on a 1,3-dioxane ring an axial methyl group on C_5 may be considered to interact with axial lone pairs on the oxygen atoms. The "size" or "steric requirement" of a lone pair is a concept which is still the subject of much controversy (54–57, 62, 63). However, it seems to be agreed that *syn*-axial interactions involving axial lone pairs on oxygen atoms are considerably smaller than those involving axial hydrogen atoms on carbon atoms (*cf.* Section 3.2.2).

The conformational preferences of methyl groups at different locations on the 1,3-dioxane ring have important consequences for the conformational stabilities of *gem*-dimethyl 1,3-dioxanes. It has been shown that 1,3-dioxane (**33**) (50–52, 64, 65), 2,2-dimethyl-1,3-dioxane (**34**) (50), 4,4-dimethyl-1,3-dioxane (**35**) (51), and 5,5-dimethyl-1,3-dioxane (**36**) (50)

---

[16] An approximate estimate (*cf.* ref. 56) of the conformational free energy of a methyl group on C_4 of a 1,3-dioxane ring may be obtained by summing one-half the conformational free energy of a methyl group on C_2 with one-half the conformational free energy of a methyl group on cyclohexane, that is, $\frac{1}{2}(3.97) + \frac{1}{2}(1.70)$, which equals 2.84 kcal mole^{-1}, and is in excellent agreement with the experimental value of 2.9 kcal mole^{-1}.

all exhibit the expected coalescence of signals in their low-temperature ^{1}H nuclear magnetic resonance spectra. From the free energies of activation $\Delta G\ddagger$ for the ring inversions listed in Table 5.8, it is evident that the $\Delta G\ddagger$

Table 5.8   The Free Energies of Activation $\Delta G\ddagger$ for 1,3-Dioxane (**33**), *2,2-Dimethyl-1,3-dioxane* (**34**), *4,4-Dimethyl-1,3-dioxane* (**35**), *and 5,5-Dimethyl-1,3-dioxane* (**36**)

Dioxane		$\Delta G\ddagger$ kcal mole^{-1}
(33)		9·7
(34)		7·8
(35)		9·1
(36)		10·5

values for the 2,2- and 4,4-dimethyl-1,3-dioxanes are smaller than those for 1,3-dioxane itself and its 5,5-dimethyl derivative. These observations have been attributed (50, 52, 54) to ground-state compression by the axial methyl groups on C_2 and C_4, which leads to a lowering of the barrier to interconversion. The fact that 2,2-dimethyl-1,3-dioxane (**34**) and 4,4-diemthyl-1,3-dioxane (**35**) exist as interconverting chair conformers has been cited as evidence that the twist-boat conformers of 1,3-dioxane must be at least 3–4 kcal mole^{-1} less stable than the chair conformer. This has been confirmed by thermochemical studies (66–68). From the thermodynamic parameters for the chair/twist-boat interconversions of cyclohexane and 1,3-dioxane (**33**) presented in Table 5.9, it is interesting to

Table 5.9   Chair/Twist-Boat Interconversions

Compound	$\Delta H^{\circ}_{C \to TB}$ kcal mole^{-1}	$\Delta S^{\circ}_{C \to TB}$ cal deg^{-1} mole^{-1}	$\Delta G^{\circ}_{C \to TB}$ kcal mole^{-1}	Ref.
Cyclohexane	5.9	3.5	4.9	63
1,3-Dioxane	7.1	4.8	5.7	68

note that ΔH° is larger[17] for 1,3-dioxane than for cyclohexane. Chiefly on account of the large interaction (ΔH°) of 8.9 kcal mole^{-1} (67, 68) between *syn*-axial methyl groups on the chair conformers of 2,2-*trans*-4,6-tetramethyl-1,3-dioxane (Figure 5.15), a twist-boat has been predicted

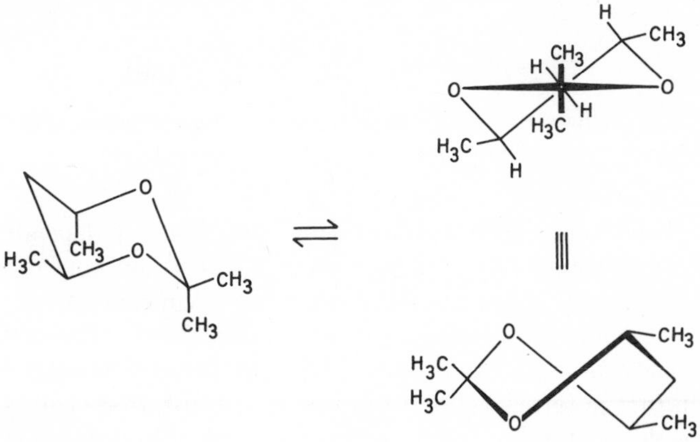

Figure 5.15   The chair/twist-boat conformational equilibrium for 2,2-*trans*-4,6-tretramethyl-1,3-dioxane.

as the predominant conformer. Indeed, thermochemical data (67, 68) and ^{1}H nuclear magnetic resonance spectroscopic data (54, 57, 71) are consistent with this prediction. We shall see later in this section, when con-

---

[17] Although in 1,3-dioxane the torsional strain is likely (63) to be about the same as, or a little less than, that in cyclohexane [*cf.* barriers of 2.7 kcal mole^{-1} for dimethyl ether (69) and 3.3 kcal mole^{-1} for propane (70)], nonbonded interactions are probably much more severe in the more compact and distorted heterocyclic ring.

sidering the conformational properties of some bicyclic acetals such as 6-deoxy-1,2:3,5-di-*O*-isopropylidene-6-nitro-α-D-glucofuranose, that 2,2-*trans*-4,6-tetramethyl-1,3-dioxane is an important model compound.

Recently, it has been found (57) that the conformational free energy of a phenyl group on C_2 of the 1,3-dioxane ring is only 3.1 kcal mole^{-1} [*cf*. a $-\Delta G^\circ_{Ph}$ value of 3.0 kcal mole^{-1} for a phenyl group on a cyclohexane ring (61)]. It is somewhat surprising to find that the conformational free energy of a phenyl group is less than that of a methyl group. This has been confirmed, however, by the observation (57) that in 2-phenyl-2,4,6-trimethyl-1,3-dioxane (Figure 5.16) the diastereomer (**37**) with the axial phenyl and equatorial methyl groups is much more stable than that (**38**) with the axial

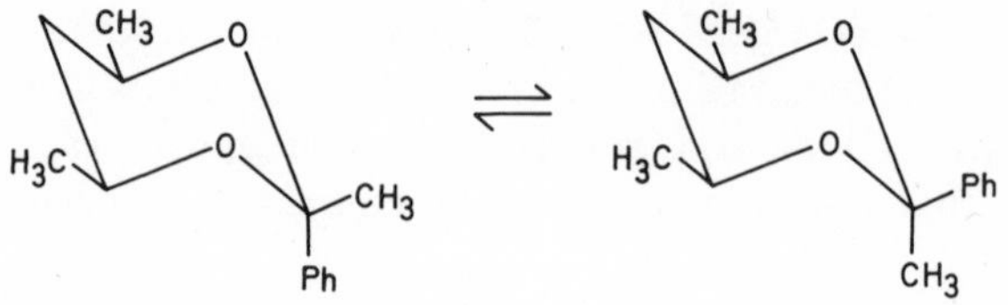

(37)   (38)

Figure 5.16   Acid-catalyzed equilibration of the two diastereomers (**37** and **38**) of 2-phenyl-2,4,6-trimethyl-1,3-dioxane (57).

methyl and equatorial phenyl groups. Since the effect is independent of the nature of substituents on the phenyl ring (57), it would appear that electronic interactions are not responsible for this phenomenon. An explanation based on the analysis of coupling constant data in ^{1}H nuclear magnetic resonance spectra and on the results of dipole moment measurements has been given (57) in terms of the stabilization of a distorted chair conformer for axial 2-phenyl-1,3-dioxane, in which the axial phenyl group is directed away from the ring.

Other factors may influence the conformational properties of 1,3-dioxane ring systems. An axial hydroxyl group on C_5 is suitably orientated (57, 72–75) to become involved in hydrogen bonding with the ring oxygen atoms (*cf*. Section 4.4). As a result, in dilute carbon tetrachloride solution, 5-hydroxy-1,3-dioxane, otherwise known as 1,3-*O*-methylene-glycerol (**39** in Figure 5.17), exists to a large extent as the chair conformer with an axial hydroxyl group which may be hydrogen-bonded to either or both ring oxygen atoms. Although illustrated as the latter in Figure 5.17, it is not known (76) whether bifurcated hydrogen bonds are present in 5-hydroxy-1,3-dioxane derivatives. However, it is significant that, as indicated by the

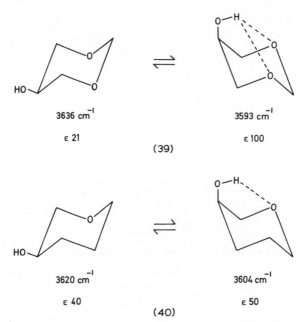

Figure 5.17   Intramolecular hydrogen bonding in 5-hydroxy-1,3-dioxane (**39**) and 3-hydroxytetrahydropyran (**40**).

relative magnitudes of the extinction coefficients ϵ, the equilibrium is displaced much more toward the hydrogen-bonded conformer in 5-hydroxy-1,3-dioxane (**39**) than it is in 3-hydroxytetrahydropyran (**40** in Figure 5.17).

Table 5.10 shows some results obtained (57, 75) on equilibration of 2-isopropyl-5-hydroxy-1,3-dioxane in three different solvents. The preference for the *syn* isomer with the axial hydroxyl group is in accordance with the finding (76) that such isomers are stabilized by intramolecular hydrogen bonding. In a hydroxylic solvent, hydrogen bonding with the solvent stabilizes the *anti* isomer with the equatorial hydroxyl group and so decreases the preference for the *syn* isomer. Examples are also known in which the preference for an axial hydroxyl group on C_5 of a 1,3-dioxane ring system influences the course of reaction. Hence, in the acid-catalyzed condensation of benzaldehyde with D-arabinitol, 1,3-*O*-benzylidene-D-arabinitol (**41**) with an axial hydroxyl group available (76) for intramolecular hydrogen bonding to the oxygen atoms in the 1,3-dioxane ring was obtained[18] (77) in high yield in preference to 3,5-*O*-benzylidene-D-arabinitol

[18] The analogous 1,3-*O*-methylene-D-arabinitol has been obtained (78) on acid-catalyzed methylenation of D-arabinitol.

Table 5.10   The Conformational Free Energy of a Hydroxyl Group on C_5 of a 1,3-Dioxane Ring System in Different Solvents (57, 75)

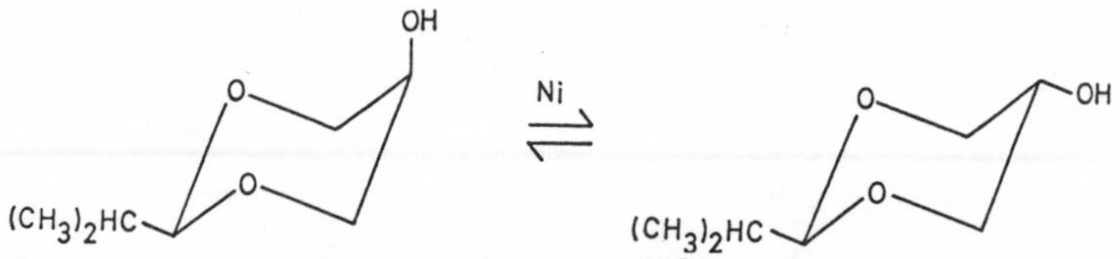

Solvent	ΔG°_{80}, kcal mole^{-1}
Cyclohexane	+0.92
Isopropyl alcohol	+0.51
t-Butyl alchol	+0.50

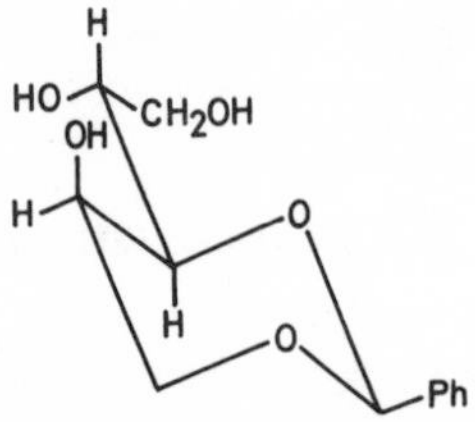

(41)

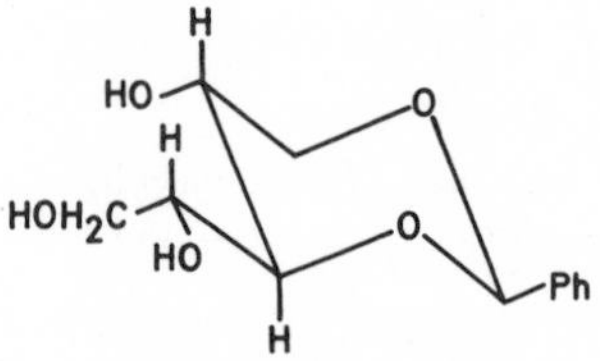

(42)

(1,3-*O*-benzylidene-D-lyxitol) (**42**) with an equatorial hydroxyl group. It is also significant that 1,3:4,6-di-*O*-methylene-galactitol (**43**) with axial hydroxyl groups on C_5 of each of the 1,3-dioxane rings was obtained (79) quantitatively from the acid-catalyzed condensation of galactitol with formaldehyde.

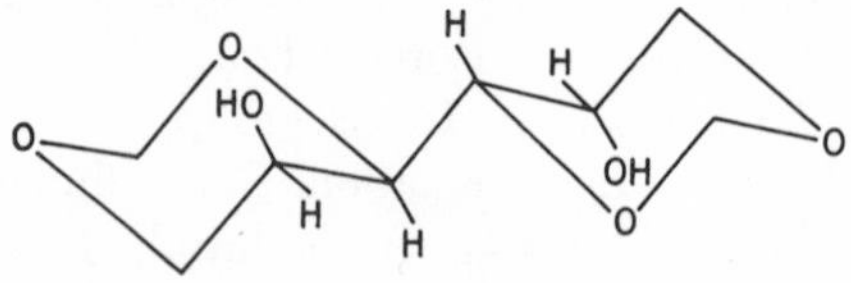

(43)

5.5.3   Monocyclic Acetals with 1,3-Dioxolane Ring Systems

There is some evidence (80–82) that 1,3-dioxolane (**44** in Figure 5.18) and 2,2-dimethyl-1,3-dioxolane (**45** in Figure 5.18) exist in puckered con-

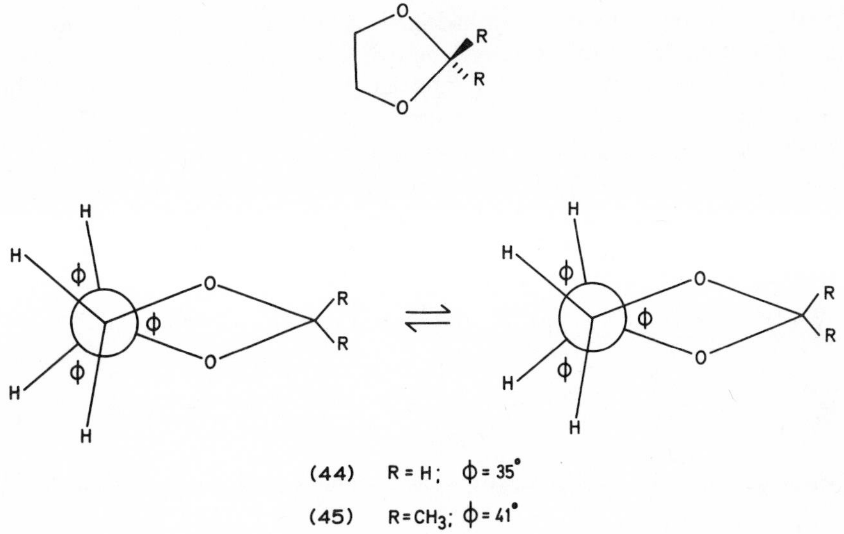

(44)   R = H; $\phi = 35°$

(45)   R = CH$_3$; $\phi = 41°$

Figure 5.18   The puckered conformations of 1,3-dioxolane (44) and 2,2-dimethyl-1,3-dioxane (45).

formations related to the envelope and twist conformations, wherein one atom and two atoms, respectively, are displaced from the plane of the other ring atoms. Although both 1,3-dioxolane (44) and its 2,2-dimethyl derivative (45) have been represented as twist conformations in Figure 5.18, this kind of representation is selected only for diagrammatic convenience. It is possible (58, 83, 84) that in some 1,3-dioxolane derivatives important minimum energy conformations lie somewhere between the envelope and the twist conformations.

Although substituents on 1,3-dioxolane rings impose (85) restrictions on pseudorotational itineraries, a whole range of conformations of about the same energy exists for most 1,3-dioxolane derivatives, and the wide conformational oscillation that occurs in the liquid phase or in solution has been called (58, 85) *pseudolibration*. The four C-methylene protons at C$_4$ and C$_5$ in 1,3-dioxolane (44) and in 2,2-dimethyl-1,3-dioxolane (45) are isochronous, since in each case the two C-methylene groups are equivalent and each pair of C-methylene protons are enantiotopic. However, coupling constant data obtained (80, 81) from satellites in their ^{1}H nuclear magnetic resonance spectra caused by ^{13}CH$_2$ groups, indicate [19] that the magnitude

---

[19] It should be mentioned that the calculation of specific torsional angles from coupling constants in five-membered rings has been criticized (84) on the basis that pseudolibration leads to rather wide conformational oscillations and that consequently coupling constants should be integrated over the whole pseudorotational itinerary.

of the torsional angle ϕ shown in Figure 5.18 is 35° in 1,3-dioxolane (**44**) and 41° in 2,2-dimethyl-1,3-dioxolane (**45**). Obviously, introduction of two methyl groups on C_2 of the 1,3-dioxolane ring causes an increase in the puckering of the ring. This observation is in accordance with the Thorpe-Ingold *gem*-dimethyl effect (86), which predicts an increase in the endo-cyclic O_1—C_2—O_3 angle when methyl groups replace the hydrogen atoms on C_2.

When aldehydes or ketones condense with alditols in the presence of an acid catalyst to yield 1,3-dioxolane derivatives, the more stable ring has (24) the substituent groups (R_1 and R_2 in Figure 5.19a) *trans* and involves

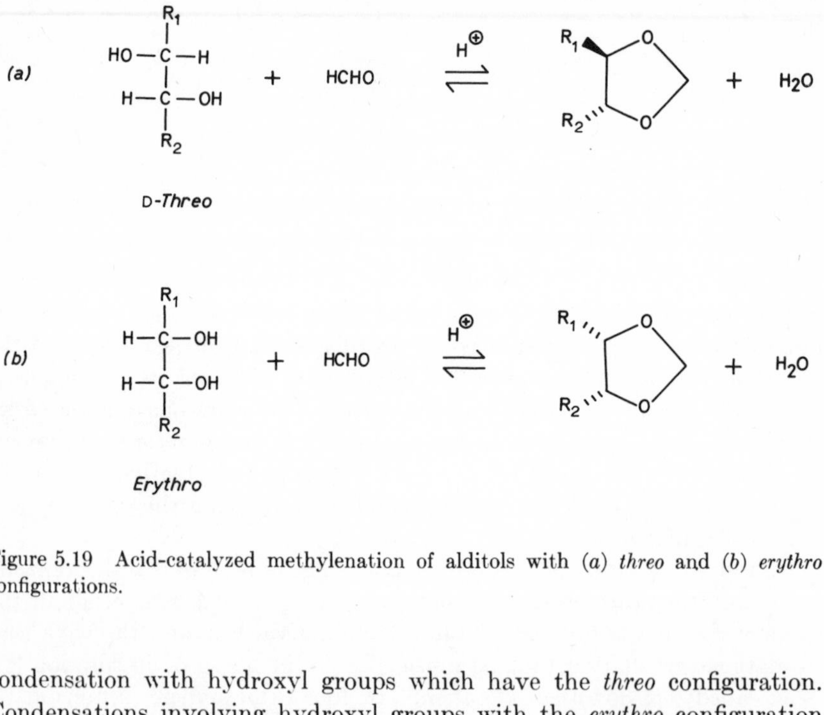

Figure 5.19   Acid-catalyzed methylenation of alditols with (*a*) *threo* and (*b*) *erythro* configurations.

condensation with hydroxyl groups which have the *threo* configuration. Condensations involving hydroxyl groups with the *erythro* configuration form less stable 1,3-dioxolane derivatives where the substituent groups (R_1 and R_2 in Figure 5.19*b*) are *cis*. This order of stability reflects the destabilization of the 1,3-dioxolane ring on account of nonbonded inter-actions between *cis*-1,2 substituents (87). Thus, it is not surprising to find that acid-catalyzed acetonation of D-mannitol with hydroxyl groups on C_3 and C_4 in the *threo* configuration affords (88) 1,2:3,4:5,6-tri-*O*-iso-propylidene-D-mannitol (**46**). The situation becomes more complex when

(46)

aldehydes condense with alditols, since the possibility of obtaining dia-stereomers arises. Thus, benzylidenation of 1,6-di-O-benzoyl-galactitol with hydroxyl groups on C_2 and C_3, and C_4 and C_5, both in the *threo* configuration, has yielded (89, 90) two of the three possible stereoisomers (**47, 48**, and **49**) of 1,6-di-O-benzoyl-2,3:4,5-di-O-benzylidene-(DL)- galacti-tol. The benzylidene-methine protons of one stereoisomer were aniso-chronous (91), and hence it was assigned to the *dl*-modification (**47**), since each enantiomer has diastereotopic benzylidene-methine protons. The benzylidene-methine protons of the other stereoisomer were isochronous; therefore it was assigned (91) to one of the *meso* forms (**48** or **49**) with enantiotopic benzylidene-methine protons.

(47)	DL-forms	R_1=H; R_2=Ph;	R_3=H;	R_4=Ph
		R_1=Ph; R_2=H;	R_3=Ph;	R_4=H
(48)		R_1=Ph; R_2=H;	R_3=H;	R_4=Ph
(49)		R_1=H; R_2=Ph;	R_3=Ph;	R_4=H

In a recent investigation of the configurational stability of 2,4-*cis*-5-trisubstituted 1,3-dioxolanes, it was shown (84, 92) that the *syn* isomers are generally thermodynamically more stable than the *anti* isomers (*cf.*

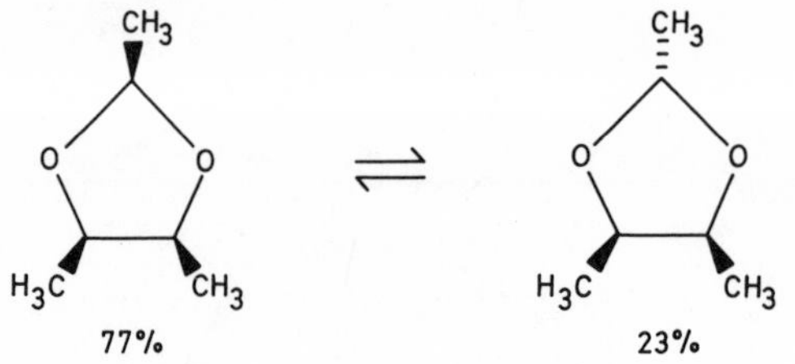

77%   23%

(50)   (51)

Figure 5.20   Acid-catalyzed equilibration of the *syn* (**50**) and *anti* (**51**) diastereomers of 2,4-*cis*-5-trimethyl-1,3-dioxolane (84,92).

ref. 93). Thus, the *syn* isomer (**50**) of 2,4-*cis*-5-trimethyl-1,3-dioxolane predominates (Figure 5.20) over the *anti* isomer (**51**) at equilibrium. This difference in stability of diastereomers has important consequences in determining the product compositions (*cf.* ref. 94) of bicyclic and tricyclic acetals with *cis*-fused dioxolane rings (see Section 5.5.6).

5.5.4   Monocyclic Acetals with 1,3-Dioxepane Ring Systems

The conformational properties of 1,3-dioxepane (**52**) and its derivatives would be expected to be rather similar to those of cycloheptane (95) (*cf.* septanoid rings in Section 3.5). The fact that 1,6-di-*O*-benzoyl-2,5-*O*-methylene-D-mannitol (**53**) with *trans* hydroxyl groups on C_3 and C_4 forms

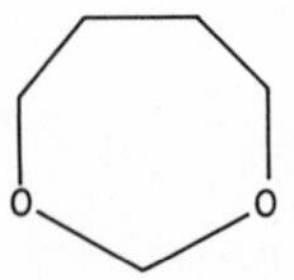

(52) 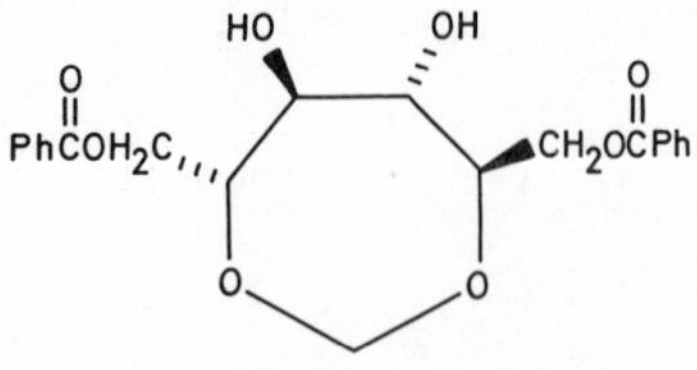   (53)

a 3,4-*O*-benzylidene derivative (96–98) and a 3,4-*O*-isopropylidene derivative (98) indicates that the 1,3-dioxepane ring is flexible enough to accommodate torsional angles between projected *trans* C-O bonds of 41°, or less, in order to form these derivatives. If it is accepted that 1,3-dioxepanes are flexible, their conformational properties may be examined as part of a chair/twist-chair pseudorotational itinerary (*cf.* Section 3.5).

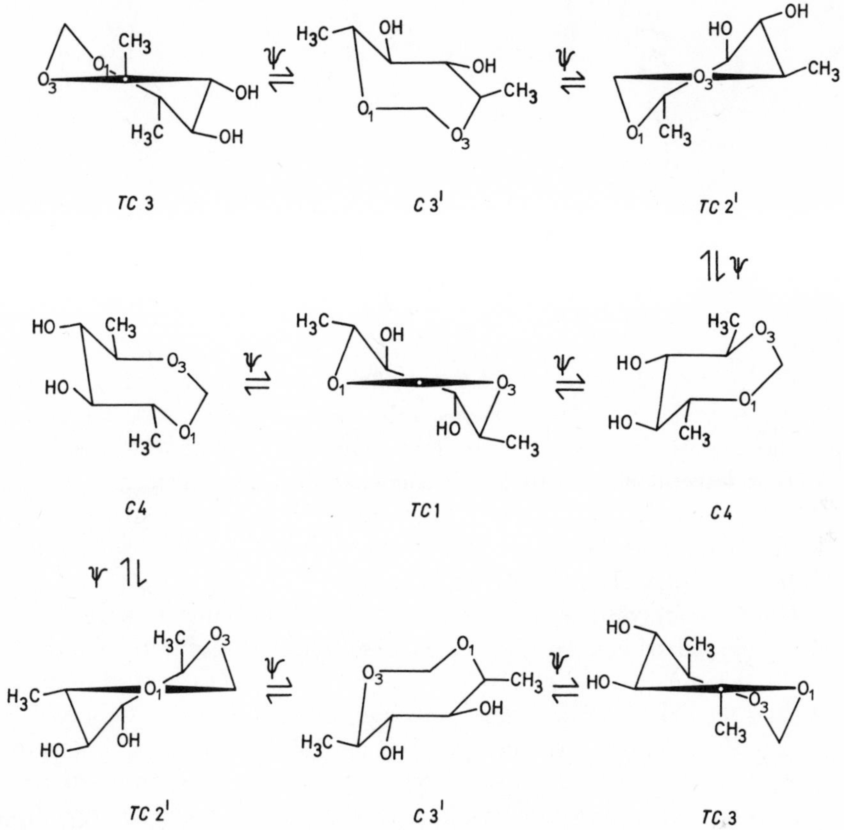

Figure 5.21   Part of the chair/twist-chair pseudorotational itinerary of 1,6-dideoxy-2,5-O-methylene-D-mannitol (**54**).

Examination of the chair/twist-chair pseudorotational itinerary (98) of 1,6-dideoxy-2,5-O-mannitol (**54**) indicates (Figures 5.21) that three twist-chair conformers (*TC*1, *TC*2′, and *TC*3) have both methyl groups and both hydroxyl groups equatorial. All other twist-chair conformers on the pseudorotational itinerary have one or more of these groups axial. Of the three "all-equatorial" twist-chair conformers, one (*TC*1) has a C_2 axis of symmetry and the other two (*TC*2′ and *TC*3) are degenerate. The prediction from conformational analysis that they are the predominant contributors to a conformational equilibrium is consistent with (98) coupling constant data obtained from the ^{1}H nuclear magnetic resonance spectrum of 1,6-dideoxy-2,5-O-methylene-D-mannitol (**54**).

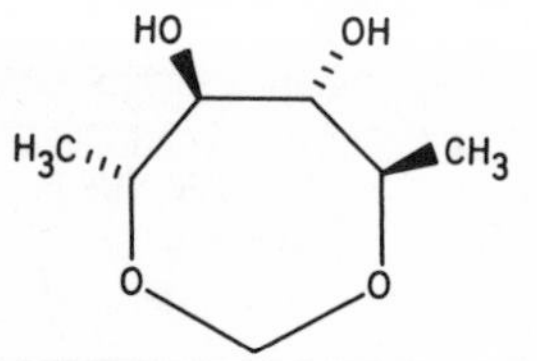

(54)

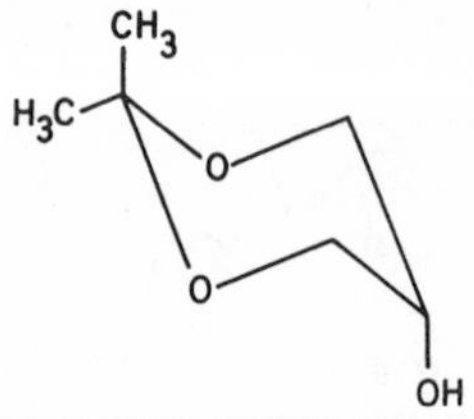

(55)

5.5.5 Acetal Ring Isomerization

The acid-catalyzed isomerization of five- and six-membered acetal rings may now be accounted for in terms of the conformational properties of these cyclic acetals. It is well known that aldehydes, including formaldehyde (99) and acetaldehyde (100), will condense with glycerol to give approximately equimolar mixtures of 1,3-dioxane and 1,3-dioxolane derivatives at equilibrium, whereas in the condensation of acetone (101) with glycerol only the 1,3-dioxolane derivative is formed.

On acid-catalyzed isomerization of each of the pure diastereomers of 1,3-*O*-ethylidene-glycerol and of 1,2-*O*-ethylidene-DL-glycerol (*cf.* Figure 5.13), identical ratios of products were obtained (102) at equilibrium. Values for $\Delta G°$, $\Delta H°$, and $\Delta S°$ were calculated from the equilibrium constants K between the 1,3-dioxanes and the 1,3-dioxolanes at various temperatures. From the values recorded in Table 5.11 for these thermodynamic parameters, it is seen that the 1,3-dioxanes have a much lower entropy than the 1,3-dioxolanes. This is not surprising, since the dioxolanes are more flexible as well as being *dl*-pairs. The large entropy difference means that the product composition is strongly temperature dependent. Thus, formation of dioxanes is less unfavorable at low temperatures, and use (102) of this fact has been made in preparing 1,3-*O*-isopropylidene-glycerol (**55**) in 2% yield by keeping 1,2-*O*-isopropylidene-DL-glycerol (**56**) with an

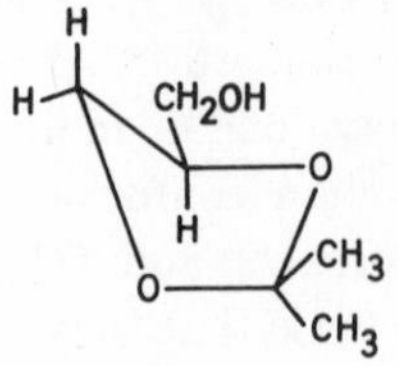

(56)

acid catalyst below 0° for several days. The high conformational free energy (3.97 kcal mole^{-1}) of a methyl group on C_2 of the 1,3-dioxane ring explains (24, 35, 54, 102) why condensation of acetone with glycerol gives the 1,3-dioxolanes almost exclusively.[20] Since this interaction is absent in 1,3-dioxane derivatives obtained on condensation of aldehydes with glycerol, about equal amounts of five- and six-membered ring acetals are formed.[21]

Table 5.11 Equilibrium Constants K and Thermodynamic Parameters for the 1,3-Dioxane/1,3-Dioxolane System (102)

Temperature, °C	K	$\Delta G°$, cal mole^{-1}	$\Delta S°$, cal deg^{-1} mole^{-1}
70	0.8913	77.7	20.2
75	1.0015	9.86	20.1
80	1.195	−135	20.3
106.5	2.371	−650	20.2

Isomerization of a 1,3-dioxane ring to a 1,3-dioxolane ring occurs readily if a *cis*-fused [3.3.0] ring system (*cf.* Sections 5.2, 5.3, and 5.4) can be adopted 103–105). Thus, it has been shown (105) that, on treatment with *p*-toluene sulfonic acid in *N,N*-dimethylformamide, 2,4-*O*-benzylidene-D-erythrose (**57**) isomerizes (Figure 5.22) to 2,3-*O*-benzylidene-D-erythrose, which in turn undergoes hemiacetal formation to give the furanose derivatives. As shown in Figure 5.22, the isomerization occurs by a mechanism (*cf.* ref. 104) which gives the diastereomer (**58**) with the phenyl group *endo* under kinetic control. Subsequently, acid-catalyzed equilibration yields some of the diastereomer (**59**) with the phenyl group *exo* at equilibrium.

[20] In addition, the dioxolane ring will be stabilized by a small *gem*-dimethyl effect (86), allow greater puckering of the ring and hence reduce the torsional strain.
[21] With fewer substituents, dioxolane rings are not destabilized with respect to dioxane rings as much as furanoid rings are destabilized relative to pyranoid rings.

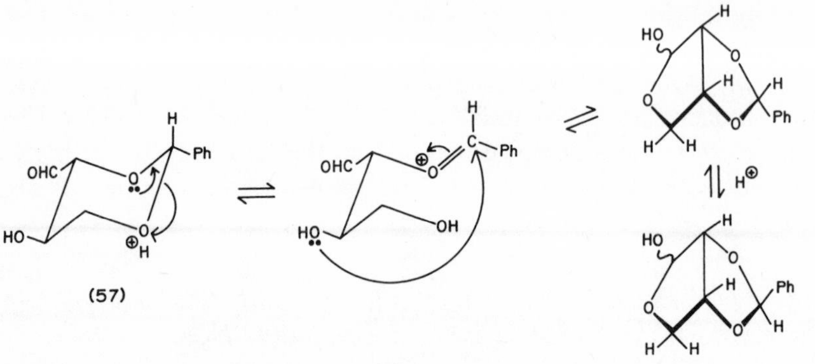

Figure 5.22   Proposed mechanism (104) for the acid-catalyzed isomerization of 2,4-*O*-benzylidene-D-erythrose (**57**) to the *endo* (**58**), and subsequently the *exo* (**59**), isomers of 2,3-*O*-benzylidene-D-erythrose.

5.5.6   Fused Five-Membered Ring Acetals

Cyclohexane-*cis*-1,2-diol is known (106) to form an *O*-isopropylidene derivative more readily than cyclohexane-*trans*-1,2-diol, which requires forcing conditions to bring about formation of its cyclic acetal. Since the torsional angle involving the *O*-isopropylidene residue at the ring junction is restricted (81) to a maximum of 41°, considerable distortion of the chair conformers of the cyclohexane-diols from the normal torsional angles between *cis*- and *trans*-projected C-O bonds is required. When it is recalled from Section 3.2.1 that the cyclohexane ring is naturally somewhat flattened and that, as a result, axial-equatorial substituents are closer together than equatorial-equatorial substituents, the fact that the *cis*-diol[22] with axial-equatorial hydroxyl groups undergoes acetonation much more readily than does the *trans*-diol with equatorial-equatorial hydroxyl groups is not surprising. Moreover, any further distortion necessary for the formation of the *O*-isopropylidene derivatives imposes less strain on the six-membered ring (*cf.* ref. 108) in the case of acetonation of the *cis*-diol than in the acetonation of the *trans*-diol.

If it is accepted that the six-membered ring in *O*-isopropylidene-cyclohexane-*cis*-1,2-diol (**60**) exists as a distorted chair conformer,[23] then, by

[22] In fact, infrared spectroscopic data on the hydrogen-bonding properties of each diol in dilute carbon tetrachloride solution indicate (107) that the *cis*-diol with a torsional angle between projected C-O bonds of 50° is even more flattened than cyclohexane itself.

[23] It is significant that 2-oxa-*cis*-hydrindane-5,6-diol with the related oxabicyclo[4.3.0]-nonane ring system exists (109) as a distorted chair conformer.

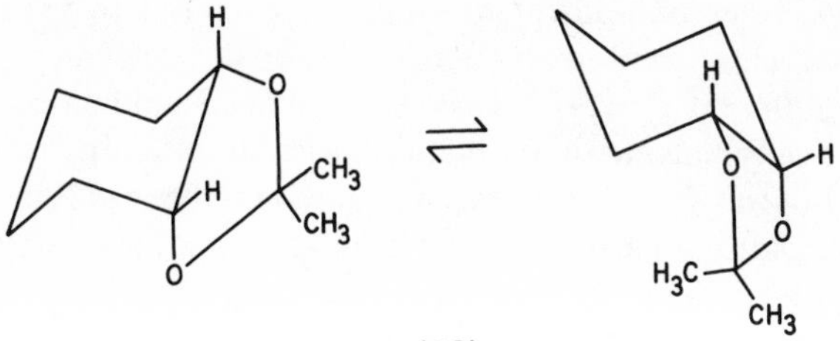

(60)

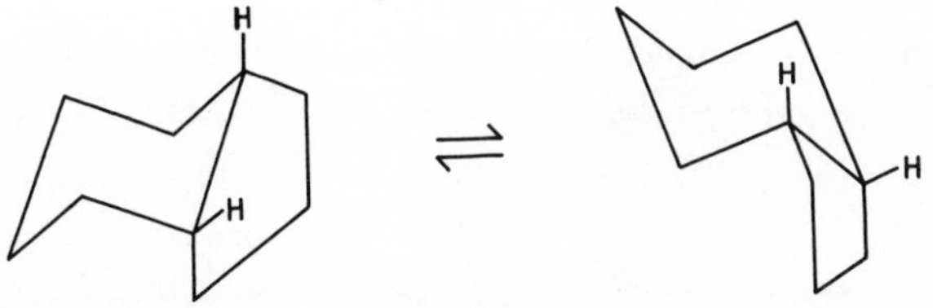

(61)

Figure 5.23   Ring inversion of *O*-isopropylidene-cyclohexane-*cis*-1,2-diol (**60**) and *cis*-hydrindan (**61**).

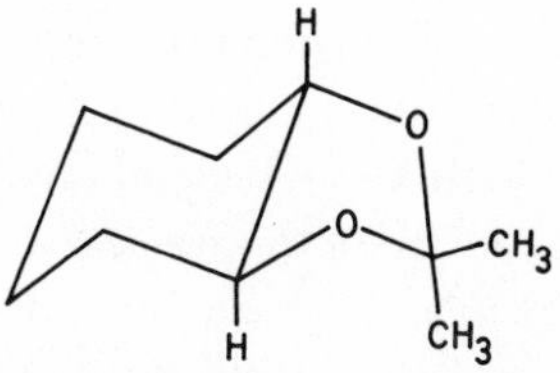

(62)

virtue of ring inversion, it must exhibit (Figure 5.23) conformational isomerism between enantiomers in a manner akin to that of *cis*-hydrindan (**61**) (110). The six-membered ring of *O*-isopropylidene-cyclohexane-*trans*-1,2-diol (**62**) probably exists as a somewhat puckered chair conformer.

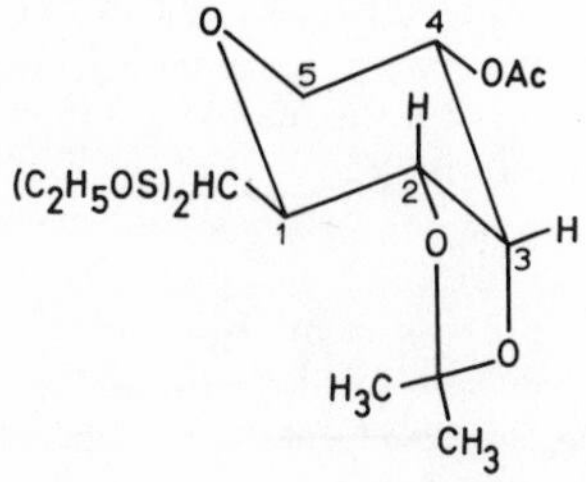

(63)

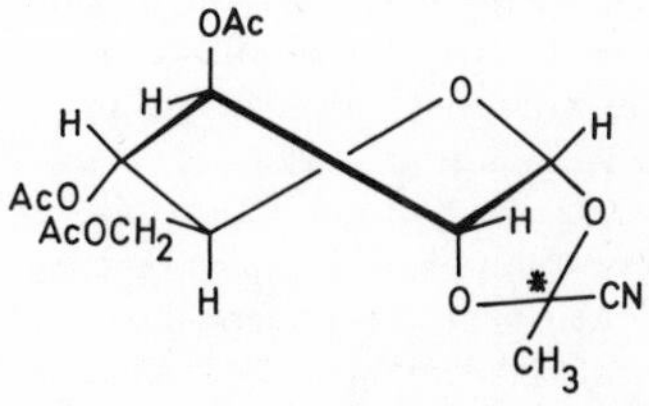

(64)

In the cases where 1,3-dioxolane rings are *cis*-fused to pyranoid rings, both distorted chair conformers and twist-boat conformers have been proposed for different pyranoid derivatives. Thus, coupling constant data from the ¹H nuclear magnetic resonance spectrum of diethylsulfonyl (4-*O*-acetyl-2,3-*O*-isopropylidene-α-D-lyxopyranosyl) methane (**63**) indicate (111) that the pyranoid ring exists as a distorted chair conformer. On the other hand, in 3,4,6-tri-*O*-acetyl-1,2-*O*-(1'-cyanoethylidene)-α-D-glucopyranose (**64**)[24] (112), coupling constant data from ¹H nuclear magnetic resonance spectroscopy indicate (114) that the pyranoid ring exists in a conformation closely related to a twist-boat conformer.[25]

A study of the intramolecular hydrogen-bonding properties of 1,2:5,6-di-*O*-isopropylidene-(−)-inositol (**65**) in dilute carbon tetrachloride solu-

(65)

tion has shown (116) that the torsional angle between the projected C-O bonds associated with the vicinal hydroxyl groups on C_3 and C_4 is *ca.* 49°. This value is consistent with the six-membered ring existing as a twist-boat conformer. It turns out that the *cis-anti-cis* arrangement with these conformational properties is a particularly stable steric arrangement, and there is some evidence that the pyranoid sugars which can assume it will do so in preference to forming *cis*-fused furanoid derivatives. Thus, coupling constant data from ¹H nuclear magnetic resonance spectroscopy indicate (117) that 1,2:3,4-di-*O*-isopropylidene-α-D-galactopyranose (**66**) and 1,2:3,4-di-*O*-isopropylidene-β-L-arabinopyranose (**67**) exist as twist-boat conformers. It is tempting to speculate that 1,2:3,4-di-*O*-isopropylidene-

[24] The configuration at the acetal carbon atom (C*) is not known. It is noteworthy that, when methyl β-L-arabinopyranoside is condensed with paraldehyde in the presence of an acid catalyst, two diastereomeric 3,4-*O*-ethylidene derivatives are obtained (113). Acid-catalyzed isomerization shows that the diastereomer with the methyl group *endo* predominates (at least 70%) at equilibrium. This is not surprising in view of the finding (84, 92) that in most 2-alkyl-4-*cis*-5-trisubstituted 1,3-dioxolanes the *syn* isomers are more stable than the *anti* isomers.

[25] Twist-boat conformers have also been postulated (115) for some branched-chain methyl glycopyranosides, including methyl 6-deoxy-2,3-*O*-isopropylidene-4-*C*-methyl-α-L-talopyranoside and methyl 6-deoxy-3,4-*O*-isopropylidene-2-*C*-methyl-α-L-galacto-pyranoside, but the evidence in these instances is less convincing.

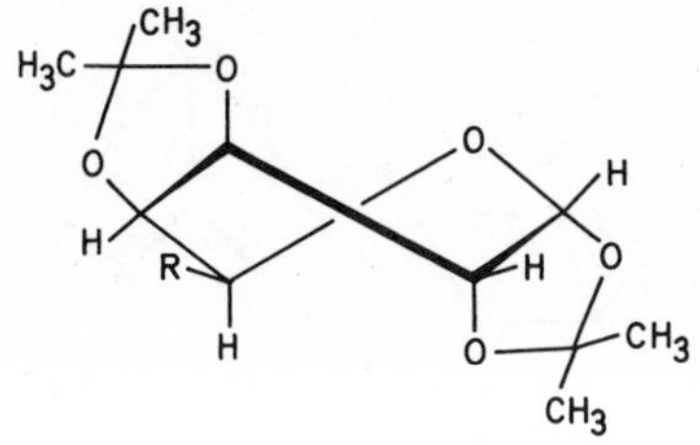

(66) R=CH₂OH

(67) R=H

β-D-altropyranose (**68**) (118) and 2,3:4,5-di-*O*-isopropylidene-β-D-fructo-pyranose (**69**) (119) may also exist as twist-boat conformers.

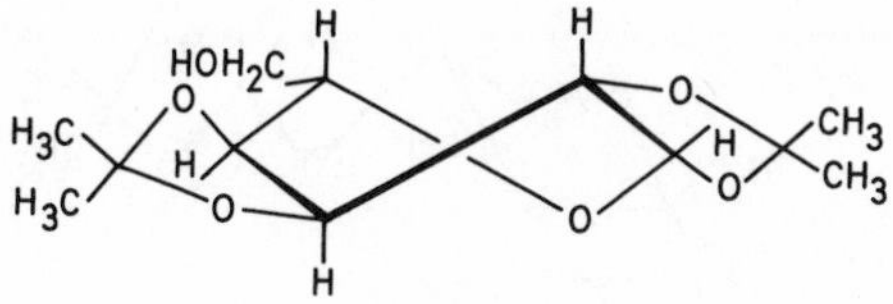

(68)

Cyclopentane-*cis*-1,2-diol forms (106) an *O*-isopropylidene derivative (**70**) readily, whereas the stereochemistry of the hydroxyl groups of the

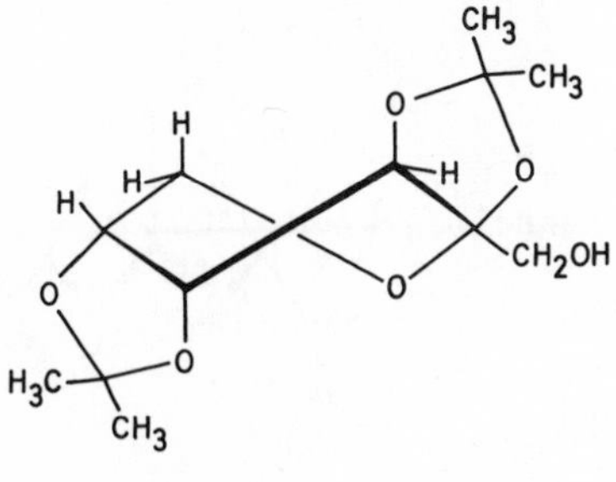

(69)

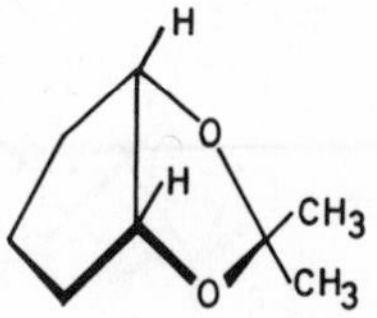

(70)

trans isomer is such that it cannot form an *O*-isopropylidene derivative without the introduction of considerable strain. In fact, cyclopentane-*trans*-1,2-diol does not form an *O*-isopropylidene derivative (106). Examples of *O*-isopropylidene rings *cis*-fused to furanoid rings occur in the 1,2:5,6-di-*O*-isopropylidene derivatives of D-glucose (**71**) (120), D-talose (**72**) (121), D-galactose (**73**) (122), and D-altrose (**74**) (118). In the case of the D-

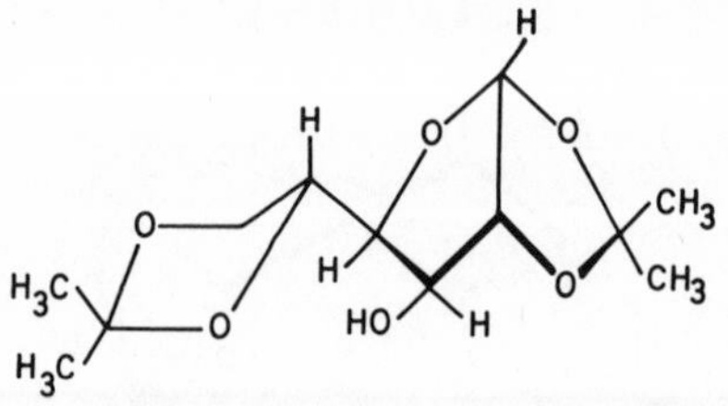

(71)

glucose and D-talose derivatives (**71** and **72**) the 5,6-*O*-isopropylidene residues have the *exo* configuration at C$_4$ of their furanoid rings, whereas

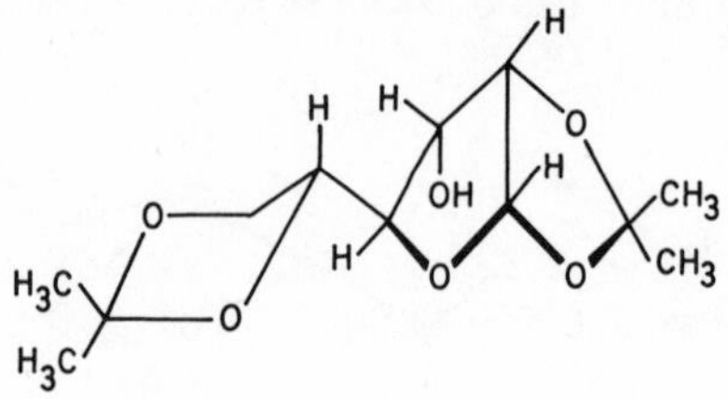

(72)

in the D-galactose and D-altrose derivatives (**73** and **74**) the 5,6-*O*-iso-propylidene residues have the *endo* configuration. The fact that 1,2:5,6-di-*O*-isopropylidene-D-galactose (**73**) has been obtained (122) only in low

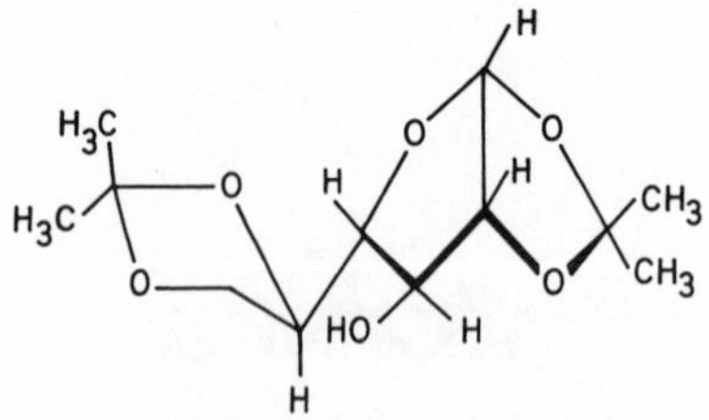

(73)

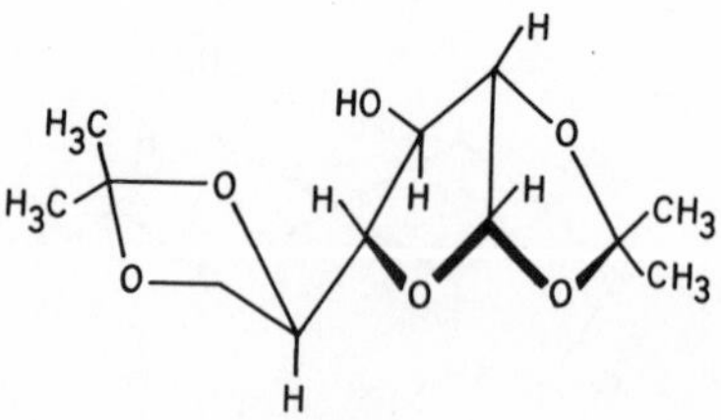

(74)

yield (3%) on acetonation of D-galactose reflects the greater stability of the 1,2:3,4-diacetal (66) with the *cis-anti-cis* arrangement. Although this steric arrangement is a particularly stable one, the 1,2:5,6-diacetal (**73**) may also be destabilized by the bulky 5,6-*O*-isopropylidene residue on C$_4$ having to assume the *endo* configuration.[26]

[26] It is noteworthy that, although *syn* diastereomers (which correspond to the 1,2:5,6-di-*O*-isopropylidene derivatives with the *endo* configuration) are generally more stable in

There is some evidence that the five-membered rings in the *cis*-fused systems are puckered, that is, they are not as represented in **70–74**. Coupling constant data from ^1H nuclear magnetic resonance spectroscopy have indicated (123) that the furanoid ring in 5,6-anhydro-1,2-*O*-isopropylidene-α-D-glucofuranose exists predominantly in the twist conformation $(^3T_2)$ shown in **75**.

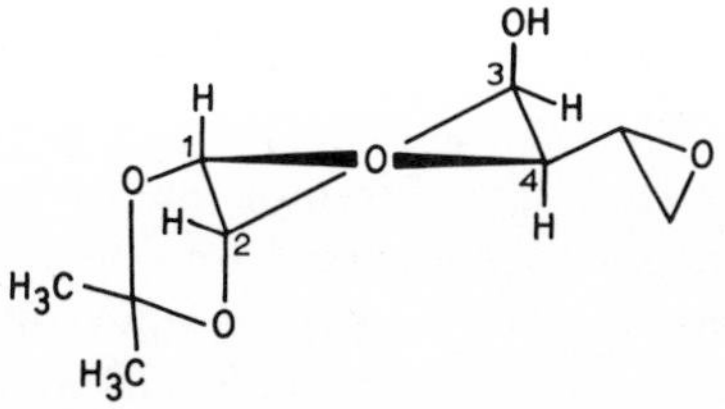

(75)

It is interesting that the acid-catalyzed condensation of D-glucose with acetone yields not only the 1,2:5,6- (**71**) and the 1,2:3,5- (see Section 5.5.7) diacetals, but also 1,2:3,4-di-*O*-isopropylidene-α-D-glucoseptanose (**76**) (1.9%) and 2,3:4,5-di-*O*-isopropylidene-D-glucoseptanose (**77**) in low

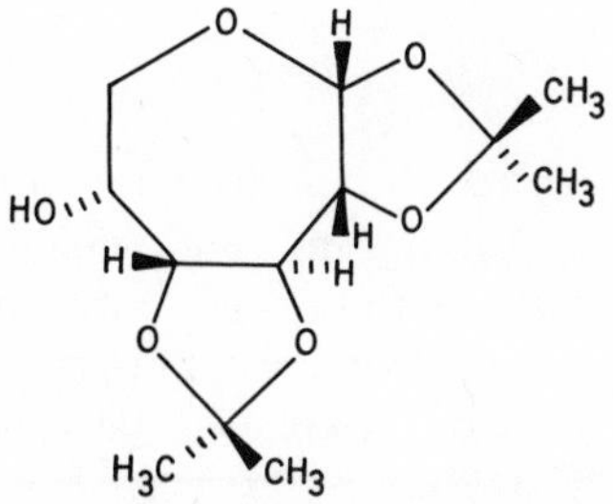

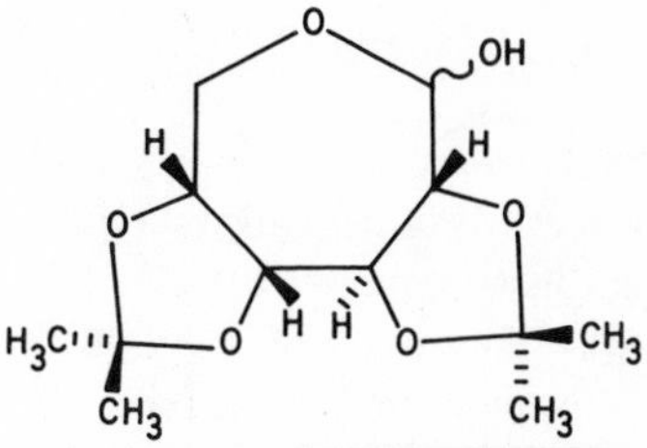

(76)   (77)

yield (124). This indicates that the diacetals with glucoseptanoid rings must be only about 1–2 kcal mole^{-1} less stable than the 1,2:5,6-diacetal

---

2,4-*cis*-5-trisubstituted 1,3-dioxolanes, in 2-*t*-butyl-4-*cis*-5-di-isopropyl-1,3-dioxolane and 2,4-*cis*-5-tri-*t*-butyl-1,3-dioxolane the *anti* diastereomers (which correspond to the 1,2:5,6-di-*O*-isopropylidene derivatives with the *exo* configuration) are favored (84, 92). By analogy, it is possible that the 1,2-diacetals having bulky 5,6-*O*-isopropylidene residues with the *exo* configuration at C$_4$ of the furanoid ring are stablized relative to diastereomers with the *endo* configuration at C$_4$. If this is the case, the 1,2:5,6-diacetals formed from D-galactose and D-altrose will be destabilized with respect to those formed from D-glucose and D-talose.

with a glucofuranoid ring. Examination of the most stable twist-chair conformers for the glucoseptanoid ring shown in Figures 3.41 and 3.42 indicates that many of them can form the 1,2:3,4- and 2,3:4,5-diacetals without imposing much strain on the septanoid ring.

5.5.7   Fused Six-Membered Ring Acetals

Condensation of D-glucose with benzaldehyde in the presence of zinc chloride and acetic acid has yielded (125) one of the four diastereomers of 1,2:3,5-di-O-benzylidene-α-D-glucofuranose in low yield (16%). If only distorted chair conformers[27] are assumed for the 1,3-dioxane rings, there are two conformations that they may assume with equatorial phenyl groups corresponding to the diastereomers (**78** and **79**)[28] with opposite

(78)   (79)

configurations at the 3,5-benzylic carbon atom. In one diastereomer (**78**) C_2 of the furanoid ring is axial on C_4 of the 1,3-dioxane ring, while in the other diastereomer (**79**) the 1,3-dioxane ring has the oxygen atom in the furanose ring axial on C_5 as well as an axial hydroxylmethyl group on C_4. Coupling constant data from ^{1}H nuclear magnetic resonance spectroscopy have indicated (126) it was the second diastereomer (**79**) with two axial groups on the 1,3-dioxane ring that was obtained from the benzylidenation (125). However, it is not known whether or not this is the more stable diastereomer.[29]

---

[27] In view of the much higher free energy of twist-boat conformers (Section 5.5.2) of 1,3-dioxane, this is a reasonable assumption. In this case, there is also some evidence (126) from ^{1}H nuclear magnetic resonance spectroscopy on which to exclude twist-boat conformers from consideration.

[28] The configuration at the 1,2-benzylic carbon atom is not known (126).

[29] The yield (16%) of the diastereomer is low; moreover, the benzylidenation may not have reached equilibrium. However, it is interesting to note that the diastereomeric 1,2-O-isopropylidene-3,5-O-(methoxymethylidene)-6-O-p-tolylsulfonyl-α-D-glucofuranoses, one with an axial and the other with an equatorial methoxyl group on C_2 of the 1,3-dioxane ring, both exist (127) in conformations analogous to that of the second diastereomer (**79**) of 1,2:3,5-di-O-benzylidene-α-D-glucofuranose.

Examination of the distorted chair conformations of the 1,3-dioxane ring of 1,2:3,5-di-*O*-isopropylidene-*α*-D-xylofuranose (**80**) (128) shows that one conformer, **A**, has a *syn*-axial interaction between substituents on C₂ and C₄ of the dioxane ring and so should be disfavored relative to the other conformer, **B**. As yet, however, no experimental data are available to examine this prediction.

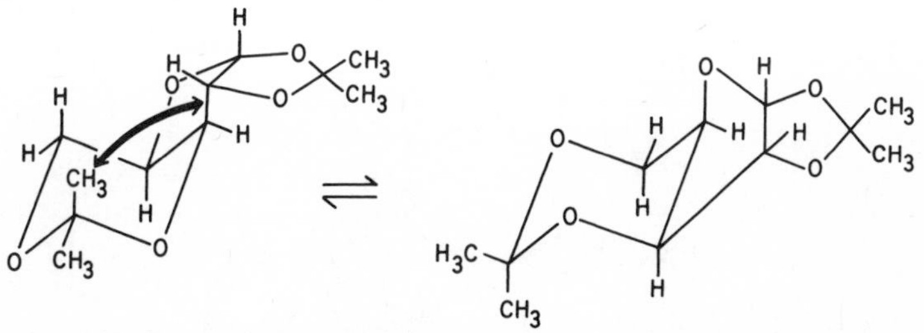

(A)   (80)   (B)

The ease of formation of 6-deoxy-1,2:3,5-di-*O*-isopropylidene-6-nitro-*β*-L-idofuranose (**81**), compared with that of 6-deoxy-1,2:3,5-di-*O*-isopropy-lidene-6-nitro-*α*-D-glucofuranose (**82**), on acid-catalyzed condensation (129) of the corresponding 1,2-*O*-isopropylidene derivatives with acetone may be explained by conformational analysis (*cf.* ref. 24). In the case of the *ido* derivative (**81**), conformer **B** will be expected to predominate over con-

(A)   (81)   (B)

former **A**, which would experience a *syn*-axial interaction within its 1,3-dioxane ring. In the *gluco* derivative (**82**), conformers **A** and **B** would each experience *syn*-axial interactions,[30] and so the 1,3-dioxane ring probably exists as the twist-boat conformer **C**. Clearly, the *gluco* derivative (**82**) is destabilized relative to the *ido* derivative (**81**), and the relative ease of formation of the latter finds an explanation.

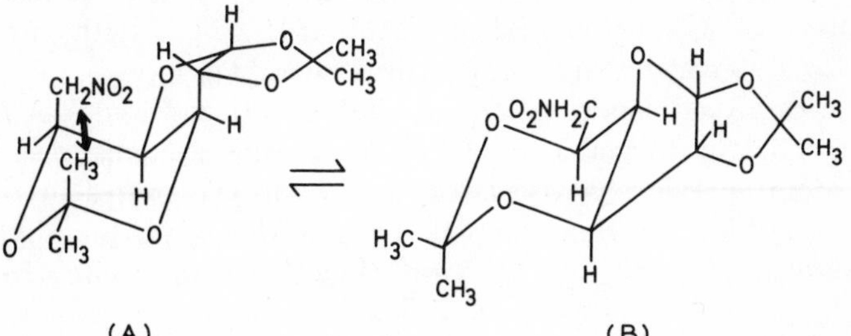

[30] The situation is analogous to that of 2,2-*trans*-4,6-tetramethyl-1,3-dioxane, which is known (57, 68, 71) to exist predominantly as a twist-boat conformer (see Section 5.5.2).

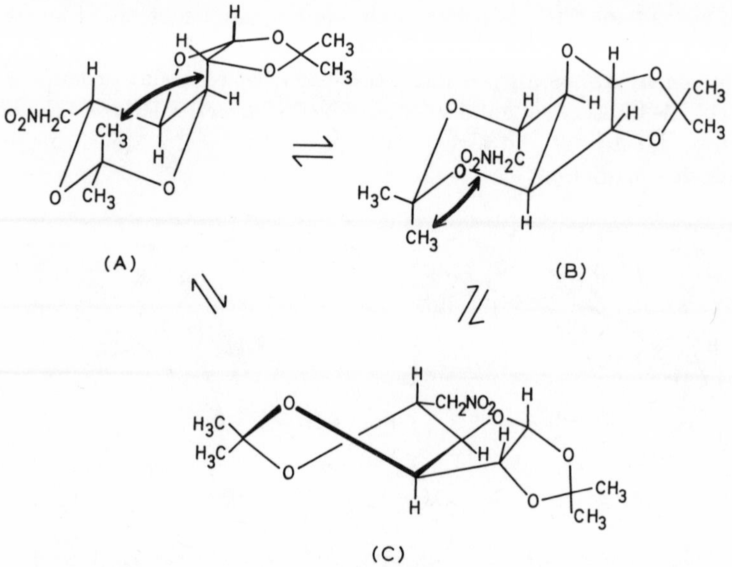

(A)   (B)

(C)

(82)

In acid-catalyzed condensations of alditols with aldehydes or ketones, *trans*-fused 1,3,6,8-tetraoxabicyclo[4.4.0]decane ring systems result when carbon atoms previously associated with hydroxyl groups in the *erythro* configuration form the ring junction. Thus, acid-catalyzed methylenation of ribitol and allitol has yielded 1,3:2,4-di-*O*-methylene-DL-ribitol (**83**) (130) and 2,4:3,5-di-*O*-methylene-allitol (**84**) (131) with *trans*-fused [4.4.0] ring systems and equatorial hydroxymethyl groups.

In acid-catalyzed condensations of alditols with aldehydes or ketones, *cis*-fused 1,3,6,8-tetraoxabicyclo[4.4.0]decane ring systems result when carbon atoms previously associated with hydroxyl groups in the *threo* configuration form the ring junction. Thus, acid-catalyzed methylenation of L-threitol has yielded (132) 1,3:2,4-di-*O*-methylene-L-threitol (**85**) with a

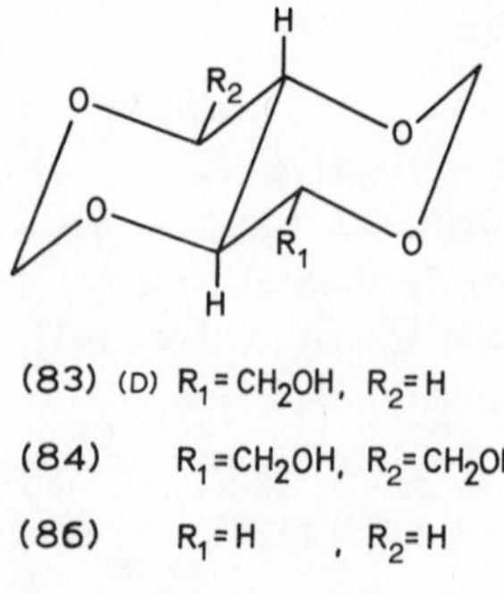

(**83**) (D) $R_1 = CH_2OH$, $R_2 = H$

(**84**) $R_1 = CH_2OH$, $R_2 = CH_2OH$

(**86**) $R_1 = H$, $R_2 = H$

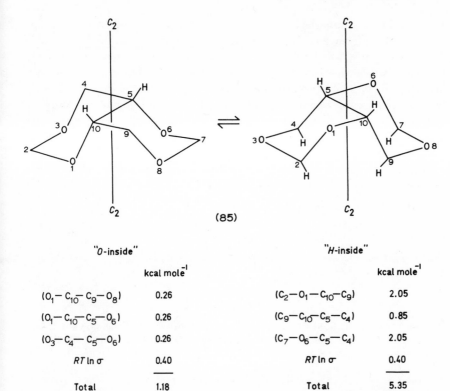

Figure 5.24 The relative free energies of the "O-inside" and "H-inside" conformers of 1,3:2,4-di-O-methylene-L-threitol (**85**). *Gauche* interactions between oxygen atoms, that is, (O_1—C_{10}—C_9—O_8), (O_1—C_{10}—C_5—O_6), and (O_3—C_4—C_5—O_6), have been made equal to one-half the conformational free energy of a hydroxyl group in aprotic solvents [$-\Delta G_{OH} = 0.52$ kcal mole^{-1} (61)]. The *gauche* interaction (C_9—C_{10}—C_5—C_4) between carbon atoms has been made equal to one-half the conformational free energy of a methyl group [$-\Delta G°_{CH_3} = 1.70$ kcal mole^{-1} (61)] on cyclohexane. The other two *gauche* interactions, (C_2—O_1—C_{10}—C_9) and (C_7—O_6—C_5—C_4), correspond to the conformational free energy of a methyl group on C_4 of a 1,3-dioxane ring [$-\Delta G°_{CH_3} = 2.9$ kcal mole^{-1} (57)] minus one-half the conformational free energy of a methyl group on cyclohexane.

cis-fused [4.4.0] ring system. Two conformers, which have been termed (24) the "O-inside" and the "H-inside" conformers, are possible for **85**, and their contribution to the conformational equilibrium shown in Figure 5.24 will be dependent on their relative free energies. The free energies of each conformer relative to a hypothetical 1,3:2,4-di-O-methylene-erythritol (**86**) with no nonbonded interactions have been calculated as detailed in

Figure 5.24. A comparison of these calculated values indicates that the "O-inside" conformer is 4.2 kcal mole^{-1} more stable than the "H-inside" conformer. Thus, 1,3:2,4-di-*O*-methylene-L-threitol (**85**) may be expected to exist, albeit entirely in solution, as the "O-inside" conformer. Indeed, it has been shown (132) from dipole moment measurements that it exists as the "O-inside" conformer to an extent of at least 90% in benzene. Coupling constant data from ^{2}H nuclear magnetic resonance spectroscopy also indicates that the 1,3:2,4-diacetal (**85**) exists predominantly as its "O-inside" conformer in chloroform.[31]

Figure 5.25 shows that 1,3:2,4-di-*O*-methylene-DL-xylitol (**87**) (134), 2,4:3,5-di-*O*-methylene-D-glucitol (**88**) (135, 136), and 2,4:3,5-di-*O*-

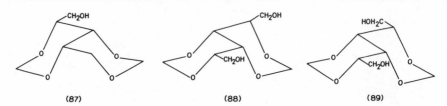

(87)   (88)   (89)

Figure 5.25   The "O-inside" conformers of 1,3:2,4-di-*O*-methylene-D-xylitol (**87**), 2,4:3,5-di-*O*-methylene-D-glucitol (**88**), and 2,4:3,5-di-*O*-methylene-L-iditol (**89**).

methylene-L-iditol (**89**) (137) must also exist as "O-inside" conformers, since the "H-inside" conformers would have axial hydroxymethyl groups "inside" experiencing very large nonbonded interactions. However, as Figure 5.26 shows, 2,4:3,5-di-*O*-methylene-D-mannitol (**90**) (136) can exist as the "O-inside" conformer with two axial hydroxymethyl groups or as the "H-inside" conformer with two equatorial hydroxymethyl groups. Comparison of the relative free energies calculated for each conformer in Figure 5.26 indicates that the "H-inside" conformer is preferred by 1.6 kcal mole^{-1}. Indeed, coupling constant data from the ^{1}H nuclear magnetic resonance spectrum of 1,6-dideoxy-2,4:3,5-di-*O*-methylene-D-mannitol show (138) that the "H-inside" conformer is the predominant contributor to the conformational equilibrium at room temperature in chloroform solution.[32] However, when the temperature is lowered to −59°, the "O-

[31] It should also be noted that acid-catalyzed benzylidenation of L-threitol gives (133) the diastereomer of 1,3:2,4-di-*O*-benzylidene-L-threitol with equatorial phenyl groups on the "O-inside" conformer.

[32] Acid-catalyzed benzylidenation of 1,6-di-*O*-benzoyl-D-mannitol gives (138) two diastereomers of 1,6-di-*O*-benzoyl-2,4:3,5-di-*O*-benzylidene-D-mannitol, one with equatorial phenyl groups on the "H-inside" conformer and the other with equatorial phenyl groups on the "O-inside" conformer.

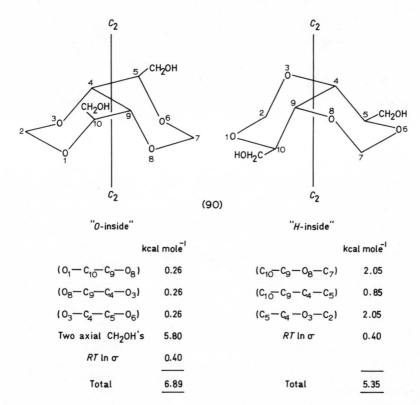

$$(90)$$

"*O*-inside"   "*H*-inside"

kcal mole^{-1} kcal mole^{-1}

$(O_1 - C_{10} - C_9 - O_8)$	0.26		$(C_{10} - C_9 - O_8 - C_7)$	2.05
$(O_8 - C_9 - C_4 - O_3)$	0.26		$(C_{10} - C_9 - C_4 - C_5)$	0.85
$(O_3 - C_4 - C_5 - O_6)$	0.26		$(C_5 - C_4 - O_3 - C_2)$	2.05
Two axial CH$_2$OH's	5.80		$RT \ln \sigma$	0.40
$RT \ln \sigma$	0.40			
Total	6.89		Total	5.35

Figure 5.26 The conformational equilibrium between the "O-inside" and "H-inside" conformers of 2,4:3,5-di-*O*-methylene-D-mannitol (**90**). The conformational free energy of the hydroxymethyl group on C_4 of the 1,3-dioxane ring system has been taken as equal to that of a methyl group. See the caption to Figure 5.24 for an explanation of the values assigned to the other interactions.

inside" conformer is preferred. The temperature dependence of this conformational equilibrium may be interpreted in terms of the "H-inside" conformer being more flexible and thus having a higher entropy than the "O-inside" conformer.

The order of stability of 2,4:3,5-di-*O*-methylene derivatives with *manno*, *gluco*, and *ido* configurations is well demonstrated (139) by the facile base-catalyzed epimerization of the 2,4:3,5-di-*O*-methylene-D-hexosaccharic acids with *manno* and *gluco* configurations to 2,4:3,5-di-*O*-methylene-L-idosaccharic acid.

As shown in Figure 5.27, acid-catalyzed condensation of D-arabinitol with formaldehyde may yield the 2,4:3,5-diacetal (**91**) with a *trans*-fused

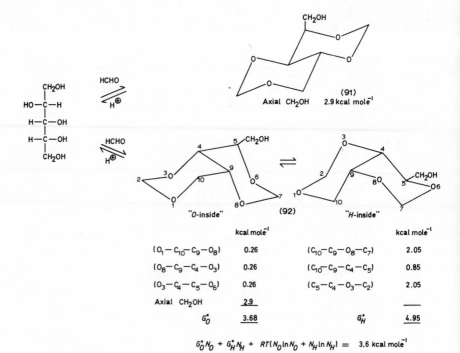

Figure 5.27 The acid-catalyzed condensation of D-arabinitol with formaldehyde. See the captions to Figures 5.24 and 5.26 for explanations of the values assigned to the various interactions.

[4.4.0] ring system and an axial hydroxymethyl group, or the 1,3:2,4-diacetal (92) with a *cis*-fused [4.4.0] ring system in which the "O-inside" conformer has an axial hydroxymethyl group and the "H-inside" conformer has an equatorial hydroxymethyl group. At equilibrium, the product composition of this methylenation will be determined by the relative free energies of the constitutional isomers (91 and 92). Although the 2,4:3,5-

diacetal (**91**) is predicted from Figure 5.27 to be 0.7 kcal mole^{-1} more stable than the 1,3:2,4-diacetal (**92**), it is the latter which has been isolated (78) in low yield (49% after three successive equilibrations of the same reaction mixture) from the acid-catalyzed methylenation of D-arabinitol.

The methyl 4,6-*O*-benzylidene-α-D-aldohexopyranosides with the *allo* (**93**), *altro* (**94**), *gluco* (**95**), and *manno* (**96**) configurations all have *trans*-

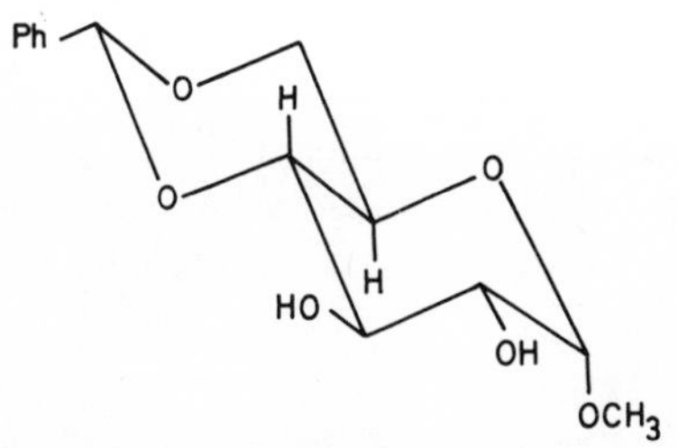

(95) 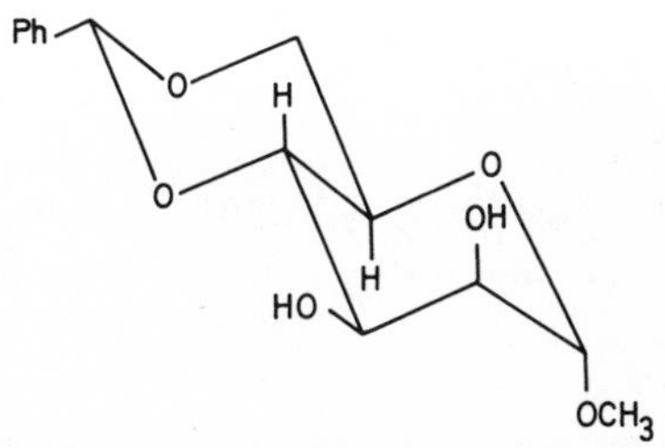   (96)

fused [4.4.0] ring systems. Coupling constant data from the ^{1}H nuclear magnetic resonance spectra of these compounds have indicated (140) that in each case the pyranoid ring exists as a chair conformer.

Base-catalyzed benzylidenation of methyl 2,3-di-*O*-methyl-α-D-gluco-pyranoside with benzylidene bromide (141) has yielded the diastereomers **97** and **98** with opposite configurations at the benzylic carbon atom. Al-

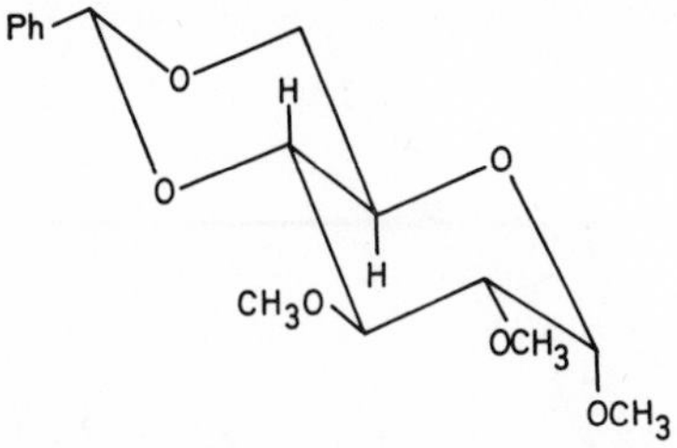

(97) 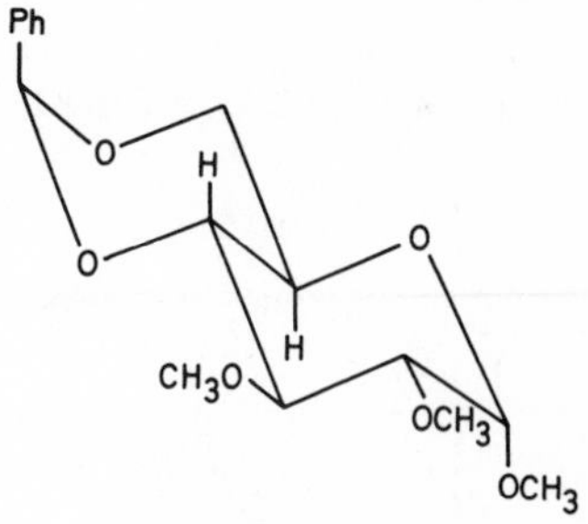   (98)

though it has been suggested (141) that the 1,3-dioxane ring of **98** might adopt a boat conformation, it seems more likely that the phenyl group will assume an axial orientation on the chair conformation, as shown in conformer **98**.[33]

[33] The conformational free energy of a phenyl group on C_2 of a 1,3-dioxane ring is only 3.1 kcal mole^{-1} (57), compared with a destabilization of 5.7 kcal mole^{-1} (68) when a 1,3-dioxane ring exists as a twist-boat conformer.

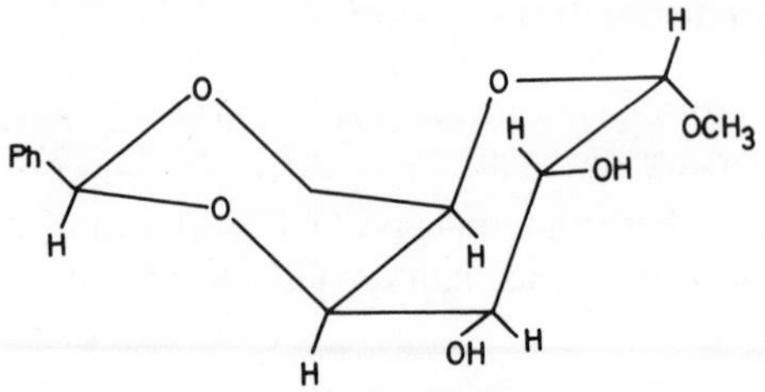

(99)

The methyl 4,6-*O*-benzylidene-α-D-aldohexopyranosides with the *galacto* (99), *gulo* (100), *ido* (101), and *talo* (102) configurations all have *cis*-fused [4.4.0] ring systems. In 99–102, they are shown as the diastereomers with

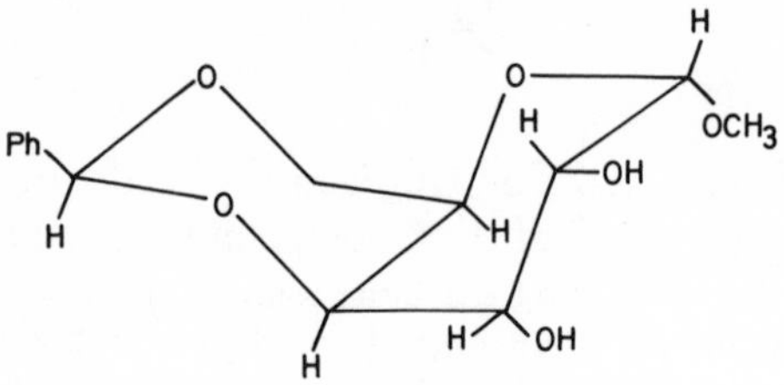

(100)

equatorial phenyl groups on the "O-inside" conformers (*cf*. ref. 24). Indeed, the methyl 4,6-*O*-benzylidene-2,3-di-*O*-di-*O*-methyl-α-D-galactopyranoside obtained on acid-catalyzed benzylidenation of methyl 2,3-di-*O*-methyl-α-

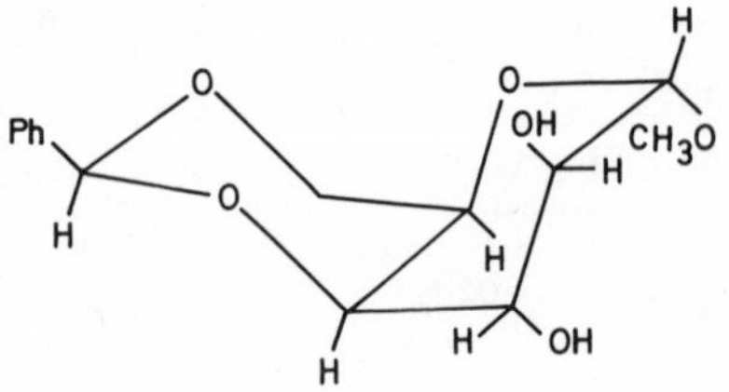

(101)

D-galactopyranoside has been found (141) to be the diastereomer corresponding to the 2,3-dimethyl ether of 99. The pyranoid ring in the 2,3-dimethyl ether of 101 has recently been reported (142), on the basis of coupling constant data in its ¹H nuclear magnetic resonance spectrum, to exist in a twist-boat conformation.

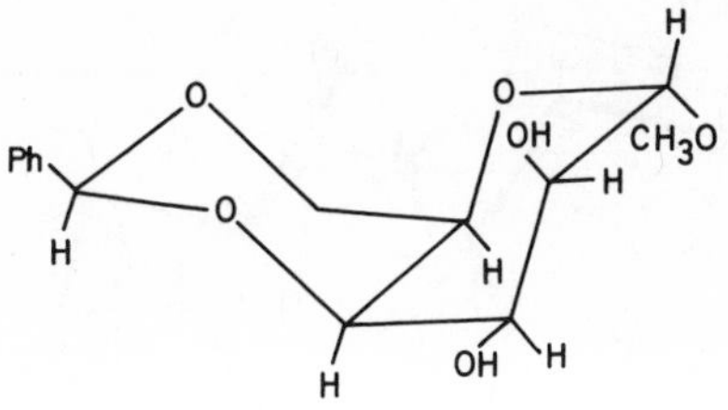

(102)

5.5.8 Fused Seven-Membered Ring Acetals

Perhaps the best-known examples of fused seven-membered ring acetals are the 1,3:2,5:4,6-tri-*O*-alkylidene derivatives (e.g., **103**, **104**, and **105**) of D-mannitol (143, 144). The *trans-anti-trans* configuration of this fused-ring system confers (*cf.* ref. 24) on these acetals their remarkable stability.

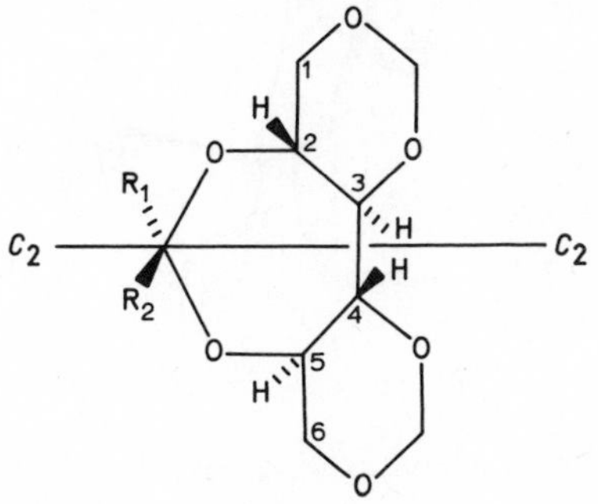

(103) $R_1 = R_2 = H$

(104) $R_1 = R_2 = CH_3$

(105) $R_1 = CH_3,\ R_2 = H$

Examination of molecular models has shown (143) that they may assume one of three conformers wherein the 1,3-dioxepane ring adopts, approximately at least, a twist-chair (*TC*), a twist-boat (*TB*), or a chair (*C*) conformation. By a process of ring inversion, the seven-membered ring may undergo an interconversion of the following type:

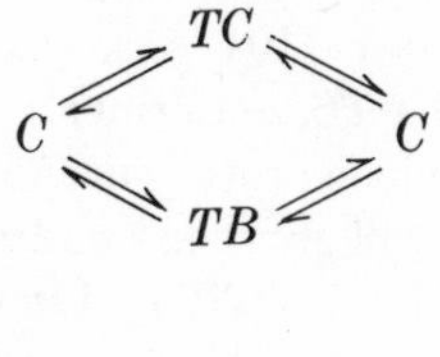

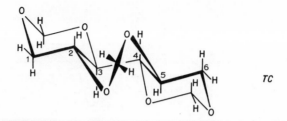

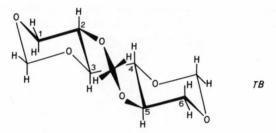

Figure 5.28   The *TC* and *TB* conformers of 1,3:2,5:4,6-tri-*O*-methylene-D-mannitol (**103**).

Here the two *C* conformations are degenerate. As shown in Figure 5.28, the *TC* and *TB* conformations of 1,3:2,5:4,6-tri-*O*-methylene-D-mannitol (**103**) have a C_2 axis of symmetry passing through the 2,5-*O*-methylene carbon atom and the centers of the C_3-C_4 bonds. As a result, the two *O*-methylene protons may be exchanged by a C_2 symmetry operation and are therefore equivalent. On the other hand, in the degenerate *C* conformations shown in Figure 5.29, the *O*-methylene protons are diastereotopic. The observation that these protons are isochronous, even down to −82°, has been cited as evidence (143) that **103** exists as either the *TC* or the *TB* conformer. Conformational analysis predicts that the *TC* conformer will be the more stable (*cf.* Section 5.5.4). It has also been shown (143) that the methyl groups of the *O*-isopropylidene residue of 2,5-*O*-isopropylidene-1,3: 4,6-di-*O*-methylene-D-mannitol (**104**) are isochronous. This derivative almost certainly exists as the *TC* conformer.

  Since the two 2,5-*O*-methylene protons in **105** are equivalent, replacement of either by a methyl group will give the same compound: 2,5-*O*-ethylidene-1,3:4,6-di-*O*-methylene-D-mannitol (**105**). Even this derivative is believed (144) to exist as a *TC* conformer, albeit slightly distorted.

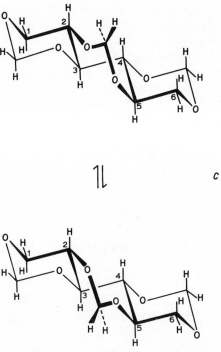

Figure 5.29   The degenerate C conformers of 1,3:2,5:4,6-tri-O-methylene-D-mannitol (**103**).

It is interesting that, although three new chiral centers are created when methyl α-D-glucopyranoside condenses with paraldehyde in the presence of sulfuric acid to give (145) methyl 4,6-O-ethylidene-2,3-O-oxyethylidene-α-D-glucopyranoside, only one diastereomer appears to be obtained (146). The conformational diagrams in Figure 5.30 show that the seven-membered

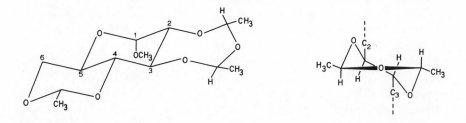

Figure 5.30   Conformational representation of methyl 4,6-O-ethylidene-2,3-oxyethylidene-α-D-glucopyranoside (**106**).

ring can readily adopt a stable *TC* conformation with equatorial methyl groups on both acetal carbon atoms. Thus, the equatorial orientations of the methyl groups on the acetal carbon atoms in Figure 5.30 define **106** as the most stable diastereomer of methyl 4,6-*O*-ethylidene-2,3-*O*-oxydiethylidene-α-D-glucopyranoside. It seems not unlikely that **106** is the diastereomer which has been prepared (145, 146).

(106)

5.6   Glycosidic Anhydride Formation

In aqueous acidic solutions, aldoses and ketoses are known (*cf.* refs. 2, 5, 24, and 147) to form internal glycosides or glycosidic anhydrides (*cf.* Section 2.10) through condensation of their lactol hydroxyl groups with other hydroxyl groups in the molecules. For hexoses and heptuloses, an equilibrium (sugar ⇌ anhydride + water) is eventually established with the 1,6-anhydrohexopyranoses and the 2,7-anhydroheptulopyranoses, respectively. Although other anhydrides (e.g., anhydrofuranoses) may be formed, they are usually of high enough free energy to ensure that their contributions at equilibrium will be small. Certainly, those potentially involving cyclic systems with three- or four-membered rings will have extremely high free energies and are not considered further.

The equilibrium free energies $G^\circ_{\text{pyranose}}$ of all the aldohexopyranoses are known (Table 3.9 in Section 3.2.4), and those for the heptulopyranoses may be obtained by analogous computational procedures. Thus, in the event that the free energy contents of the anhydropyranoses could be calculated, the proportions of each anhydride at equilibrium would be predictable. However, since the magnitudes of the interactions involving the anhydro bridge are unknown, this approach is not possible and another one has been devised (147). In this second approach, the reaction is assumed to proceed in two stages:

1. The $^4C_1$ and $^1C_4$ conformers of the α- and β-anomers, that is, the forms present at equilibrium, are converted into the $^1C_4$ conformer of the β-D-anomer or the $^4C_1$ conformer of the β-L-anomer.

2. The 1,6- or the 2,7-anhydride is formed as shown in Figure 5.31.

Free energy changes are associated with each stage in the reaction. This approach involves the postulation of a hypothetical reaction sequence. However, since we are interested in the free energies of the reactant and

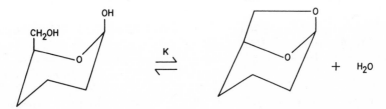

Figure 5.31   The formation of 1,6- or 2,7-anhydrides.

the product, the actual course of the reaction is immaterial. The free energy change $\Delta G°$ associated with stage 1 may be obtained for the D-hexoses from the difference between $G°_{^1C_4}$ for the β-anomer and $G°_{\text{pyranose}}$, listed in Tables 3.6 and 3.9, respectively, in Section 3.2.4. The values obtained for $\Delta G°$ are recorded in Table 5.12. The results of similar calculations on the D-heptuloses are summarized in Table 5.13. The free energy change associated with the formation of the anhydride in stage 2 is assumed to be

Table 5.12   The Equilibrium Proportions of 1,6-Anhydro-hexopyranoses at 100° (147)

Hexose	$G°_{^1C_4(\beta)}$[a]	$G°_{\text{pyranose}}$[b]	$\Delta G°$	$\Delta G°_A$	Anhydride (mole), % Theory	Anhydride (mole), % Experimental
D-Idose	5.35	3.4	1.95	−0.85	76	86
D-Altrose	5.35	2.95	2.4	−0.4	63	65.5
D-Gulose	5.45	2.85	2.6	−0.2	59	65
D-Allose	6.05	2.85	3.2	+0.4	37	14
D-Talose	8.0	3.3	4.7	+1.9	7.2	2.8
D-Mannose	7.65	2.25	5.4	+2.6	2.9	0.8
D-Galactose	7.75	2.25	5.5	+2.7	2.6	0.8
D-Glucose	8.0	1.8	6.2	+3.4	1.0	0.2

[a] From Table 3.6 in Section 3.2.4.
[b] From Table 3.9 in Section 3.2.4.

the same for diastereomers, that is, K has a constant value for the hexoses, and a different but constant value for the heptuloses. It has been found (147) that the best agreement with the experimental results is obtained when ΔG_F° has the value of -2.8 kcal mole^{-1} for hexoses and -3.25 kcal mole^{-1} for heptuloses. With the use of these values, the free energy change ΔG_A° on anhydride formation may be obtained by summing ΔG° and ΔG_F° Values for ΔG_A° are recorded in Tables 5.12 and 5.13 for the hexoses and heptuloses, respectively, along with the theoretical mole percentages of

Table 5.13   The Equilibrium Proportions of 2,7-Anhydro-heptylopyranoses at 100° (147)

Heptulose	$G^\circ_{{}^1C_4(\beta)}$	$G^\circ_{\text{pyranose}}$	ΔG°	ΔG_A°	Anhydride, (mole) %	
					Theory	Experimental
D-*Ido*-	5.8	4.7	1.1	-2.15	94.5	96
D-*Altro*-	5.8	4.05	1.75	-1.5	88.5	90
L-*Gulo*-	5.9[a]	4.35	1.55	-1.7	91	91.5
D-*Allo*-	6.5	4.3	2.2	-1.05	80	51.5
D-*Talo*-	8.45	3.95	4.5	$+1.25$	15.5	...
D-*Manno*-	8.1	2.9	5.2	$+1.95$	6.8	9.0
L-*Galacto*-	8.2[a]	3.25	4.95	$+1.75$	9.2	...
D-*Gluco*-	8.45	2.8	5.65	$+2.4$	4.0	2.1

[a] $G^\circ_{{}^4C_1(\beta)}$

anhydrides calculated from the equilibrium constants deduced from ΔG_A° at 100°.[34]

The theoretical mole percentages may be compared with the experimental values obtained[35] from equilibrations carried out in aqueous acidic solutions at 100°. In general, the agreement is quite good, and at least the order of stability of 1,6- and 2,7-anhydrides with hexo configurations is predicted. The sequence is the same for both and decreases in the following order:

ido > *altro* ≃ *gulo* > *allo* > *talo* > *manno* ≃ *galacto* > *gluco*

From Figure 5.32, it may be seen that when agreement between theory and experiment is not so good, as in the case of the *allo, talo, manno,*

[34] It should be noted that the values for $G^\circ_{\text{pyranose}}$ were calculated from data obtained at either 22° or 25°. The use of such $G^\circ_{\text{pyranose}}$ values in calculating equilbrium proportions at 100° must introduce some error (147).

[35] The compositions at equilibrium were determined (147) by gas-liquid chromatography of the acetylated mixtures in the case of the hexoses, and by gas-liquid chromatography of the trimethylsilylated mixtures in the case of the heptuloses.

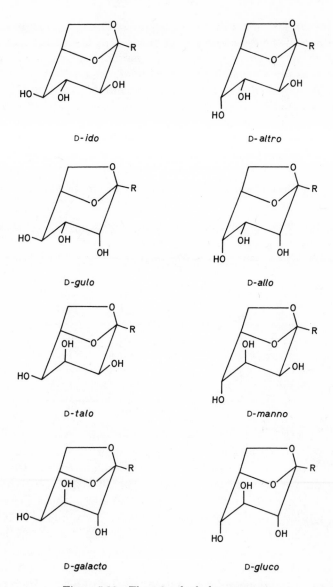

Figure 5.32 The 1,6-anhydrohexopyranoses.

galacto, and *gluco* configurations, there are *syn*-axial interactions in the $^1C_4$ conformers of the β-D-anomers and in the anhydrides. The assumption that the free energy change (ΔG_F°) on formation of these anhydrides will be the same as for the configurations without *syn*-axial interactions (i.e., the *ido, altro,* and *gulo*) is probably not valid.[36] The destabilizing influence of an axial hydroxyl group on C$_3$ interacting with the anhydro bridge has been investigated by studying (147, 148) the proportions of 1,6-anhydro-3-deoxy-D-hexopyranoses in equilibrium at 100° with their corresponding 3-deoxy-D-hexopyranoses. The results, which are summarized in Table 5.14, show that the extents of anhydro formation are intermediate (147) between those of the two related hexoses epimeric at C$_3$.

Table 5.14   The Equilibrium Proportions of 1,6-Anhydro-3-deoxyhexopyranoses at 100° (147)

3-Deoxy-hexose	$G^\circ_{^1C_4(\beta)}$	$G^\circ_{\text{pyranose}}$	ΔG°	ΔG_A°	Anhydride, (mole) %	
					Theory	Experimental
D-*Lyxo*-	4.65	2.45	2.2	−0.6	69	76.5
D-*Arabino*-	4.65	1.55	3.1	+0.3	40	47.5
D-*Xylo*-	4.75	1.55	3.2	+0.4	37	44.5
D-*Ribo*-	5.35	1.1	4.25	+2.45	12.5	10.5

In the case of some hexoses, 1,6-anhydrofuranoses exist at equilibrium in approximately equimolar amounts with their 1,6-anhydropyranoses. Thus, it has been found that 1,6-anhydro-α-D-talofuranose (**107**) (2.5%) (147), 1,6-anhydro-α-D-galactofuranose (**109**) (0.95%) (149), and 1,6-anhydro-β-D-glucofuranose (**111**) (0.17%) (150), as shown in Figure 5.33, are in equilibrium with their respective 1,6-anhydropyranoses (**108, 110,** and **112,** respectively). It should be noted that both 1,6-anhydrides have the same ring system, namely, the dioxabicyclo[3.2.1]octane, and that for aldohexoses with the *talo, galacto,* and *gluco* configurations the 1,6-anhydrofuranoses are of the same order of stability as their 1,6-anhydropyranoses.

It is possible that aldohexoses and aldopentoses could form 1,5-anhydrofuranoses (1,4-anhydropyranoses) with a dioxabicyclo[2.2.1]heptane ring system. In fact, after acid-catalyzed equilibration, aqueous solutions of

---

[36] The *syn*-axial interaction between O$_1$ and C$_6$ in the $^1C_4$ (D) conformer is common to all the β-anomers and therefore has not been considered in making this statement.

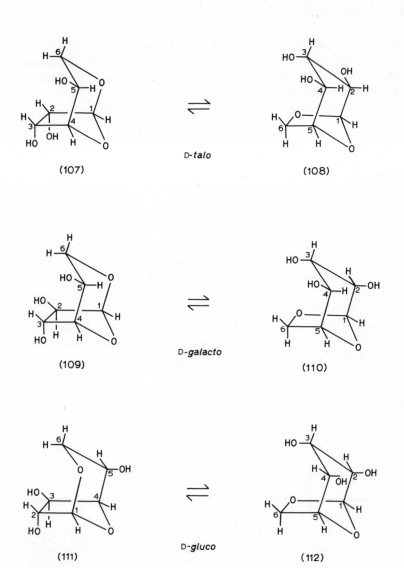

Figure 5.33 Some 1,6-anhydrohexofuranoses in equilibrium with their 1,6-anhydro-hexopyranoses.

galactose may contain (149) small amounts of 1,5-anhydro-β-D-galacto-
furanose (**113**). Generally speaking, however, favorable conditions for
the isomerization to furanose forms are required to induce their formation.
Thus, when D-ribose is allowed to react with benzaldehyde in the presence
of an acid catalyst, the two diastereomers of 2,3-*O*-benzylidene-1,5-anhydro-

(113)

β-D-ribofuranose (**114**) are found (151, 152) in equilibrium with the three
diastereomers of di-(2,3-*O*-benzylidene)-β-D-ribofuranose 1,5′:1′,5-dianhy-
dride (**115**). These products are presumably formed from the diastereomers
of 2,3-*O*-benzylidene-D-ribose, reaction intermediates in which the ribose
moieties prefer to assume β-furanose forms (*cf.* Section 5.2).

(114)   (115)

It should be noted that heptoses may form 1,7-anhydropyranoses with a
dioxabicyclo[3.3.1]nonane ring system, as well as 1,6-anhydropyranoses, on
acid-catalyzed equilibration in aqueous solutions. Thus, at equilibrium,

D-*glycero*-D-*gulo*heptose contains (147) 1,6-anhydro-D-*glycero*-D-*gulo*hepto-pyranose (8.9%)[37] (**116**) and 1,7-anhydro-D-*glycero*-D-*gulo*heptopyranose (66.0%) (**117**). As indicated in Figure 5.34, the interaction between C_3 and C_7 in **117** may be sufficiently large to encourage the 1,3-dioxane ring to exist, partially at least, in a boat conformation.[38]

In addition to forming glycosidic anhydrides through intramolecular condensation, aldoses and ketoses may undergo intermolecular condensation in aqueous acidic solutions to form oligosaccharides of dianhydrides [*cf.* the formation of di-(2,3-*O*-benzylidene)-β-D-ribofuranose 1,5′:1′,5-dianhydride]. Thus, one of the major products of refluxing an aqueous acidic solution of L-arabinose is (154) 3-*O*-β-L-arabinopyranosyl-L-arabinose (**3**). This process is sometimes referred to (e.g., ref. 155) as *acid reversion*, and its possible occurrence must be considered when assessing the primary structural significance of disaccharides present in small amounts in poly-saccharide hydrolyzates.[39] For example, when inulin, which is a food reserve polysaccharide composed primarily of β(2→1)-linked D-fructo-furanose residues, and found in the tubers of plants. such as the artichoke and the dahlia, is subjected to acid hydrolysis, fructose dianhydrides, including 1′,2-anhydro-[1-(α-D-fructofuranosyl)]-β-D-fructofuranose (**34** in Section 3.4), are found (156) to be present in the polysaccharide hydroly-zate.

[37] The low percentage compared with that of 1,6-anhydro-D-gulopyranose (Table 5.12) is probably a result of some destabilization caused by the *endo* hydroxymethyl group on C_6.

[38] Recently, the 1,3-dioxane ring in the preferred conformers of some 2,4-dioxabicyclo [3.3.1]nonane (**A**) derivatives has been shown (153) to adopt a boat conformation:

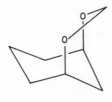

(A)

[39] The isolation and characterization of small fragments such as disaccharides and oligosaccharides after partial acid hydrolysis of a polysaccharide constitute the method of primary structural analysis known as *linkage analysis*. The identification of disac-charides which are acid reversion products may lead to erroneous primary structural conclusions. Since disaccharides arising from acid reversion are equilibrium-controlled products, they will not be destroyed on prolonged acid hydrolysis. This criterion may be employed in their initial identification.

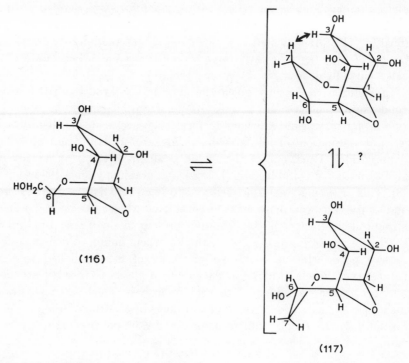

Figure 5.34   Equilibrium between 1,6-anhydro-D-*glycero*-D-*gulo*heptopyranose (**116**) and
1,7-anhydro-D-*glycero*-D-*gulo*heptopyranose (**117**).

5.7   Conclusion

It has been the purpose of this chapter, and indeed of this book, to attempt to high-light the important role that isomerism plays among the carbohydrates. The fact that constitutional, configurational, and conformational isomerisms are often superimposed on each other would almost seem to confer on the carbohydrates a unique status among organic compounds.

References

1. F. Shafizadeh, *Advan. Carbohydrate Chem.*, **13**, 9 (1958).
2. E. L. Eliel, N. L. Allinger, S. J. Angyal, and G. A. Morrison, *Conformational Analysis*, Wiley-Interscience, New York, 1965, p. 422.
3. B. Capon, *Chem. Rev.*, **69**, 407 (1969).

4. W. Pigman and H. S. Isbell, *Advan. Carbohydrate Chem.*, **23**, 11 (1968); *Advan. Carbohydrate Chem. Biochem.*, **24**, 13 (1969).

5. S. J. Angyal, *Angew. Chem. Intern. Ed.*, **8**, 157 (1969).

6. S. J. Angyal and V. A. Pickles, *Carbohydrate Res.*, **4**, 269 (1967).

7. R. U. Lemieux and J. D. Stevens, *Can. J. Chem.*, **44**, 249 (1966).

8. M. Rudrum and D. F. Shaw, *J. Chem. Soc.*, 52 (1965).

9. W. Mackie and A. S. Perlin, *Can. J. Chem.*, **44**, 2039 (1966).

10. A. S. Perlin, *Can. J. Chem.*, **44**, 539 (1966).

11. R. Kuhn, H. Trischmann, and I. Löw, *Angew. Chem.*, **67**, 32 (1955); R. Kuhn and H. Grassner, *Ann.*, **610**, 122 (1957).

12. C. C. Sweeley, R. Bentley, M. Makita, and W. W. Wells, *J. Am. Chem. Soc.*, **85**, 2497 (1963); R. Bentley and N. Botlock, *Anal. Biochem.*, **20**, 312 (1967).

13. R. S. Shallenberger and T. E. Acree, *Carbohydrate Res.*, **1**, 495 (1965); T. E. Acree, R. S. Shallenberger, and L. R. Mattick, *Carbohydrate Res.*, **6**, 498 (1968); C. Y. Lee, T. E. Acree, and R. S. Shallenberger, *Carboyhdrate Res.*, **9**, 356 (1969); T. E. Acree, R. S. Shallenberger, C. Y. Lee, and J. W. Einset, *Carbohydrate Res.*, **10**, 355 (1969).

14. R. U. Lemieux and A. A. Pavia, *Can. J. Chem.*, **47**, 4441 (1969).

15. M. A. Kabayama and D. Patterson, *Can. J. Chem.*, **36**, 563 (1958).

16. D. M. W. Anderson, Sir Edmund Hirst, and J. F. Stoddart, *J. Chem. Soc.*, C, p. 1476 (1967).

17. D. Y. Curtin, *Record Chem. Progr. Kresege-Hooker Sci. Lib.*, **15**, 111 (1954).

18. E. L. Eliel, *Stereochemistry of Carbon Compounds*, McGraw-Hill, New York, 1962, pp. 151, 237.

19. M. Mazurek and A. S. Perlin, *Can. J. Chem.*, **41**, 2403 (1963).

20. A. S. Perlin, *Can. J. Chem.*, **42**, 1365 (1964).

21. A. S. Perlin, *Can. J. Chem.*, **42**, 2365 (1964).

22. A. S. Perlin and E. von Rudloff, *Can. J. Chem.*, **43**, 2071 (1965).

23. S. J. Angyal, V. A. Pickles, and R. Ahluwalia, *Carbohydrate Res.*, **3**, 300 (1967).

24. J. A. Mills, *Advan. Carbohydrate Chem.*, **10**, 1 (1955).

25. A. B. Foster, W. G. Overend, M. Stacey, and G. Vaughan, *J. Chem. Soc.*, p. 3367 (1954).

26. W. N. Haworth, L. N. Owen, and F. Smith, *J. Chem. Soc.*, p. 88 (1941).

27. C. T. Bishop and F. P. Cooper, *Can. J. Chem.*, **41**, 2743 (1963).

28. V. Smirnyagin and C. T. Bishop, *Can. J. Chem.*, **46**, 3085 (1968).

29. W. N. Haworth, J. Jackson, and F. Smith, *J. Chem. Soc.*, p. 620 (1940).

30. A. B. Foster, W. G. Overend, and G. Vaughan, *J. Chem. Soc.*, p. 3625 (1954).

31. R. U. Lemieux, in *Molecular Rearrangements*, ed. P. de Mayo, Wiley-Interscience, New York, 1963, p. 713.

32. L. Hough and A. C. Richardson, in *Rodd's Chemistry of Carbon Compounds*, Vol. 1F, Ch. 23, ed. S. Coffey, Elsevier, Amsterdam, 1967, p. 337.

33. Ref. 2, p. 413.

34. G. R. Barker, T. M. Noone, D. C. C. Smith, and J. W. Spoors, *J. Chem. Soc.*, p. 1327 (1955).

35. H. C. Brown, J. H. Brewster, and H. Shechter, *J. Am. Chem. Soc.*, **76**, 467 (1954).

36. S. R. Carter, W. N. Haworth, and R. A. Robinson, *J. Chem. Soc.*, p. 2125 (1930).

37. M. L. Hackert and R. A. Jacobson, *Chem. Comm.*, p. 1179 (1969).

38. H. D. K. Drew and W. N. Haworth, *J. Chem. Soc.*, p. 775 (1927).

39. N. L. Allinger, J. Allinger, and N. A. Le Bel, *J. Am. Chem. Soc.*, **82**, 2926 (1960).

40. G. A. Jeffrey and S. H. Kim, *Chem. Comm.*, p. 211 (1966).

41. D. S. Noyce and L. J. Dolby, *J. Org. Chem.*, **26**, 3619 (1961).

42. F. Smith, *J. Chem. Soc.*, p. 584 (1955).
43. H. L. Frush and H. S. Isbell, *J. Res. Natl. Bur. Std.*, **37**, 1, 321 (1946).
44. D. Heslop and F. Smith, *J. Chem. Soc.*, pp. 574, 577, 637 (1944).
45. Y. Imai and Y. Hirasaka, *J. Pharm. Soc. Japan*, **80**, 1139 (1960).
46. Ref. 2, p. 249.
47. M. Hanack, *Conformational Theory*, Academic, New York, 1965, p. 308.
48. J. E. Anderson, *Quart. Rev.*, **19**, 426 (1967).
49. F. G. Riddell, *Quart. Rev.*, **19**, 364 (1967).
50. J. E. Anderson and J. C. D. Brand, *Trans.* Faraday Soc., **62**, 39 (1965).
51. J. E. Anderson and F. G. Riddell, *Tetrahedron Letters*, p. 2017 (1967).
52. F. G. Riddell and M. J. T. Robinson, *Tetrahedron*, **23**, 3417 (1967).
53. K. Pihlaja and J. Heikkla, *Acta Chem. Scand.*, **21**, 2390 (1967).
54. E. L. Eliel and Sr. M. C. Knoeber, *J. Am. Chem. Soc.*, **90**, 3444 (1968).
55. E. L. Eliel, *Kem. Tidskr.*, **81**, 6/7, 22 (1969).
56. E. L. Eliel, *Accounts Chem. Res.*, **3**, 1 (1970).
57. E. L. Eliel, Plenary Lecture on *Insights gained from Conformational Analysis on Heterocyclic Systems* at International Symposium on Conformational Analysis, Brussels, September, 1969; *Pure Appl. Chem.*, forthcoming publication.
58. C. Romers, C. Altona, H. R. Buys, and E. Havinga, in *Topics in Stereochemistry*, Vol. 4, ed. E. L. Eliel and N. L. Allinger, Wiley-Interscience, New York, 1969, p. 39.
59. H. R. Buys, *Rec. Trav. Chim. Pays-Bas*, **88**, 1003 (1969).
60. A. J. deKok and C. Romers, *Rec. Trav. Chim. Pays-Bas*, **89**, 313 (1970).
61. J. A. Hirsch, in *Topics in Stereochemistry*, Vol. 1, ed. E. L. Eliel and N. L. Allinger, Wiley-Interscience, New York, 1967, p. 199.
62. N. L. Allinger and J. C. Tai, *J. Am. Chem. Soc.*, **87**, 1227 (1965).
63. E. L. Eliel and R. O. Hutchins, *J. Am. Chem. Soc.*, **91**, 2703 (1969).
64. H. Friebolin, S. Kabuss, W. Maier, and A. Lüttringhaus, *Tetrahedron Letters*, p. 683 (1962); H. G. Schmidt, H. Friebolin, and R. Mecke, *Spectrochim. Acta*, **22**, 623 (1966).
65. B. Pedersen and T. Schaug, *Acta Chem. Scand.*, **22**, 1705 (1968).
66. K. Pihlaja and J. Heikkila, *Acta Chem. Scand.*, **21**, 2430 (1967).
67. K. Pihlaja, *Acta Chem. Scand.*, **22**, 716 (1968).
68. K. Pihlaja and S. Luoma, *Acta Chem. Scand.*, **22**, 2401 (1968).
69. F. A. French and R. S. Rasmussen, *J. Chem. Phys.*, **14**, 389 (1946); U. Blakis, P. H. Kasai, and R. J. Meyers, in *J. Chem. Phys.*, **38**, 2735 (1963).
70. K. S. Pitzer, *J. Chem. Phys.*, **12**, 310 (1944).
71. D. Tavernier and M. Anteunis, *Bull. Soc. Chim. Belges*, **76**, 157 (1967).
72. S. A. Barker, J. S. Brimacombe, A. B. Foster, D. H. Whiffen, and G. Zweifel, *Tetrahedron*, **7**, 10 (1959).
73. N. Baggett, M. A. Bukhari, A. B. Foster, J. Lehmann, and J. M. Webber, *J. Chem. Soc.*, p. 457 (1963).
74. S. A. Barker, A. B. Foster, A. H. Haines, J. Lehmann, J. M. Webber, and G. Zweifel, *J. Chem. Soc.*, p. 4161 (1963).
75. E. L. Eliel and M. Kaloustain, *Chem. Comm.*, p. 290 (1970).
76. N. Baggett, J. S. Brimacombe, A. B. Foster, M. Stacey, and D. H. Whiffen, *J. Chem. Soc.*, p. 2574 (1960).
77. W. T. Haskins, R. M. Hann, and C. S. Hudson, *J. Am. Chem. Soc.*, **65**, 1663 (1943).
78. E. Zissis and N. K. Richtmeyer, *J. Am. Chem. Soc.*, **76**, 5515 (1954).
79. R. M. Hann, W. T. Haskins, and C. S. Hudson, *J. Am. Chem. Soc.*, **64**, 986 (1942).
80. N. Sheppard and J. J. Turner, *Proc. Roy. Soc. (London)*, Series A, **252**, 506 (1959).

81. R. U. Lemieux, J. D. Stevens, and R. R. Fraser, *Can. J. Chem.*, **40**, 1955 (1962).
82. M. Anteunis and F. Alderweireldt, *Bull. Soc. Chim. Belges*, **73**, 889 (1964); F. Alderweireldt and M. Anteunis, *Bull. Soc. Chim. Belges*, **74**, 488 (1965).
83. C. Altona and A. P. M. van der Veck, *Tetrahedron*, **24**, 4377 (1968).
84. W. E. Willy, G. Binsch, and E. L. Eliel, *J. Am. Chem. Soc.*, **92**, 5394 (1970).
85. C. Altona, H. R. Buys, and E. Havinga, *Rec. Trav. Chim. Pays-Bas*, **85**, 973 (1966).
86. C. K. Ingold and J. F. Thorpe, *J. Chem. Soc.*, p. 1318 (1928).
87. J. A. Mills, *Chem. Ind.*, p. 633 (1954).
88. L. F. Wiggins, *J. Chem. Soc.*, p. 13 (1946).
89. W. T. Haskins, R. M. Hann, and C. S. Hudson, *J. Am. Chem. Soc.*, **64**, 136, 137 (1942).
90. H. Zinner and W. Thielebeule, *Chem. Ber.*, **93**, 2791 (1960).
91. N. Baggett, K. W. Buck, A. B. Foster, M. H. Randall, and J. M. Webber, *J. Chem. Soc.*, p. 3394 (1965).
92. E. L. Eliel and W. E. Willy, *Tetrahedron Letters*, p. 1775 (1969).
93. S. A. Barker, E. J. Bourne, R. M. Pinkard, M. Stacey, and D. H. Whiffen, *J. Chem. Soc.*, p. 3232 (1958); B. E. Leggetter and R. K. Brown, *Can. J. Chem.*, **43**, 1030 (1965).
94. N. Baggett, J. M. Duxbury, A. B. Foster, and J. M. Webber, *J. Chem. Soc.*, C, p. 208 (1966).
95. (a) J. B. Hendrickson, *J. Am. Chem. Soc.*, **83**, 4537 (1961); (b) **84**, 3355 (1962); (c) *Tetrahedron*, **19**, 1387 (1963); (d) *J. Am. Chem. Soc.*, **89**, 7036 (1967); (e) **89**, 7043 (1967); (f) **89**, 7047 (1967).
96. A. T. Ness, R. M. Hann, and C. S. Hudson, *J. Am. Chem. Soc.*, **65**, 2215 (1943).
97. B. Wickberg, *Acta Chem. Scand.*, **12**, 1187 (1958).
98. J. F. Stoddart and W. A. Szarek, *J. Chem. Soc.*, B, p. 437 (1971).
99. H. Hibbert and N. M. Carter, *J. Am. Chem. Soc.*, **50**, 3120 (1928).
100. H. S. Hill and H. Hibbert, *J. Am. Chem. Soc.*, **45**, 3117 (1923); H. S. Hill, H. C. Hill, and H. Hibbert, *J. Am. Chem. Soc.*, **50**, 2242 (1928).
101. H. Hibbert and J. G. Morazain, *Can. J. Res.*, **2**, 35, 214 (1930).
102. G. Aksnes, P. Albriktsen, and P. Juvvik, *Acta Chem. Scand.*, **19**, 920 (1965).
103. C. E. Ballou, *J. Am. Chem. Soc.*, **82**, 2585 (1960).
104. F. S. Al-Jeboury, N. Baggett, A. B. Foster, and J. M. Webber, *Chem. Comm.*, p. 222 (1965).
105. N. Baggett, K. W. Buck, A. B. Foster, B. H. Rees, and J. M. Webber, *J. Chem. Soc.*, C, p. 212 (1966).
106. W. R. Christian, C. J. Gogek, and C. B. Purves, *Can. J. Chem.*, **29**, 911 (1951).
107. L. P. Kuhn, *J. Am. Chem. Soc.*, **76**, 4323 (1954).
108. S. J. Angyal and C. G. Macdonald, *J. Chem. Soc.*, 686 (1952).
109. E. L. Eliel and C. Pillar, *J. Am. Chem. Soc.*, **77**, 3600 (1955).
110. W. B. Monitz and J. A. Dixon, *J. Am. Chem. Soc.*, **83**, 1671 (1961).
111. L. D. Hall, L. Hough, K. A. McLauchlan, and K. Pachler, *Chem. Ind.*, p. 1465 (1962).
112. B. Coxon and H. G. Fletcher, Jr., *J. Am. Chem. Soc.*, **85**, 2637 (1963).
113. J. G. Buchanan and A. R. Edgar, *Chem. Comm.*, p. 29 (1967).
114. B. Coxon and L. D. Hall, *Tetrahedron*, **20**, 1685 (1964).
115. R. D. King and W. G. Overend, *Carbohydrate Res.*, **9**, 423 (1969).
116. S. J. Angyal and R. M. Hoskinson, *J. Chem. Soc.*, p. 2991 (1962).
117. C. Cone and L. Hough, *Carbohydrate Res.*, **1**, 1 (1965).
118. F. H. Newth and L. F. Wiggins, *J. Chem. Soc.*, p. 1734 (1950).

119. D. H. Brauns and H. L. Frush, *J. Res. Natl. Bur. Std.*, **6**, 449 (1931).
120. A. N. de Belder, *Advan. Carbohydrate Chem.*, **20**, 220 (1965).
121. J. S. Brimacombe and P. A. Gent., *Carbohydrate Res.*, **9**, 231 (1969).
122. D. C. DeJongh and K. Biemann, *J. Am. Chem. Soc.*, **86**, 67 (1964).
123. R. J. Abraham, L. D. Hall, L. Hough, and K. A. McLauchlan, *J. Chem. Soc.*, p. 3699 (1962).
124. J. D. Stevens, *Chem. Comm.*, p. 1140 (1969); J. Jackobs and M. Sundaralingam, *Chem. Comm.*, p. 157 (1970).
125. H. B. Wood, Jr., H. W. Diehl, and H. G. Fletcher, Jr., *J. Am. Chem. Soc.*, **79**, 3862 (1957).
126. B. Coxon, *Carbohydrate Res.*, **8**, 125 (1968).
127. B. Coxon, *Carbohydrate Res.*, **12**, 313 (1970).
128. W. N. Haworth and C. R. Porter, *J. Chem. Soc.*, p. 611 (1928).
129. J. M. Grosheintz and H. O. L. Fischer, *J. Am. Chem. Soc.*, **70**, 1476 (1948).
130. R. M. Hann and C. S. Hudson, *J. Am. Chem. Soc.*, **66**, 1906 (1944).
131. M. L. Wolfrom, B. W. Lew, and R. M. Goepp, *J. Am. Chem. Soc.*, **68**, 1443 (1946).
132. R. U. Lemieux and J. Howard, *Can. J. Chem.*, **41**, 393 (1963).
133. A. B. Foster, A. H. Haines, and J. Lehmann, *J. Chem. Soc.*, p. 5011 (1961).
134. R. M. Hann, A. T. Ness, and C. S. Hudson, *J. Am. Chem. Soc.*, **66**, 670 (1944).
135. R. M. Hann, J. K. Wolfe, and C. S. Hudson, *J. Am. Chem. Soc.*, **66**, 1898 (1944).
136. W. N. Haworth and L. F. Wiggins, *J. Chem. Soc.*, p. 58 (1944).
137. R. M. Hann and C. S. Hudson, *J. Am. Chem. Soc.*, **67**, 602 (1945).
138. D. M. Kilburn, M. Sc. Thesis, Queen's University, Kingston, Canada, 1969.
139. W. N. Haworth, W. G. N. Jones, M. Stacey, and L. F. Wiggins, *J. Chem. Soc.*, p. 61 (1944).
140. B. Coxon, *Tetrahedron*, **21**, 3481 (1965).
141. N. Baggett, J. M. Duxbury, A. B. Foster, and J. M. Webber, *Carbohydrate Res.*, **1**, 22 (1965).
142. S. J. Angyal, *Aust. J. Chem.*, **21**, 2737 (1968).
143. T. B. Grindley, J. F. Stoddart, and W. A. Szarek, *J. Chem. Soc.*, B, p. 172 (1969).
144. T. B. Grindley, J. F. Stoddart, and W. A. Szarek, *J. Chem. Soc.*, B, p. 623 (1969).
145. H. Appel, W. N. Haworth, E. G. Cox, and F. J. Llewellyn, *J. Chem. Soc.*, p. 793 (1938).
146. E. G. Ansell and J. Honeyman, *J. Chem. Soc.*, p. 2778 (1952).
147. S. J. Angyal and K. Dawes, *Aust. J. Chem.*, **21**, 2747 (1968).
148. J. W. Pratt and N. K. Richtmeyer, *J. Am. Chem. Soc.*, **79**, 2597 (1957).
149. N. K. Richtmeyer, *Arch. Biochem. Biophys.*, **78**, 376 (1958).
150. S. Peat, W. J. Whelan, T. E. Edwards, and O. Owen, *J. Chem. Soc.*, p. 586 (1958).
151. E. Vis and H. G. Fletcher, Jr., *J. Am. Chem. Soc.*, **79**, 1182 (1957).
152. T. B. Grindley, J. F. Stoddart, and W. A. Szarek, Unpublished results.
153. R. J. Bishop, L. E. Sutton, M. J. T. Robinson, and N. W. J. Pumphrey, *Tetrahedron*, **25**, 1417 (1969).
154. J. K. N. Jones and D. H. Ball, *J. Chem. Soc.*, p. 27 (1958)
155. W. J. Whelan, *Ann. Rev. Biochem.*, **29**, 105 (1960).
156. E. J. McDonald, *Advan. Carbohydrate Chem.*, **2**, 253 (1946).

Author Index

Numbers in parentheses are reference numbers to the author's work; numbers in *italics* indicate the pages on which the full references appear.

A

Abraham, R. J., 101(122), *122*, 207(123), *232*

Acree, T. E., 167(13), *229*

Adkins, H., 26(13), *46*

Ahluwahlia, R., 64(37), *119*, 133(28), *156*, 169, 170(23), *229*

Aksnes, G., 200, 201(102), *231*

Albriktsen, P., 200, 201(102), *231*

Alderweireldt, F., 194, 195(82), *231*

Al-Jeboury, F. S., 201, 202(104), *231*

Allen, L. C., 48(3), 85(3), *118*

Allinger, J., 74(63), *120*, 179(39), *229*

Allinger, N. L., 6(34), *8*, 37(25), *46*, 47, 50(1), 59(21), 60, 67(1), 74(63), 81, 93(1), *118*, *120*, 123(1, 2), 127(17), 147-153(77), *155*, *156*, *157*, 158(2), 173(33), 179(39), 187(46), 189(62), 220(2), *228-230*

Altona, C., 50, 54(10), 73(60-62), 81(10), 84(10, 84), 87(10), *119-121*, 146(71, 72), *157*, 187, 188(58), 195(83, 85), *230*, *231*

Amaral, D., 34, 35(22), *46*

Anderson, C. B., 66(42), 68(51), 70(53), 72(55), 74(51), 76(71, 72), 81(55), *119*, *120*

Anderson, D. M. W., 168(16), *229*

Anderson, J. E., 187, 189, 190(48, 50, 51), *230*

Anderson, N. S., 44, 45(30), *46*, 109-118 (135), 113, 114(146), 114, 115(147),

116(150), *122*

Anet, E. F. L. J., 32(21), *46*, 105-108(127), *122*

Anet, F. A. L., 145(70), *157*

Angyal, S. J., 6(34), *8*, 32(20), 37(25), *46*, 47, 50(1), 59-72(21-23), 60(1), 61(31), 63(34), 67(1, 48), 76, 77(23), 81(1), 87 (22), 89-92(21-23), 93(1), 94, 95(103), 100, 101(23, 117), *118-122*, 123(1, 2), 127(17), 133(28, 33), 135(40), 140(32), 147-153(77), *155-157*, 158(2), 159-165 (5, 6), 169, 170(23), 170, 171(5), 173 (33), 175(5), 187(46), 202(108), 204 (116), 216(142), 220(2, 5, 147), 221-224 (147), *228-232*

Ansell, E. G., 220(146), *232*

Anteunis, M., 142(60), *157*, 191(71), 194, 195(82), 209(71), *230*, *231*

Aoki, K., 82(81), *121*

Appel, H., 219, 220(145), *232*

Arigoni, D., 1(9), *7*

Aroney, M. J., 85(89), *121*

Asensio, C., 34, 35(12), *46*

Aspinall, G. O., 6(35), *8*

Avigad, G., 34, 35(22), *46*

Azarnia, N., 95, 97(107), *121*

B

Baggett, N., 128(20), 133(29), *156*, 192, 193(73, 76), 197(91), 198(94), 201, 202 (104, 105), 215, 216(141), *230*, *231*

Subject Index

A

librium proportions of, 224
3,6-Anhydro-2,4-di-*O*-methyl-D-hexanoic
acids, δ-lactonization of, 184, 185
1',2-Anhydro-[1-(α-D-fructofuranosyl)]-β-D-
fructofuranose, 101, 102, 227
1,5-Anhydrofuranoses, 224, 226
1,6-Anhydrofuranoses, 224
1,5-Anhydro-β-D-galactofuranose, 226
1,6-Anhydro-α-D-galactofuranose, 224, 225
3,6-Anhydro-D-galactose, dimethyl acetal
of, 177
1,6-Anhydro-β-D-glucofuranose, 224, 225
3,6-Anhydro-D-glucose, 170
1,6-Anhydro-D-*glycero*-D-*gulo*heptopyranose, 227, 228
1,7-Anhydro-D-*glycero*-D-*gulo*heptopyranose, 227, 228
2,7-Anhydroheptulopyranoses, equilibrium
proportions of, 222
formation of, 220, 221
1,6-Anhydrohexopyranoses, equilibrium
proportions of, 221
formation of, 220, 221, 223
1,6-Anhydro-β-D-idopyranose, 39
5,6-Anhydro-1,2-*O*-isopropylidene-α-D-
glucofuranose, 207
1,6-Anhydro-α-D-talofuranose, 224, 225
1,6-Anhydro-2,3,4-tri-*O*-acetyl-β-D-galacto-
pyranose, long range coupling in, 142
1,6-Anhydro-2,3,4-tri-*O*-acetyl-β-D-gluco-
pyranose, long range coupling in, 142
1,6-Anhydro-2,3,4-tri-*O*-acetyl-β-D-manno-
pyranose, long range coupling in, 142
1,4-Anhydro-2,3,6-tri-*O*-methyl-β-D-galacto-
pyranose, conformation of, 92, 93
Anisochronous, definition of, 16
Anomeric center, 32
effect, 6, 68, 106, 172
dipole-dipole interactions associated
with, 81
interpretation in terms of lone pairs,
81-84
origin of, 81
quantitative definition of, 68, 69, 70
quantitative estimations of, 81
quantum mechanical explanation of,
85-87
stereoelectronic explanation of, 84, 85
Anomerization, 32
Anomers, nomenclature of, 32

3-*O*-β-L-Arabinopyrosyl-L-arabinose, 168,
227
Asymmetric, definition of, 10
Atropisomers, 4
Axial substituents, 50
destabilizing effects of, 59

B

1,3-*O*-Benzylidene-D-arabinitol, 193, 194
2,3-*O*-Benzylidene-D-erythrose, diastereomers of, 201, 202
2,4-*O*-Benzylidene-D-erythrose, 201, 202
2,3-*O*-Benzylidene-1,5-β-D-ribofuranose,
226
Bond-angle-bending strain, 48
Bond deformation, strain associated with,
48
Branched polysaccharides, 41, 43
2-Bromo-4-methyltetrahydropyean, 72, 73
2-Bromotetrahydropyran, 73, 81
n-Butane, 2
potential energy profile for, 3
γ-Butyrolactone, 177, 178

C

C_2 conformation of cyclopentane, 98
C_S conformation of cyclopentane, 97
Cahn-Ingold-Prelog convention, 17, 18, 19
ι-Carrageenan, double helix for, 115-117
gelation by, 118
optical rotatory properties of, 155
primary structure of, 114, 115
X-ray diffraction studies on, 115, 116
κ-Carrageenan, gelation by, 118
optical rotatory properties of, 155
primary structure of, 44, 45, 113-115
X-ray diffraction studies on, 115, 116
λ-Carrageenan, primary structure of, 114,
115
X-ray diffraction studies on, 116
Cellobiose, 40
conformation of, 109-113
Cellulose, conformation of, 109-113
Chiral carbon atom, 1
Chiral, definition of, 10
Chloromethoxymethane, anomeric effect in,
84, 85
2-Chloro-4-methyltetrahydropyran, 72, 73

DATE DUE

GAYLORD			PRINTED IN U.S.A.